*How to Live Longer and Feel Better*

*How to Live Longer and Feel Better*

# Linus Pauling

Oregon State University Press
Corvallis

*To Arthur M. Sackler*

**Library of Congress Cataloging-in-Publication Data**
Pauling, Linus, 1901-
  How to live longer and feel better / Linus Pauling.— First OSU Press ed.
    p. cm.
  Originally published: New York : W.Y. Freeman, 1986.
  Includes bibliographical references and index.
  ISBN-13: 978-0-87071-096-4 (alk. paper)
  ISBN-10: 0-87071-096-6 (alk. paper)
  1. Orthomolecular therapy.  I. Title.
  RM235.5.P38 2006
  615.5—dc22

                                                                2006000253


⊗ This paper meets the requirements of ANSI/NISO Z39.48-1992
(Permanence of Paper).

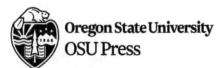

**Oregon State University**
**OSU Press**

**Oregon State University Press**
121 The Valley Library
Corvallis OR 97331
541-737-3166 • fax 541-737-3170
www.osupress.oregonstate.edu

# Contents

# Introduction

## to Oregon State University Press edition

*by Melinda Gormley*

> What should we strive for?
> Happiness—to lead a good life, as long as possible; and to avoid
>   suffering.
> The new nutrition can lead to elongations of the period of well-being.
> —LINUS PAULING, note to self, undated

Human suffering troubled Linus Pauling. In an effort to alleviate the amount of suffering in the world, Pauling actively campaigned on a grand scale for various causes. The two most notable were his work for peace and health; he attempted not only to educate people about the scientific and technical basis behind each issue, but also to suggest solutions. In the note to himself quoted above, Pauling essentially sketched out his objective in writing *How to Live Longer and Feel Better*: the improvement of our health and well-being through a dietary regimen.

In *How to Live Longer and Feel Better,* Pauling synthesized information on vitamins and nutrition that he had been gathering for over twenty years. This book represents the culmination of his efforts—a compilation of information previously mentioned in three books, numerous articles, and many speeches. *How to Live Longer and Feel Better* became a *New York Times* bestseller immediately after its publication in 1986 and was translated into numerous other languages. In this book Pauling promotes orthomolecular medicine, a term he coined to describe his approach to obtaining optimal health through proper intake of vitamins and other nutrients.

Linus Pauling had a phenomenal career as a scientist and political activist. His life spanned most of the twentieth century, and he was acknowledged as one of the most important scientists of the century. He won two unshared Nobel Prizes—the 1954 Nobel Prize in Chemistry and the 1962 Nobel Peace Prize—the only person to have done so, as noted by many who have written about him. Pauling also received many other awards and accolades, including some fifty honorary degrees, the National Medal of Science, the National Academy of Science Medal in Chemical Sciences, the Pasteur Medal, the Priestley Medal, and the Presidential Medal for Merit.

Born in 1901 in Portland, Oregon, Pauling grew up mainly in the rural area of Condon, Oregon. His father, Herman Pauling, was a respected pharmacist and businessman who prepared many medicines in his store, where Linus was exposed to this medicinal chemistry as a youngster. Herman Pauling died at the age of thirty-three, when Linus was only ten years old. Pauling's mother, Lucy Isabelle Pauling, suffered from chronic mental and physical ailments, primarily bouts of depression and exhaustion. Her health continued to deteriorate over time; in 1926, Pauling and his wife were in Europe on a Guggenheim Fellowship when she died of pernicious anemia, which is caused by a deficiency of vitamin $B_{12}$, and characterized by neurological problems and loss of normal mental function, resulting, ultimately, in death. The pharmacological interests of his father and mental and physical illnesses of his mother, more than likely, had some influence upon Pauling's later endeavors in medicine.

Scientific subjects intrigued Pauling from an early age, and he cultivated his interest by collecting and labeling insects and minerals. Pauling himself said that his interest in the chemical sciences stemmed from his best friend, Lloyd Jeffress, who introduced him to chemistry when they were in high school. Pauling set up a laboratory in the basement, where he performed chemical experiments.

Pauling's entire life and career were spent on the West Coast of the United States. He studied Chemical Engineering at Oregon Agricultural College (since renamed Oregon State University) as an undergraduate student from 1917 to 1922. After graduating, Pauling went to the West Coast's newly established academic center for science, the California Institute of Technology (Caltech) in Pasadena, where he received his Doctor of Philosophy degree in chemistry (with a minor in mathematics and physics) in 1927, and remained as a chemistry professor. Ten years later, at the age of thirty-six, he accepted the position of director and chairman of Caltech's Department of Chemistry. Pauling stayed at Caltech until 1963; for the next six years he held various positions in Santa Barbara and San Diego, becoming Professor of Chemistry at Stanford University in 1969. In 1973

Pauling decided to start his own institute, named the Linus Pauling Institute of Science and Medicine. Located adjacent to Stanford University, the Linus Pauling Institute focused its research on orthomolecular medicine and received the bulk of Pauling's attention for the remaining twenty years of his life. This institute continues to conduct orthomolecular research today, having relocated to Oregon State University in 1996.

Pauling's scientific work encompassed a variety of chemical subjects, most of which overlapped with other disciplines, such as physics, biology, medicine, and psychology. As his first major scientific accomplishment, Pauling established the nature of the chemical bond in a series of seven influential papers written between 1931 and 1933. Using quantum chemistry, which fuses physics, mathematics, and chemistry, Pauling developed rules to explain how electrons interact to form the three-dimensional structures of chemical elements and compounds. Building on this intimate knowledge of structures, Pauling continued to seek fundamental chemical configurations throughout his life. This knowledge of molecular structure coupled with his ability to cross disciplinary boundaries contributed to his success as a scientist.

Pauling's chemical interests in biology, medicine, and psychology have independent origins, but are ultimately related because his work in these fields developed one from another. He became fascinated with organic chemistry in the early 1930s after having gained a competent background in inorganic chemistry. From then until he left Caltech thirty years later, Pauling and his colleagues investigated proteins, searching for their chemical structures and properties. Pauling contributed greatly to knowledge of the fundamental structures of proteins when he suggested a few primary configurations, including the alpha-helix, gamma-helix, and pleated sheets. The most significant of these fundamental structures is the alpha-helix, which Pauling sketched out in 1948 and published a few years later in 1951 along with the others.

One protein that greatly intrigued Pauling and stimulated his interest in medicine and psychology was hemoglobin. When Pauling started working with organic molecules in the early 1930s, he specifically called attention to hemoglobin as a potential research topic, and by 1935 he had written his first article on the macromolecule. Over the next ten years, Pauling continued to analyze hemoglobin's properties and structure. These investigations included analysis of both parts of hemoglobin, the iron-containing heme and its protein portion, the globin. While working for the United States government's Office of Scientific Research and Development during World War II he developed oxypolygelatin, a synthetic blood substitute that was intended to be used in place of human blood during blood transfusions. However, it proved unnecessary because sufficient blood donors eradicated the need for a synthetic substitute. Pauling also worked on hemoglobin's magnetic properties with Charles D. Coryell and its denaturation with biochemist Alfred Mirsky, as well as devising an apparatus for the Office of Scientific Research and Development that detected the levels of oxygen in the air based on its magnetic properties. This oxygen meter was widely used by the military in airplanes and submarines.

Building on his work with chemical structures of organic molecules, Pauling became interested in immunology as a result of a conversation in 1936 with immunologist Karl Landsteiner. Landsteiner, a pioneer in the field, had been awarded the 1930 Nobel Prize in Medicine for determining that humans have different blood types. Based on what he had learned from Landsteiner, Pauling developed a theory about the structure, formation, and interaction of antibodies and antigens. He continued to conduct research on immunochemical topics throughout the 1940s, his first venture into medical topics.

Hemoglobin remained a research interest for Pauling throughout his life. In the late 1940s his intimate knowledge of hemoglobin allowed him to contribute significantly to the medical problem of sickle-cell anemia. Sickle-cell anemia—a deadly hereditary disease of the blood that primarily afflicts people of African descent—is so named because the red blood cells of those with the disease are crescent shaped instead of disk shaped. Those affected suffer from a variety of symptoms because the red blood cells' ability to transport adequate amounts of oxygen through the body is impaired.

Pauling and his collaborators, Harvey A. Itano, S. J. Singer, and Ibert C. Wells, united experimental chemistry and clinical medicine in their seminal paper, "Sickle Cell Anemia, a Molecular Disease," which was published in *Science* in November 1949. Their laboratory experiments showed that an abnormal hemoglobin molecule that twists, or sickles, the red blood cells in de-oxygenated venous blood causes sickle-cell anemia. This was the first discovery of a disease caused by an abnormal molecule and ushered in the era of molecular medicine. A healthy person has two dominant alleles, whereas a person suffering from sickle-cell anemia has two recessive alleles for the disease. Those suffering from sickle-cell trait, a less debilitating form of the disease, are heterozygous and therefore have one dominant and one recessive allele.

Pauling and his collaborators coined the term "molecular disease" in their article. According to Pauling's various definitions, a molecular disease is a hereditary ailment in which the presence of abnormal molecules in the human body causes physical or mental illness. Pauling considered the creation of a clear definition of molecular disease to be an important, original contribution to understanding the relationship between molecules and sickness. In the years following the publication of this article, Pauling turned his attention to molecular diseases and their treatment. For example, he and Harvey A. Itano, a medical doctor and chemist by training, tried to find a cure for sickle-cell anemia by introducing an agent that would inhibit the conversion of the red blood cells from their normal discus shape to a misshapen crescent, but were unsuccessful.

In 1953 Pauling added mental deficiencies to his concept of molecular disease. Perhaps his mother's madness and premature death caused by $B_{12}$ deficiency underlaid this interest. Also, at about this time, Pauling's eldest son, Linus Jr., began a residency in psychiatry, which undoubtedly prompted Pauling to consider the nature of mental illness. He studied phenylketonuria, a hereditary disease that causes physical and mental disabilities shortly after birth. Excess levels of accumulated phenylalanine cause the mental manifestations of phenylketonuria. Like sickle-cell anemia, it is a genetic disease that manifests itself in a person who is homozygous recessive for the ailment. Pauling hoped to rectify the body's imbalance by introducing artificial enzymes as therapy, but this work produced little of therapeutic value to match the grand scale of his expectations.

Pauling's concept of molecular diseases stimulated his subsequent research activities, especially his work with vitamins and in nutrition. He believed that molecular diseases could be cured by introducing substances that would induce or inhibit chemical reactions in the human body. When Pauling coined the terms "orthomolecular medicine" and "orthomolecular psychiatry," he was defining a particular approach to the treatment of molecular diseases with physical and mental manifestations. As Pauling describes in this book, the use of orthomolecular medicine and orthomolecular psychiatry is contrasted with drug therapies, which, although effective in many cases, are fraught with issues of toxicity and undesirable side effects.

Two examples of orthomolecular therapies that Pauling frequently discussed are treating diabetes with insulin and treating phenylketonuria with a diet low in phenylalanine. He was familiar with both illnesses. In the early 1920s, when he attended Caltech as a graduate student, researchers there were investigating the relationship between insulin and diabetes. Although Pauling was not directly connected to this research, it is likely that he learned enough to pique his interest and spur him to follow the relevant research, and he linked his definition of molecular disease to diabetes as early as 1953.

As his knowledge of the subject increased, Pauling realized that renal specialist Dr. Thomas Addis had successfully administered an orthomolecular treatment to cure his own bout of nephritis in the early 1940s. Also known as Bright's disease, nephritis develops when the kidneys fail to adequately filter substances, causing them to build up in the body. Addis told Pauling that his kidneys needed rest and instructed him to follow a strict diet low in protein and salt, and to consume plenty of water and supplementary vitamins and minerals. After about six months of rest and the restricted diet, Pauling regained his energy. To ensure that the disease did not recur, Ava Helen, Pauling's wife, kept him on the diet for about fifteen years. In a biographical memoir that he wrote about Addis, Pauling acknowledged that Addis had cured his nephritis using an orthomolecular approach.

In the 1960s, Pauling learned of the work of Abram Hoffer and Humphry Osmond, who used high doses of the B vitamin niacin to treat schizophrenia. In 1964 Pauling read Hoffer's book, *Niacin Therapy in Psychiatry*. About one year later, biochemist Irwin Stone informed Pauling that he could increase his longevity by taking large doses of vitamin C. Pauling was astonished that simple substances needed in minute amounts to prevent deficiency diseases could have therapeutic application in unrelated diseases when given in very large amounts. These incidents captured Pauling's curiosity and he immediately began to learn more about vitamins and nutrition and to vociferously advocate their use in maintaining optimal health. Vitamin C, also called ascorbic acid, became his primary topic when discussing the benefits of good nutrition and vitamin supplementation. Many people, unfamiliar with Pauling's earlier scientific career, tend to associate his name with this more recent endeavor—a thirty-year campaign promoting vitamin C.

Pauling enjoyed speaking about the attributes of vitamin C and did so in a vast range of media, such as books, articles, speeches, and interviews, throughout the rest of his life. In an effort to circulate his findings among the scientific and medical communities, Pauling wrote articles in academic journals, including *Science, Proceedings of the National Academy of Sciences,* and *Journal of the American Medical Association.* In hopes of reaching a wider audience, he allowed his statements to appear in popular publications, such as *Let's Live,* a magazine about health and preventive medicine, and *Harper's Bazaar,* a woman's magazine. Also, many newspaper reporters summarized his viewpoints after having attended one of his lectures.

In writing *How to Live Longer and Feel Better* Pauling not only compiled his broad scientific knowledge with almost twenty years of research on nutrition and vitamins, but also incorporated his extensive experience of writing for popular audiences. His earliest book for the general public, *No More War!*, was published in 1958. In this book Pauling promotes world peace through an end to nuclear warfare and atomic bomb testing. His book explains the science behind atomic weaponry and nuclear fallout and substantiates his call for peace by discussing the detrimental effects of radiation, such as genetic mutations that may cause birth defects and cancer. Pauling revised *No More War!* for a twenty-fifth anniversary volume in the early 1980s by writing addenda to each chapter and a new introduction. Following its publication, Pauling started work on *How to Live Longer and Feel Better.*

Pauling had written three books on the health benefits of taking large doses of vitamin C prior to this one. The first of these, *Vitamin C and the Common Cold,* took him only two months to write and was published in 1970. Jane E. Brody of *The New York Times* evaluated the book's success by reporting that pharmacies across the United States had witnessed a significant increase in vitamin C sales. Pauling revised this book a few years later, incorporating additional chapters on influenza, and in 1976 published *Vitamin C, the Common Cold and the Flu. How to Live Longer and Feel Better* draws from these previous books and also integrates information from a book Pauling co-authored with Dr. Ewan Cameron in the late 1970s titled *Cancer and Vitamin C.*

Pauling's long collaboration with Cameron began in 1970. They believed that supplemental vitamin C might inhibit the growth of solid tumors in several ways. Years later, research at the Linus Pauling Institute of Science and Medicine found that vitamin C and its derivates, due to certain structural features of the molecules, are selectively toxic to many types of cancer cells. More recently, research has shown that vitamin C is selectively toxic to cancer cells through the generation of hydrogen peroxide. These may be the principal anticancer mechanisms for vitamin C.

Pauling stated that his writing frenzy in the early 1980s developed from a need to keep busy after the death of his wife, Ava Helen. Ava Helen and Linus Pauling met at Oregon Agricultural College in January 1922 and married in June 1923. The Paulings traveled together often and influenced each other greatly. Linus Pauling attributed his desire to speak against nuclear warfare to Ava Helen's urging. Dr. Addis believed that Ava Helen had saved Pauling's life by helping him recover from nephritis. Ava Helen was diagnosed in 1976 with stomach cancer. Pauling made sure that she took ten grams of vitamin C per day, and her health improved. When she finally succumbed to cancer in 1981, Pauling noted that they should have started her vitamin C therapy earlier and in greater doses. Following her death, Pauling lost his ability to concentrate, but eventually threw himself into work as a way to cope with her loss.

*How to Live Longer and Feel Better* appealed to a diverse audience and offers a simple dietary regimen for improved health, which Pauling lays out in the first section. He provides the main tenets of the book in chapter one and a twelve-step checklist on the first couple of pages of chapter two. One attractive aspect of Pauling's program is his belief that anyone can improve their health and happiness through a few "simple and inexpensive measures," as he states in the first sentence of this book. Another appealing element is Pauling's positive perspective, a tactic he used in his other opinion pieces and campaign statements. When writing about nuclear weapons, Pauling highlighted peace and humanity. In writing this book, he focused on longevity and prevention and treatment of disease, as the title suggests. In the final chapter, "A Happy Life and a Better World," Pauling presented ideas for implementation at an individual level and then explained how the individual contributes to the universal, providing the big picture and beseeching the reader to be cognizant of a global consciousness.

Throughout this book, Pauling tells anecdotes about people who have successfully implemented his regimen. Pauling learned of these successes because many people wrote to him describing their experiences after following his advice. Pauling received hundreds, perhaps thousands, of letters in response to his earlier books and talks on vitamin C and nutrition, and he continued to receive such letters after the publication of *How to Live Longer and Feel Better*. Pauling customarily responded in some way to each letter that he received. Despite such strong support for his vitamin C work, he faced many struggles and setbacks in getting his ideas accepted. To Pauling's dismay the medical establishment did not embrace his promotion of vitamin C. Some doctors denied the veracity of Pauling's assertions and belittled his credentials by noting that he did not have a medical degree. Others simply ignored him. Pauling confronted his detractors by advancing logical arguments and sensible hypotheses. When Pauling wrote *Vitamin C and the Common Cold* he did not anticipate such a reaction from the medical community. In his next book, *Vitamin C, the Common Cold, and the Flu,* Pauling added a chapter addressing the medical establishment. He then expanded it for this book.

Pauling also had problems obtaining funding for the research conducted at the Linus Pauling Institute of Science and Medicine. A constant supporter of Pauling's nutritional campaign was Dr. Arthur M. Sackler, an internationally renowned art collector and philanthropist, and the person to whom Pauling dedicated this book. Sackler not only bolstered Pauling's endeavors through monetary assistance, but also provided him with emotional support. The two men had been close friends since the early 1970s and they had many common scientific interests. Sackler, a medical physician by training, wrote a weekly international column in a newspaper he founded and published called *Medical Tribune*. In his columns he presented his medical opinions and health advocacy, which included alerting the public to the health concerns associated with cigarette smoking, alcoholism, and drug abuse. In a few of his columns, Sackler wrote admiringly about Pauling and his accomplishments as a scientist, nutritionist, and humanitarian. Pauling described Sackler as a "physician, scientific researcher, art collector, and medical publisher" and returned the compliments by referring to Sackler as "upright and honorable" and of excellent character. Together, Pauling and Sackler addressed those in opposition to the therapeutic benefits of vitamins by submitting articles to medical journals, such as the *Journal of the American Medical Association*. If Pauling could not get his article published in one of the academic journals, then Sackler published it in his *Medical Tribune*. Additionally Pauling, Sackler, Albert Szent-Györgyi, and two other men started the Foundation for Nutritional Advancement. As explained by Pauling in this book, Szent-Györgyi isolated vitamin C in the late 1920s and was awarded the Nobel Prize for Physiology and Medicine in 1937 for his work with vitamin C. Pauling and Szent-Györgyi shared similar opinions on the value of supplemental vitamin C.

As stated by many of those who reviewed Pauling's book, he was its best advertisement. Pauling, in his eighties, appeared vibrant and energetic on the book's cover, endured the demands of the book tour with ease, and continued to conduct radio and television interviews.

Linus Pauling received many awards and honors for his research and advocacy of orthomolecular medicine. He continued to receive accolades and honors throughout the 1980s and 1990s and even into the twenty-first century. In 1991 Pauling received a certificate of recognition at the Second World Congress on Vitamin C and the Immune System, and in 2001 he was inducted into the Natural Health Hall of Fame by *Natural Health Magazine*.

In the final years of his life, Pauling continued to promote vitamin C and conduct research at the Linus Pauling Institute of Science and Medicine. He also envisioned writing a new, enlarged edition of this book that would bring it up to date and increase its length, but his own ill health prevented this. By this time Pauling had known for almost a year that he had prostate cancer; he had been diagnosed in December 1991. Many critics asked Pauling why he got cancer, since he had taken vitamin C for so long; he replied that his high intake may have postponed his inevitable illness for twenty years or so, since most elderly men have abnormal or cancerous prostate cells. Heeding his own advice, Pauling combated his cancer by taking vitamin C and other nutrients, in addition to conventional and experimental therapy. Although he eventually succumbed to the cancer at the age of ninety-three, Pauling remained mentally acute and active over the last few years of his life.

*How to Live Longer and Feel Better*

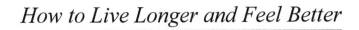

# Introduction

This book discusses some simple and inexpensive measures that you can take to lead a better and longer life, with greater enjoyment and fewer illnesses. The most important recommendation is that some vitamins be taken every day to supplement the vitamins that you get in your food. The best amounts of the supplementary vitamins and the best way to take them are discussed in the first chapters of the book, and the reasons for taking them are discussed in the following chapters.

I am a scientist, a chemist, physicist, crystallographer, molecular biologist, and medical researcher. Twenty years ago, I became interested in the vitamins. I discovered that the science of nutrition had stopped developing. The old professors of nutrition who had helped to develop this science fifty years ago seemed to be so well satisfied with their accomplishments that they ignored the new discoveries that were being made in biochemistry, molecular biology, and medicine, including vitamins and other nutrients. Although a new science of nutrition was being developed, these old professors of nutrition continued to teach their students the old ideas, many of them wrong, such as that no person in ordinary health needs to take supplementary vitamins and that all that you need to do for good nutrition is to eat some of each of the "four foods" each day.

As a result of this poor teaching, many nutritionists and dieticians today still practice the old nutrition, with the result that the American people are not as healthy as they should be. Physicians also contribute to this problem. Most of them have received only a small amount of instruction in nutrition (most of it, of course, out of date) in medical school, and since then have been kept so busy in their care of their patients as not to have time to follow the new developments about vitamins and other nutrients.

When I discovered that the new developments in the field of nutrition were being ignored I became so interested that for twenty years most of my effort has been devoted to research and education in this field. I have been fortunate in this work to have had and to continue to have the collaboration of many able scientific and medical investigators in Stanford University and Linus Pauling Institute of Science and Medicine.

Fifteen years ago many people were already convinced, on the basis of their own experience, that an increased intake of vitamin C provides some protection against the common cold, even though most physicians and authorities in the field of nutrition continued to describe vitamin C as having no value in controlling the common cold or any other disease except its specific deficiency disease, scurvy. When I examined the medical literature I found that a number of excellent studies had been carried out, and that most of them showed that vitamin C does have value in controlling the common cold. My concern about the failure of the medical authorities to pay the deserved attention to the existing evidence caused me to write my book *Vitamin C and the Common Cold.*

When this book was published it received favorable comment from some reviewers, but was quite strongly criticized by others. The discussion that followed stimulated a number of investigators, including Professor George Beaton, head of the Department of Nutrition in the School of Hygiene of the University of Toronto, to begin controlled trials. These trials all supported the conclusion that vitamin C has value in controlling the common cold. As a result, the medical and nutritional authorities could no longer claim that vitamin C has no value in connection with the common cold, although they may contend that the amount of protection provided by it is not great enough to justify the bother and expense of taking the vitamin.

In the course of my continued studies of vitamin C I learned that this vitamin exerts a general antiviral action and provides some protection not only against the common cold but also against other viral diseases, including influenza, mononucleosis, hepatitis, and herpes. The common cold is a nuisance, but it is not very dangerous. Only rarely does it lead to complications that cause death. Influenza (the flu), on the other hand, is a very serious and dangerous disease. In the great influenza pandemic of 1918-1919 the disease was contracted by about 85 percent of the population in all countries and killed about 1 percent, including many healthy young adults—the estimated total number of deaths being about 20 million. An outbreak of influenza in early 1976 with a virus similar to that of the 1918-1919 pandemic also caused great concern. It is important to know that a good intake of vitamin C can improve your general health in such a way as to provide significant protection against these diseases. In addition, good intakes of vitamin C and other vitamins can improve your general health in such a way as to increase your enjoyment of life and can help in controlling heart disease, cancer, and other diseases and in slowing down the process of aging. All of these questions are discussed in this book.

I hope that the book will help many people to avoid serious illness and will enable them to lead and enjoy healthier and longer lives.

I thank Mrs. Dorothy Munro, Mrs. Corrine Gorham, Mrs. Ruth Reynolds, Dr. Ewan Cameron, Dr. Zelek Herman. Dr. Linus Pauling, Jr., Dr. Crellin Pauling, Dr. Kay Pauling, Dr. Armand Hammer, Mr. Ryoichi Sasakawa, and Dr. Emile Zuckerlandl for their help. I am grateful to Dr. Abram Hoffer, Dr. Humphry Osmond, and Dr. Irwin Stone for having aroused my interest in vitamins about twenty years ago, and to Linda Chaput and her associates in W. H. Freeman and Company for their help in the publication of this book. I am especially grateful to my friend Gerard Piel for his continued encouragement and his contributions to the book.

Linus Pauling<br>
Linus Pauling Institute of Science and Medicine<br>
440 Page Mill Road<br>
Palo Alto, California 94306<br>
September 1, 1985

# I
# *THE REGIMEN*

# 1

## *Good Nutrition for a Good Life*

I believe that you can, by taking some simple and inexpensive measures, lead a longer life and extend your years of well-being. My most important recommendation is that you take vitamins every day in optimum amounts to supplement the vitamins that you receive in your food. Those optimum amounts are much larger than the minimum supplemental intake usually recommended by physicians and old-fashioned nutritionists. The intake of vitamin C they advise, for example, is not much larger than that necessary to prevent the dietary-deficiency disease scurvy. My advice that you take larger amounts of C and other vitamins is predicated upon new and better understanding of the role of these nutrients—they are not drugs—in the chemical reactions of life. The usefulness of the larger supplemental intakes indicated by this understanding has been invariably confirmed by such clinical trials as have been run and by the first pioneering studies in the new epidemiology of health.

By the proper intakes of vitamins and other nutrients and by following a few other healthful practices from youth or middle age on, you can, I believe, extend your life and years of well-being by twenty-five or even thirty-five years. A benefit of increasing the length of the period of well-being is that the fraction of one's life during which one is happy becomes greater. Youth is a time of unhappiness; young people, striving to find their places in the world, live under great stress. The deterioration in health as the result of age usually makes the period before death a time of unhappiness again. There is evidence that there is less unhappiness associated with death at an advanced age than at an early age.

For such reasons it is sensible to take the health measures that will increase the length of the period of well-being and the life span. If you are already old when you begin taking vitamin supplements in the proper amounts and following other practices that improve your health, you can expect the control of the process of aging to be less, but it may still amount to fifteen or twenty years.

For most of the statements in the following chapters I give reference to the published reports of the observations on which the statements are based. It is not possible, however, for me to substantiate in the same way the foregoing statements of my beliefs about the increase in the length of the period of well-being and the length of life. I have formed these beliefs on the basis of my knowledge of a great many observations about the effects of vitamins in varying amounts on animals and human beings under various conditions of good or poor health, including some significant epidemiological studies. There is, however, no single study to which I can point as showing with high statistical significance that the amounts of benefit is as great as I believe it to be. One complication. discussed in a later chapter, is that human beings differ from one another; they show a pronounced biochemical individuality. It is far easier to obtain reliable information about the factors determining the health of guinea pigs or monkeys than of human beings, and I have relied to some extent on the studies made on these and other animal species.

I am, for example, impressed by the fact that the Committee on the Feeding of Laboratory Animals of the U.S. National Academy of Sciences-National Research Council recommends far more vitamin C for monkeys than the Food and Nutrition Board of the same U.S. National Academy of Sciences-National Research Council reommends for human beings. I am sure that the first committee has worked hard to find the optimum intake for the monkeys, the amount that puts them in the best of health. The second committee has not made any effort to find the optimum intake of vitamin C or of any other vitamin for the American people. In its Recommended Daily Allowances, so well publicized that they are referred to on breakfast-cereal boxes by the initials RDA, the committee rations the vitamins at not much above the minimum daily intake required to prevent the particular deficiency disease that is associated with each of them.

No evidence compels the conclusion that the minimum required intake of any vitamin comes close to the optimum intake that sustains good health. The best supplementary amounts of the vitamins and the best way to take them I discuss in the first chapters of this book, and the reasons for taking them in the chapters that follow. As you will see, I think that vitamin C is the most important in the sense that the value of increasing the intake of this vitamin beyond that supplied by an ordinary diet is greater than for the other vitamins, but the other vitamins are also important.

When it comes to concern about health, an important question is the extent to which a person in the United States should depend on his or her physician. At the present time the main job of the physician is to try to cure the patient when he or she appears in the office with a specific illness. The physician usually does not make any great effort to prevent the illness or to strive to put the person consulting him or her in the best of health.

A remarkable book has been published recently (1984) by Dr. Eugene D. Robin, professor of medicine and physiology in Stanford Medical School. Its title is *Matters of Life and Death: Risks vs. Benefits of Medical Care.* In it the author discusses the drawbacks of present-day medicine as well as its strengths. His thesis is that there are "serious flaws in the basic processes by which diagnostic and therapeutic measures are introduced and used in medicine" and that "potential or actual patients can reduce the risks and increase the benefits of their medical care if they are familiar with the flaws in medicine." Robin writes that if you pay attention to your own health and do not see the "doctor as God," you can avoid serious errors in your own care. "You will be advised," he says, "to consult doctors only when you believe that you are truly ill. By restricting your medical encounters to those that are absolutely necessary you will be avoiding the risks inherent in most diagnostic and therapeutic procedures."

"This advice," Robin says, "tends to slight an important function that doctors have assumed in our society: dealing with patients whose main problem is an unhappy life. It is your privilege to consult a doctor for that purpose, but you should know that few doctors have high cure rates for unhappy lives, so that the chances of obtaining real help are small. Moreover, your visit may start a series of potentially dangerous medical tests and treatments. If, as a result of reading this book, you see that *even a decision to consult a doctor* is a serious and potentially risky one, that it requires some estimate of potential risks as well as potential benefits, you will have spent your time well.

"You will be cautioned to *avoid hospitalization* unless you are seriously ill and only a hospital has the facilities for your treatment. Many hospitalizations are unnecessary. Hospitals can be dangerous places."

Robin does not discuss vitamins in his book. This omission is probably the result of his having no more knowledge about vitamins than most other physicians have. If he knew more about vitamins, he might have warned his readers to be careful about accepting their doctor's advice about vitamins and other aspects of nutrition, because most physicians and surgeons received little instruction in this field in medical school and have picked up much misinformation since their graduation.

It is particularly important that you not let your doctor stop your vitamin supplements when you are hospitalized. That is when you have the greatest need for them.

In April 1970, I wrote to Dr. Albert Szent-Györgyi, the man who first separated ascorbic acid, which is another name for vitamin C, from the plant and animal tissues in which it occurs. I asked his opinion about vitamin C, especially with relation to the optimum rate of intake. He gave me permission to quote part of his answering letter, as follows. "As to ascorbic acid, right from the beginning I felt that the medical profession misled the public. If you don't take ascorbic acid with your food you get scurvy, so the medical profession said that if you don't get scurvy you are all right. I think that this is a very grave error. Scurvy is not the first sign of the deficiency but a premortal syndrome, and for full health you need much more, very much more. I am taking, myself, about 1 g a day. This does not mean that this is really the optimum dose because we do not know what full health really means and how much ascorbic acid you need for it. What I can tell you is that one can take any amount of ascorbic acid without the least danger."

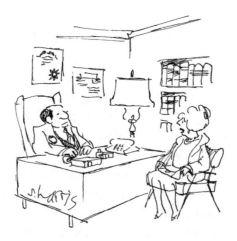

"I'D LIKE SOME OF THAT PREVENTIVE MEDICINE I'VE HEARD SO MUCH ABOUT."

The medical profession and the powerful medical institutions and enterprises in this country have taken to calling themselves the health profession, health centers, and health companies. This is a misnomer for what is really the sickness industry. I like the definition of health set out in the constitution of the World Health Organization, which states "Health is a state of complete physical, mental, and social well-being and not merely the absence of disease and infirmity."

The World Health Organization constitution goes on to say, "The enjoyment of the highest attainable standard of health is one of the fundamental rights of every human being without regard to race, religion, political belief and economic or social condition." This is a right that only a minority of the world population can yet enjoy. It is a right open to the lucky people of this country who have the material wealth to make it real. It is a right that is open to you. All that you need to do is to assert it by sensible behavior. What is more, thanks to the new science of nutrition, you can today multiply the benefits of healthy habits by taking, every day, the optimum amounts of the essential vitamins.

No one knows the state of health of a person better than the person himself or herself. It is important to think about one's health and to act in such a way as to improve it.

# 2

## *A Regimen for Better Health*

The measures that you take to improve your health and prolong your life should not be so burdensome and disagreeable as to interfere seriously with the quality of your life and make it difficult for you to continue with the regimen day after day, year after year. Compliance is very important. The regimen described in the following paragraphs is of such a nature that you should be able to adhere to it rigorously, day after day, for the rest of your life.

The regimen does not include every health measure of which I have knowledge. Moreover, it does not take into account the special nutritional needs of individuals. For example, persons with a tendency toward arthritis might benefit by increases in vitamin C, niacinamide, and vitamin $B_6$. The regimen is instead an average or basic one, which should benefit nearly every person in the United States. Additional benefits may result from changes made in response to biochemical individuality. The steps of the regimen are as follows:

1.  Take vitamin C every day,† 6 grams (g) to 18 g (6000 to 18,000 milligrams [mg]), or more. Do not miss a single day.
2.  Take vitamin E every day,† 400 IU, 800 IU, or 1600 IU.*
3.  Take one or two Super-B tablets every day, to provide good amounts of the B vitamins.
4.  Take a 25,000 IU vitamin A tablet every day.†
5.  Take a mineral supplement every day, such as one tablet of the Bronson vitamin-mineral formula, which provides 100 mg of calcium, 18 mg of iron, 0.15 mg of iodine, 1 mg of copper, 25 mg of magnesium, 3 mg

---

†This symbol is used to alert readers to an annotation in the Afterword. Readers are urged to check these annotations, since many of them involve updated information.

*IU stands for International Unit, the quantity of a vitamin (or other substance) specified in accordance with an international convention adopted by the World Health Organization.

of manganese, 15 mg of zinc, 0.015 mg of molybdenum, 0.015 mg of chromium, and 0.015 mg of selenium.

6. Keep your intake of ordinary sugar (sucrose, raw sugar, brown sugar, honey) to 50 pounds per year, which is half the present U.S. average. Do not add sugar to tea or coffee. Do not eat high-sugar foods. Avoid sweet desserts. Do not drink soft drinks.

7. Except for avoiding sugar, eat what you like—but not too much of any one food. Eggs and meat are good foods. Also, you should eat some vegetables and fruits. Do not eat so much food as to become obese.

8. Drink plenty of water every day.

9. Keep active; take some exercise. Do not at any time exert yourself physically to an extent far beyond what you are accustomed to.

10. Drink alcoholic beverages only in moderation.

11. DO NOT SMOKE CIGARETTES.

12. Avoid stress. Work at a job that you like. Be happy with your family.

The main feature of this regimen is the vitamin supplements. Taking them need not be burdensome. It is easy to get in the habit of taking your vitamins every day, and it is important to do so.

The great advantage of this regimen over other proposed methods of prolonging life and improving health is that it is firmly based on the new science of nutrition that has been developed only during recent years. The greatest difference between this new science and the old nutrition is the recognition that vitamins taken in the optimum amounts have far greater value than when taken in the usually recommended small amounts, shown in the table on page 11. Moreover, with the optimum intake of supplementary vitamins there is no longer so much need to stress other dietary measures, such as decreasing the intake of animal fat and not eating eggs. The regimen that I recommend permits compliance, day after day, year after year. A burdensome or disagreeable regimen will not be followed by many people. The quality of life is enhanced when one is liberated from these dietary restrictions.

The discovery of vitamins three quarters of a century ago and the recognition that they are essential elements of a healthy diet was one of the most important contributions to health ever made. Of equal importance was the recognition about twenty years ago that the optimum intakes of several

**Recommended daily adult intakes of vitamins**

|  | RDA† | Williams | Allen* | Leibovitz** | This book |
|---|---|---|---|---|---|
| Vitamin C | 60 mg | 2500 mg | 1500 mg | 2500 mg | 1000-18,000 mg |
| Vitamin E | 10 IU | 400 IU | 600 IU | 300 IU | 800 IU |
| Vitamin A | 5000 IU | 15,000 IU | 15,000 IU | 20,000 IU | 20,000-40,000 IU |
| Vitamin K | none | 100 mg | none | none | none |
| Vitamin D | 400 IU | 400 IU | 300 IU | 800 IU | 800 IU |
| Thiamine, $B_1$ | 1.5 mg | 20 mg | 300 mg | 100 mg | 50-100 mg |
| Riboflavin, $B_2$ | 1.7 mg | 20 mg | 200 mg | 100 mg | 50-100 mg |
| Niacinamide, $B_3$ | 18 mg | 200 mg | 750 mg | 300 mg | 300-600 mg |
| Pyridoxine, $B_6$ | 2.2 mg | 30 mg | 350 mg | 100 mg | 50-100 mg |
| Cobalamin, $B_{12}$ | 0.003 mg | 0.09 mg | 1 mg | 0.1 mg | 0.1-0.2 mg |
| Folacin | 0.4 mg | 0.4 mg | 0.4 mg | 0.4 mg | 0.4-0.8 mg |
| Pantothenic acid | none | 150 mg | 500 mg | 200 mg | 100-200 mg |

\* Harrell et al., 1981  \*\* Leibovitz, 1984

of the vitamins, far larger than the usually recommended intakes, lead to further improvement in health, greater protection against many diseases, and had great value as an adjunct to the appropriate conventional therapy in the treatment of diseases. The principal way in which vitamin C and other vitamins function is by strengthening the natural protective mechanisms of the human body, especially the immune system, and by increasing the effectiveness of enzymes in catalyzing biochemical reactions.

The optimum daily amounts of vitamins are far larger than the amounts that can be obtained in food, even by selecting foods for their high vitamin content. The only way to obtain the amounts of vitamins that put you in the best of health is to take vitamin supplements. For example, to obtain the 18,000 mg of vitamin C that I take each day I would have to drink more than 200 large glasses of orange juice.

To secure my recommended intakes of supplementary vitamins and minerals, shown in the table above, I take only four tablets a day. These are one 800-IU vitamin E capsule, one Super-B tablet, one vitamin and mineral tablet, and one 25,000-IU vitamin A capsule. I take them in the evening. I take much of my vitamin C in the morning, before breakfast, 12 g (three level teaspoonfuls) of pure crystalline ascorbic acid either dissolved in orange juice to buffer it or in water with a small amount of baking soda (sodium hydrogen carbonate) added to make an effervescent drink. Vitamin C may also be taken as sodium ascorbate or calcium ascorbate. If I feel tired later in the day or feel that I have been exposed to a cold virus, I take a few 1-g tablets or another spoonful of ascorbic acid.

**Recommended daily allowances (RDA)†**

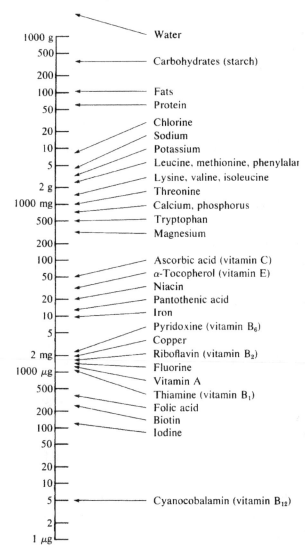

| | |
|---|---|
| 1000 g | Water |
| 500 | |
| 200 | Carbohydrates (starch) |
| 100 | Fats |
| 50 | Protein |
| 20 | Chlorine |
| | Sodium |
| 10 | Potassium |
| 5 | Leucine, methionine, phenylalar |
| | Lysine, valine, isoleucine |
| 2 g | Threonine |
| 1000 mg | Calcium, phosphorus |
| 500 | Tryptophan |
| | Magnesium |
| 200 | |
| 100 | Ascorbic acid (vitamin C) |
| 50 | α-Tocopherol (vitamin E) |
| | Niacin |
| 20 | Pantothenic acid |
| 10 | Iron |
| 5 | Pyridoxine (vitamin B$_6$) |
| | Copper |
| 2 mg | Riboflavin (vitamin B$_2$) |
| 1000 μg | Fluorine |
| 500 | Vitamin A |
| | Thiamine (vitamin B$_1$) |
| 200 | Folic acid |
| 100 | Biotin |
| 50 | Iodine |
| 20 | |
| 10 | |
| 5 | Cyanocobalamin (vitamin B$_{12}$) |
| 2 | |
| 1 μg | |

These allowances, set by the Food and Nutrition Board of the U.S. National Academy of Sciences-National Research Council, specify for adult males the amounts of thirty-three nutrients needed for preventing overt manifestation of deficiency disease in most persons. The list includes four macronutrients—water, carbohydrates, fats, and protein—and twenty-nine micronutrients to be taken daily in food and supplements. The RDA for vitamins typically fall short of the optimum intakes required for the best of health. Other nutrients, probably or possibly required, not shown here, are the essential fatty acids, para-aminobenzoic acid (PABA), choline, vitamin D, vitamin K, selenium, chromium, manganese, cobalt, nickel, zinc. molybdenum, vanadium, tin, and silicon.

At this writing, in the year 1985, the four tablets I take every day plus the 18 g of vitamin C (L-ascorbic acid, fine crystals) cost me by mail order, postage paid, the total sum of 41 cents a day. If I were to take, instead, the six tablets of the Roger J. Williams Fortified Insurance Formula, offered in the Bronson catalog, containing somewhat smaller amounts of these nutrients plus some others, the cost would be 37 cents a day. Thus these vitamin-mineral supplements, which can mean the difference for you between ordinary poor health and really good health, need cost you only as much as one small chocolate bar.

Even if, as a cancer patient, you were to take 50 g of vitamin C per day, it would cost only 78 cents, and with the other vitamins and minerals only $1.00 altogether, a negligible cost in comparison with the other expenses for a patient's care.

The values of the RDA given in the table on page 10 are those for adult males from the 1980 edition of the Recommended Dietary Allowances; the values for women and children are somewhat different. The Williams values are for the Fortified Insurance Formula of Professor Roger J. Williams; the Williams tablets also contain para-aminobenzoic acid, biotin, choline, inositol, rutin, and eleven minerals (calcium, magnesium, phosphorus, iron, zinc, copper, manganese, chromium, molybdenum, iodine, and selenium). The Allen formula also contains eight minerals. Brian Leibovitz (in his book *Carnitine*) also recommends biotin, choline, inositol, bioflavonoids, and ten minerals.

The essential minerals differ from the vitamins in that overdoses of minerals may be harmful. Do not increase your vitamin intake by taking a large number of vitamin-mineral tablets. Limit your mineral intake to the recommended amounts.

It is important not to stop the vitamin supplements, even for a single day. We know that there is a rebound effect† on stopping the intake of vitamin C, such as to increase temporarily the risk of disease. There may be similar rebound effects also for the other water-soluble vitamins, although none has been reported.

In general, the sensible way to buy vitamins is to check the prices and to buy the cheapest. It is required by the Food and Drug Administration (FDA) that the contents be stated on the label. There are probably a few unscrupulous companies, but usually the label can be relied on.

The range of prices for essentially the same items is far larger for vitamins than for most consumer goods, such as beefsteak or a television set. When I began checking the prices of vitamins fifteen years ago, I found that one company was selling a solution of vitamin C said to be specially prepared for old people at one thousand times the price of ordinary vitamin C, and another company was selling vitamin C tablets at one hundred times the ordinary price. I no longer find such tremendous overpricing, but if you do not check you might pay five times or even ten times the proper amount.

The catalog of a reliable company can be used as a reference standard, or you may check the advertisements in *Prevention* magazine.

It is wise not to buy vitamins from a salesman and not to buy from a company that does not have a price list that would permit you to compare prices.

Sometimes the effort is made to charge a higher price by using names that have little significance, such as Rose Hips Vitamin C (ordinary vitamin C with a little rose-hip powder added), chelated vitamins and minerals, "natural" vitamins,† etc. Also, brands prescribed by a physician may cost four times as much as the proper price.

Most vitamin preparations are stable. Ascorbic acid in the form of fine crystals or crystalline powder kept in a brown or opaque white bottle is stable indefinitely and can be kept for years. Dry tablets are also reasonably stable and can be kept for years in a brown or opaque white bottle. Solutions of ascorbic acid may be oxidized when exposed to air and light. A solution of ascorbic acid in water may, however, be kept for several days in a refrigerator without significant oxidation.

You may have to use some care not to be taken in by unscrupulous companies. After I had recommended pure vitamin-C crystals or powder in my book *Vitamin C and the Common Cold* I saw an advertisement for "Vitamin C Powder" at a price just under $10 per kilogram (kg). I bought a bottle from the company, which was based in Kansas City, Missouri, and found in small print on the label the statement, "Each level tablespoonful contains 500 mg of ascorbic acid." A level tablespoonful is about 14 g. Accordingly the preparation contains only 36 g of ascorbic acid in 1000 g of powder; only one twenty-eighth of the powder is ascorbic acid, and the price is $280 per kilogram of vitamin C, not $10. I wrote to the FDA about this misrepresentation and received in reply a statement that the FDA could do nothing about the matter. I then wrote to the Federal Trade Commission, which issued a cease-and-desist order on the company.

The most important part of my recommended regimen is to take the optimum amounts of the vitamins every day. This need not, as I have shown, involve swallowing more than a half-dozen tablets a day. My main other recommendation about diet (see Chapter 6) is to decrease your intake of sucrose (ordinary sugar, including raw sugar, brown sugar, syrup, and honey). You can improve your health significantly by reducing your sugar intake to half the U.S. average of 100 pounds per year, and you can do it by never putting sugar in tea or coffee, avoiding soft drinks, and eating sweet desserts and candy only rarely.

As to your diet otherwise, I think that you should for the most part eat what you like, rather than try to follow a restrictive diet that you have trouble conforming to and that does not add to your pleasure in life. Eat the foods that you like (except the high-sugar foods), but do not eat such large amounts as to make you overweight.

It is a good idea not to eat large amounts of meat. One quarter of a pound of meat provides 25 g of protein, about half the recommended amount per day. If your high intake of vitamin C keeps your serum cholesterol below 200 mg per deciliter (dl), there is no need for you to take special care to eliminate animal fat from your diet or to avoid drinking milk and eating eggs, both of which are good foods.

About 10 percent of adult Europeans and most Asians and Africans have digestive problems when they drink milk. At the end of infancy they stop making lactase, which is an enzyme involved in digesting milk sugar (lactose). Milk is a good food, especially as a source of calcium (about 500 mg per pint). The lactase-deficient person can, however, eat cheese, which is also high in calcium.

Even though a major reason for eating fruits and vegetables is to obtain vitamins, and this need may be satisfied by taking vitamin supplements, it is a good idea to include fruits and vegetables in the diet.

A moderate amount of regular exercise is good; also sleeping seven or eight hours a night, avoiding stressful situations, having an occupation that you like, and in general, enjoying life.

It is wise not to rely entirely upon dietary supplements for other essential nutrients, although they can be obtained as such in tablet and in other forms. "Essential" in this usage designates substances not manufactured in the body: certain amino acids and fats and many of the vitamins. The essential amino acids are not required as a dietary supplement if an adequate supply of protein is ingested. Moreover, although it is believed that the most important essential nutrients for humans are known, there is still the possibility that some have remained undiscovered. For this reason I agree with the first recommendation of the specialists in nutrition that everyone should eat a balanced diet, with a good amount of green vegetables, well prepared, and fresh fruits, such as oranges and grapefruit.

Since human beings show biochemical individuality, there is the possibility that a person may respond in an unusual way to an increased intake of vitamin C. Because vitamin C is required as an essential nutrient, and all of our ancestors tolerated it for millions of years, it is very unlikely that anyone would have a serious allergic response to it. There is, however, a slight possibility of allergy to the filler, if tablets are taken in preference to the powder, which is pure crystalline ascorbic acid. It is, of course, wise to increase or decrease the daily intake of this nutrient gradually.

A few months of experience should be enough to tell you whether the amount of ascorbic acid that you are ingesting approximates the desirable amount, the amount that provides protection against the common cold. That amount in the nutrition of older people can also reduce the misery of arthritis and carpal tunnel syndrome and many other ailments. If you take 1 g per day and find that you have developed two or three colds during the winter season, it would be wise to try taking a larger daily quantity.

Also, if you are exposed to a cold, by having been in contact with a person suffering from a cold, or if you have become chilled by exposure or tired by overwork or lack of sleep, it would be wise to increase the amount of vitamin C ingested.

It is wise to carry some 1000-mg tablets of ascorbic acid with you at all times. At the first sign that a cold is developing, the first feeling of scratchiness of the throat, presence of mucus in the nose, or muscle pain or general malaise, begin the treatment by swallowing two or more 1000-mg tablets. Continue the treatment for several hours by taking an additional two tablets or more every hour.

If the symptoms disappear quickly after the first or second dose of ascorbic acid, you may feel safe returning to your usual regimen. If, however, the symptoms continue, the regimen should be continued, with the ingestion of 10 g to 20 g of ascorbic acid per day. The physician Edme Régnier has pointed out (1968) that his observations indicate that when a cold is suppressed or averted by the use of an adequate amount of vitamin C the viral infection does not disappear at once but remains suppressed, and that it is accordingly important that the vitamin-C regimen be continued for an adequate period of time.

It may be worthwhile to help control a cold by the topical application of a solution of sodium ascorbate, made by dissolving 3.1 g of sodium ascorbate in 100 milliliters (ml) of water. Braenden (1973), who has reported success in curing most colds or markedly alleviating the symptoms by this method, recommends introducing twenty drops of this solution into each nostril with an eye dropper. He has pointed out that in this way a local concentration of ascorbate a thousand times the value produced by oral administration can be reached.

Ascorbic acid is inexpensive and harmless, even when it is ingested in large amounts. A common cold, when it develops, may involve serious discomfort and suffering, inconvenience, reduced efficiency, and even disability for some days. Moreover, it may lead to the complications of more serious infections. It is accordingly better to overestimate the amount of ascorbic acid needed to control the cold than to underestimate it. It may be desirable to increase the intake to the bowel tolerance limit, as discussed in Chapter 14. You must remember, too, to be on the lookout for the first symptoms of the cold and to be prepared to take immediate action. If you wait a day, or even a few hours, and if you take too small an amount of the vitamin, the cold may reach the stage where it cannot be stopped.

It is fortunate that vitamins are so cheap that even the high-potency supplements can be afforded by nearly every person in this country. My own rather large intake costs less than a can of soft drink, such as root beer, each day.

You should develop a simple regimen about your supplementary vitamins, such that you do not forget to take them. Also, you should develop good habits about moderate exercise, eating healthful foods that appeal to you, avoiding sucrose, not smoking, drinking large amounts of water, and drinking alcoholic liquors only in moderation, in such a way as not to be a burden to you but rather a pleasure, so that you have no trouble in continuing the regimen. The goal is to lead a good and satisfying life, free to as great an extent as possible from the suffering caused by poor health.

As the value of the optimum intakes of supplementary vitamins becomes known, it may well be recognized that the last period of the twentieth century, as well as the first period, has involved discoveries about vitamins that have not only already led to great improvement in human health and well-being but also can lead to even greater improvement in the future.

# 3

## *The Old Nutrition and the New*

The world of today is different from that of one hundred years ago. We now have a much greater understanding of nature than our grandparents had. We have entered the atomic age, the electronic age, the nuclear age, the age of jet planes, television, and modern medicine and its wonder drugs. For the good of our health, we should also recognize that this is the age of vitamins.

The world has been changed by the discoveries made by scientists. Sometimes the changes have occurred rapidly. For example, the fission of the nuclei of uranium atoms was discovered in 1938; and by 1945, after a crash program, nuclear bombs had been devised, constructed, and used in war. Insulin was discovered by Sir F. G. Banting, C. H. Best, J. J. R. McLeod, and J. B. Collip in 1922, and within a couple of years thousands of diabetic patients were being kept alive and in reasonably good health by injection of this hormone. Sometimes, however, there is a surprising delay. One of the best known examples is penicillin. This important substance was discovered in 1929 by Alexander Fleming, who showed that it exerted antibacterial action, but it began to be used therapeutically only in 1941, by W. H. Florey and E. B. Chain.

An older example is the delay in accepting the idea that childbed fever could be prevented by having the doctor wash his hands after delivering one infant before going to the next one. The American writer and physician Oliver Wendell Holmes in 1843 published an article on the contagiousness of this disease. It brought him bitter personal abuse. In 1847 the Hungarian physician Ignaz Philipp Semmelweis recommended that physicians wash their hands in chlorinated water between deliveries. In his clinic in Vienna and then in Budapest he himself was able to reduce the puerperal mortality rate from the terrible value of 16 percent to 1 percent. Reactionary physicians nonetheless rejected his idea for years. He became embittered and insane before he died in 1865.

The discovery of vitamins during the first third of the twentieth century and the recognition that they are essential elements of a healthy diet was one of the most important contributions to health ever made. Of equal importance was the recognition, about twenty years ago, that the optimum intakes of several of the vitamins, far larger than the usually recommended intakes, lead to further improvement in health, greater protection against many diseases, and enhanced effectiveness in the therapy of diseases. The potency of vitamin C and other vitamins is explained by the new understanding that they function principally by strengthening the natural protective mechanisms of the body, especially the immune system. The nutritional establishment has shown itself to be, however, as sluggish in recognizing this discovery as the medical establishment was in its response to Holmes and Semmelweis.

As early as 1937 Albert Szent-Györgyi, the scientist who isolated vitamin C, had said that vitamins, used in the proper way, could have fantastic results in improving human health. Yet even now, a half century later, the old-fashioned nutritionists, speaking with the authority of the Food and Nutrition Board of the U.S. National Academy of Sciences-National Research Council, continue to ignore the evidence about the value of the optimum intakes of these important substances. They persist in recommending no more than the minimum supplementary intakes, established by clinical experience a half century and more ago, necessary to prevent the diseases associated with deficiency of the vitamins in the diet. Their recommendations stand in the way of wider popular understanding and practice of the new nutrition.

The optimum intakes of the vitamins shown in the table in Chapter 2 and urged in this book are also based upon evidence from clinical trials and experience. That evidence is illuminated by understanding gained through the powerful new methods of molecular biology; we know and are learning to know better just what role each vitamin molecule plays in the chemistry of the body. Thus, by the classic interaction of clinic and laboratory, molecular biology explains what the clinic finds, and the clinic confirms the optimum intakes commended by molecular biology.

My interest in the question of the nature of life and the structure of the characteristic molecules in the human body and other living organisms began in 1929. That was when Thomas Hunt Morgan and most of the younger men who had collaborated with him in locating Mendel's gene, the basis of heredity, in the chromosomes in the nucleus of the cell came from

Columbia University to the California Institute of Technology to organize the new Division of Biological Sciences. I had been trained in physics and chemistry. With my interest now drawn to genetics, I formulated a theory of the phenomenon of crossing-over of chromosomes, which I presented at a biology symposium but did not publish in a scientific journal. Then in 1935 I began, with my students and other collaborators, to study the structure and properties of hemoglobin and other proteins, the structure of antibodies and the nature of immunological reactions, and the abnormal structures of protein molecules that show up in sickle-cell anemia and other molecular diseases.

In 1963 I decided to investigate the molecular basis of mental disease. During the next ten years my associates and I, with the support of grants from the Ford Foundation and the National Institute of Mental Health, carried out studies of the biochemistry and molecular basis of mental retardation and schizophrenia, as well as of the phenomenon of general anesthesia (Pauling, 1961). It was this work that led me to become interested in vitamins.

In 1964 I read the reports of two psychiatrists, Dr. Humphry Osmond and Dr. Abram Hoffer, who were working in Saskatoon, Saskatchewan, Canada. I read with astonishment that they were giving as much as 50 grams per day of a vitamin ($B_3$, either niacin or niacinamide) to some patients with acute schizophrenia. I knew that this vitamin is required in the amount of 5 milligrams (mg) per day to prevent the deficiency disease pellagra, which seventy years ago was causing hundreds of thousands of people to suffer from diarrhea, dermatitis, and dementia, and then to die.

What astonished me was the very low toxicity of a substance that has such very great physiological power. A little pinch, 5 mg, every day, is enough to keep a person from dying of pellagra, but it is so lacking in toxicity that ten thousand times as much can be taken without harm. Vitamin C is equally lacking in toxicity. The difference between these substances and drugs led me to coin the word *orthomolecular* to describe them (see Chapter 11).

The fact that a deficiency in the intake of vitamin $B_3$ leads to the mental illness associated with pellagra caused me to check the medical literature. I found that persons with a deficiency in vitamin $B_{12}$ usually become psychotic even before they become anemic. Mental disturbances, I found, are also associated with deficiencies of vitamin C (depression), vitamin $B_1$ (depression), vitamin $B_6$ (convulsions), folic acid, and biotin, and there is evidence that mental function and behavior are also affected by changes in the amounts in the brain of any of a number of other substances that are normally present (Chapter 20).

My interest in the vitamins was focused on vitamin C about twenty years ago by a letter I received from a biochemist named Irwin Stone. I had met him when I addressed a dinner meeting in New York City the previous month. He began his letter by reminding me that I had expressed in my lecture a desire to live for the next fifteen or twenty years. Saying that he would like to see me remain in good health for the next fifty years, he was sending me a description of his high-level vitamin-C regimen, which he had developed during the preceding three decades. My wife and I began to follow the regimen recommended by Stone. We noticed an increased feeling of well-being, and especially a striking decrease in the number of colds that we caught, and in their severity.

In the introduction to my book *Vitamin C and the Cormmon Cold* (1970), I wrote: "Dr. Stone was, of course, exaggerating. I estimate that complete control of the common cold and associated disorders would increase the average life expectancy by two or three years. The improvement in the general state of health resulting from ingesting the optimum amount of ascorbic acid might lead to an equal additional increase in life expectancy."

It is my opinion now, after an additional fifteen years of study in this field, that for most people the improvement in health and longevity associated with the ingestion of the optimum amount of vitamin C probably lies in the range of twenty to twenty-five years of well-being, with an additional increase from the optimum intake of other vitamins. As I have already conceded, I can cite no reference for this estimate, but some of the reasons I believe in it are given in the following chapters of this book.

During the period 1966 to 1970 I gradually became aware of the existence of an extraordinary contradiction between the opinions of different people about the value of vitamin C in preventing and ameliorating the common cold. Many people believe that vitamin C helps prevent colds; on the other hand, most physicians at that time denied that this vitamin has much value in that regard. For example, in the discussion of the treatment of the common cold in his excellent book *Health* (1970) Dr. Benjamin A. Kogan made the following statement: "Research has shown that vitamin C, in the form of fruit juice, however pleasant, is useless in preventing or shortening colds." Dr. John M. Adams did not mention vitamin C in his book *Viruses and Colds: the Modern Plague* (1967). More recent books by physicians contain statements such as the following, from *What You Should Know about Health Care before You Call a Doctor* by G. T. Johnson (1975): "I would again, however, like to stress that there is no evidence to support the contention that vitamin C prevents the common cold and only shaky evidence to suggest that it may lessen the effects of colds."

In the *Book of Health* of the American Health Foundation (1981), edited by Dr. Ernst L. Wynder, readers are advised against taking massive doses of a particular vitamin and are told that "The evidence that taking a huge quantity [of vitamin C]—1,000 milligrams a day or more—will avert the common cold is tenuous." There is a suggestion of a little progress, however, in the statement on page 578 that "Some studies indicate that relatively large doses of vitamin C can reduce the duration of the symptoms, although the results remain controversial."

I found myself embroiled in controversy on this question by an article about vitamin C in the magazine *Mademoiselle* in November 1969. I was quoted as supporting the use of large amounts of vitamin C. Dr. Fredrick J. Stare, then head of the department of nutrition at the Harvard School of Public Health, who was described by *Mademoiselle* as "one of the country's Big Names in nutrition," was thereupon invoked to refute my opinion. He was quoted as saying, "Vitamin C and colds—that was disproved twenty years ago. I'll tell you about just one very careful study. Of five thousand students at the University of Minnesota, half were given large doses of C, half a placebo. Their medical histories were followed for two years—and no difference was found in the frequency, severity, or duration of their colds. And yes, stores of C are depleted in massive, lingering infection—not in week-long colds."

The study to which Dr. Stare was referring had been carried out by Cowan, Diehl, and Baker; the article describing their results was published in 1942 (see Chapter 13). When I read this article, I found that the study involved only about four hundred students, rather than five thousand, and it was continued for half a year, not two years, and it involved use of only

200 mg of vitamin C per day, which is not a large dose. Moreover, the investigators reported that the students receiving the vitamin C had 31 percent fewer days of illness per subject than those who did not receive the vitamin.

The fact that Stare, as well as the investigators themselves, had not considered a decrease by 31 percent in the days of illness to be significant suggested to me that an examination of the medical literature might provide more information about this matter. I found in the August 1967 issue of the journal *Nutrition Reviews* a brief, unsigned article in which a number of studies of vitamin C and the common cold were mentioned. The conclusion reported was that "there is no conclusive evidence that ascorbic acid has any protective effect against, or any therapeutic effect on, the course of the common cold in healthy people not depleted of ascorbic acid. There is also no evidence for a general antiviral, or symptomatic prophylactic effect of ascorbic acid." It is no coincidence that Dr. Fredrick J. Stare was listed at this time as editor of *Nutrition Reviews.*

I examined the reports mentioned in this article and found that my own conclusions, on the basis of the studies themselves, were almost entirely different from those expressed in the article. Like the Cowan, Diehl, and Baker study, they showed a difference between the subjects given vitamin C and the control subjects in accordance with my argument for vitamin C, the difference tending to increase with the size of the dose of the vitamin administered.

We may ask why the physicians and authorities on nutrition have remained so lacking in enthusiasm about a substance that was reported four decades ago to decrease the amount of illness with colds by 31 percent, when taken regularly in rather small daily amounts. I surmise that several factors have contributed to this lack of enthusiasm. In the search for a drug to combat a disease the effort is usually made to find one that is 100 percent effective. (I must say that I do not understand, however, why Cowan, Diehl, and Baker did not repeat their study with use of larger amounts of vitamin C per day.) Also, there seems to have existed a feeling that the intake of vitamin C should be kept as small as possible, even though this vitamin is known to have extremely low toxicity. This attitude is, of course, proper for drugs, substances not normally present in the human body and almost always rather highly toxic, but it does not apply to vitamin C. Another factor has probably been the lack of interest on the part of the drug companies in a natural substance that is available at a low price and cannot be patented. This is a pity; for here is a substance that holds the possibility of eliminating the common cold from human experience.

An old friend of mine, René Dubos, pointed out in one of his books that it is not the viruses and bacteria we are exposed to that kill us—something else kills us. When there is an epidemic, some people die and other people do not die. What is the difference between them? It is this difference that kills. I believe that often it is too little vitamin C that permits some people to succumb.

The common cold, and influenza as well, are infections by viruses that circulate, sometimes in epidemics, throughout the world. They rapidly die out, however, in a small, isolated population. If the incidence of colds and influenza could be decreased enough throughout the world—as it might be by the use of vitamin C for prevention and therapy—these diseases would disappear. I foresee achievement of this goal, perhaps within a decade or two, in some parts of the world. Some period of quarantine of travelers might be needed, so long as a major part of the world's people are poverty-stricken and especially subject to infectious diseases because of malnutrition, including lack of ascorbic acid in the proper amount.

To achieve this goal a change in the attitude of the public and of patients may be required. A person with a cold or the flu should feel that he or she should go into isolation in order not to spread the virus to other people, and social pressure should operate to help him or her to act in such a way as not to harm others. We have recently experienced a change in feeling about the "right" of cigarette smokers to pollute the atmosphere and distress nonsmokers. A similar change in feeling about the "right" of people to spread their viruses and infect others, so long as they themselves are able to stagger about, would benefit the world.

After twenty years of research and public education in the new nutrition, I believe that I can detect some progress in the attitude of the medical profession toward the new nutrition's findings and recommendations. Despite the intransigence of official opinion, I see the attitude of practicing physicians toward ascorbic acid and the other vitamins undergoing significant change. They are responding to the new evidence that has been gathered. some of which I review in this book. It is being more widely recognized that the intake of vitamins, and of some nonessential nutritional factors as well, can be varied in such a way as to produce a significant improvement in general health and a decrease in the incidence and severity of disease.

Ultimately, it will be common knowledge that the optimum daily intakes of vitamins are far larger than what can be had in food, even by selecting foods for their high vitamin content. The major reason argued for eating fruits and vegetables is to obtain vitamins.

The availability of vitamins does not mean that you should not include fruits and vegetables in your diet. It is true that for more than eighty years science-fiction writers have been writing about a world of the future in which people would not eat ordinary food but instead would swallow a tablet or two each day. We have now gone part-way toward this goal in that the need to eat large amounts of fruits and vegetables in order to have enough vitamins to keep us alive has been eliminated. By taking a few vitamin tablets we can obtain not only the minimum requirement that may be furnished by the natural foods eaten in sufficient quantity but the optimum intake that puts and keeps us in the best of health. We may ask how much further modern nutritional science and molecular biology might take us. The answer is that our nutritional needs can never be met by a few tablets per day. A rather large amount of fuel is required to provide the energy to keep us warm and to run the biochemical processes in our bodies that permit us to function and to work. That requirement comes to about 2500 kilocalories of food energy per day. To obtain this much food energy, about 1 pound, dry weight, of starch or the sugar glucose must be ingested. What is more, the body requires certain fats it does not itself manufacture, and it must be supplied with protein to replace the protein of its principal working parts as they wear out in the course of a day. A diet of this sort is available, as will be discussed in the next chapter, and it consists of much more than a few tablets.

# 4

## *Proteins, Fats, Carbohydrates, and Water*

Living organisms require daily intake of nutrients, substances from outside the body that, ingested and assimilated in the tissues, permit growth and preserve good health, provide energy, and replace loss. Certain substances are required in large amounts. These are the macronutrients; they are four in number: proteins, fats, carbohydrates, and water. Other substances, the micronutrients, are required in small amounts: certain minerals, the vitamins, and the essential fats and essential amino acids (building blocks of protein). The latter are called essential because the organism does not manufacture them, although it manufactures other fats and amino acids.

In this chapter, in a book otherwise concerned with one class of micronutrients, we consider the macronutrients, taking them in the order in which they are listed above.

The human body contains tens of thousands of different proteins, which serve different purposes. Hair and fingernails consist of fibers of a protein called keratin; muscle is composed of fibers of myosin and actin. Another fibrous protein, collagen, strengthens the skin, blood vessels, bones, teeth, and the intercellular cement that holds the cells in various organs and tissues together. Globular proteins, in solution in the body fluids, serve as enzymes to speed up the chemical reactions that are essential to life. Certain proteins serve other special functions. Hemoglobin, for example, the red protein in the red cells of the blood, carries molecules of oxygen from the lungs to the other parts of the body, where it is used to burn molecules of food in order to provide energy.

Proteins are long chains of amino-acid residues. There are more than twenty different amino acids. The nature of the protein is determined by the sequence of these different amino acids in the chain. Amino acids are rather small molecules, consisting of between ten and twenty-six atoms of hydrogen, carbon, nitrogen, oxygen, and sulfur; at least one of the atoms is nitrogen.

Most protein chains contain a few hundred amino-acid residues. The molecule of adult hemoglobin contains four chains, two with 140 residues and two with 146 residues each. As might be expected for structural molecules, proteins are characterized by the arrangement of their component amino acids in the three dimensions of space as well as by the sequence of the residues in the chain. The simplest, natural three-dimensional structure assumed by a chain of identical asymmetrical amino acids, bonded head to toe at the same angle, is the so-called alpha helix. In hair, the keratin chains are coiled in the alpha helix, like a spring. In a globular protein such as hemoglobin or the digestive enzyme trypsin, there are straight segments, alpha-helix coils, but the chain folds back on itself to become nearly spherical. In silk, as another example, the chains are stretched out to nearly their maximum length.

The amino-acid sequence for the same proteins in different animals is different. All mammals have hemoglobin in the red cells of their blood, but the hemoglobin molecules are different in their amino-acid sequence. Because of the difference in the blood proteins (and also the blood carbohydrates) of different animals we cannot safely transfuse blood from another species of animal into a human being. As Dr. Karl Landsteiner discovered in 1900, the blood of different human beings also may be different in such a way as to make transfusion of blood from one person to another dangerous to the recipient, unless tests have shown that the two persons have the same blood type.

When the food that we eat is digested in the stomach and intestines the protein molecules are broken down by the digestive enzymes into their component amino acids. The protein molecules in the food (from meat, fish, vegetables, grains, cheese, and milk) are so large that they cannot pass through the intestinal walls into the bloodstream, but the small molecules of the amino acids and of glucose from the breakdown of the long carbohydrate chains of starch can pass through. The blood carries these small molecules to the tissues throughout the body. They enter the cells, and the amino acids are then reassembled into long chains with the sequences that are characteristic of human proteins, under the guidance of the molecules of deoxyribonucleic acid (DNA) in the nuclei of our tissue cells that determine our nature.

Our bodies are continually wearing out and being renewed. For example, our red cells live only about one month. They are then broken down, and the hemoglobin molecules are split into amino acids. Some of the amino acids are used to make new protein molecules, but some are oxidized to water, carbon dioxide, and nitrogen-containing urea, which is excreted in the urine. Because some of the amino acids are used as fuel in this way, our bodies can keep in amino-acid balance (usually called nitrogen balance) only by adding some amino acids; that is, by eating some protein. With too small an intake of protein a child will stop growing, and a child or adult may die of protein starvation, even when the intake of fat and carbohydrate is adequate. Protein starvation is called kwashiorkor (from an African word in a region with a high-corn diet). Marasmus is energy starvation, and marasmus-kwashiorkor involves both deficiencies in the diet. These diseases cause many deaths in the overpopulated and underdeveloped countries and some in the affluent countries.

The amount of protein required for amino-acid balance for an adult is proportional to body weight. It is about 0.45 grams (g) per kilogram (kg), 0.20 g per pound. The Food and Nutrition Board recommends 30 percent larger amounts, 0.26 g per pound for adults. Infants need about 1.0 g per pound, young children about 0.60 g per pound, older children and adolescents 0.50 or 0.40 g per pound.

Most adult Americans ingest two or three times the recommended amount of proteins. The excess not required for building new protein molecules is burned, for energy, along with the fats and carbohydrates, and probably no harm is done by the excess intake to people in reasonably good health. A high intake of protein means that a large amount of urea must be excreted in the urine. The excretion of urea requires work by the kidney, and increased intake of protein increases the burden on the kidney. People with impaired kidney function, such as those with only one kidney or who have suffered damage from nephritis, can avert further kidney damage by limiting protein to the amino-acid-balance level. Care must be taken not to go below this level.

Although all of the amino acids are present in the proteins in the human body, not all of them need to be in the food because most of them are manufactured by the body. Those that must be obtained in the food, the essential amino acids, are histidine, leucine, isoleucine, lysine, methionine, phenylalanine, threonine, tryptophan, and valine. The amounts required for an adult young man range from 0.50 g per day for tryptophan to 2.20 g per day for leucine, methionine. and phenylalanine. These amounts are provided by a mixed diet including animal protein (meat, fish, eggs) but not by a vegetarian diet, which may be especially low in lysine and methionine.

Everybody knows what fat is—hog fat (lard) and beef or sheep fat (tallow). It has a greasy feel, is insoluble in water, and is an important constituent of foods and of the human body. Its chemical nature was discovered about 1820 by the French chemist Michel Eugene Chevreul, who died in 1889, at age 103. (I assume that he was not fat, or he would not have lived so long.) The Roman author Pliny the Elder mentions in his book on natural history that the Germans were making a soap solution by boiling fat with the ashes of plants (potash). In 1779 the Swedish chemist K. W. Scheele discovered that a detergent solution contained not only soap, the potassium salt of a fatty acid, but also an oily, sweet-tasting, water-soluble liquid that we now call glycerine or glycerol.

Chevreul discovered that ordinary fats consist of glycerol with three molecules of a fatty acid attached. A representative fat is glyceryl tripalmitate: its atomic composition is diagrammed this way:

$$H_2C\text{—}OOC(CH_2)_{14}CH_3$$
$$|$$
$$HC\text{—}OOC(CH_2)_{14}CH_3$$
$$|$$
$$H_2C\text{—}OOC(CH_2)_{14}CH_3$$

This fat is said to be "saturated" by hydrogen (H) because hydrogen atoms occupy the four bonds of each carbon (C) atom that are not attached to other carbon atoms or to oxygen (O). Other saturated fats have a smaller or larger number of $CH_2$ groups in the hydrocarbon side chains. Unsaturated fats have fewer hydrogen atoms; that is, they are not saturated with hydrogen. There are more unsaturated side chains in liquid fats (oils) than in solid fats.

These fat molecules are called triglycerides. When you receive a report on the analysis of your blood, there may be values for total cholesterol, HDL, LDL, and triglycerides. The amount of triglycerides is nothing other than the amount of fat in the blood plasma. Cholesterol, HDL, and LDL are molecules made by the processing of fat.

Fat is an important constituent of the diet as a source of metabolic energy. It also has value in helping to move the fat-soluble vitamins across the intestinal wall into the bloodstream.

In 1929 it was discovered that young rats show slow growth, kidney deterioration, and infertility on a diet containing only saturated fats. Between 1930 and 1956 different investigators discovered seven unsaturated fatty acids that are necessary, essential, in small amounts for normal growth and life for rats and other animals. Presumably human beings also require intake of these essential fatty acids. Only a few observations have been made on human beings on a very low fat diet; they showed an abnormal basal metabolism rate, increased incidence of infections, and a tendency to dermatitis. It is believed that a diet containing the usual amount of fat provides sufficient amounts of the essential fatty acids. There is some evidence, however, that an increased intake of two of them, linoleic acid and gamma-linolenic acid, may have protective value against atherosclerosis and cancer.

Carbohydrates were given this name because chemists noticed that these substances (various sugars, starch, glycogen, and cellulose) have formulas $C + H_2O$, that is, hydrated carbon. For example, glucose and fructose are $C_6H_{12}O_6$, sucrose is $C_{12}H_{22}O_{11}$. In fact, there are no water molecules in these substances; instead, there are carbon atoms and one or two hydrogen atoms attached to them along with the oxygen atoms and hydroxyl groups (OH).

Starch is the principal carbohydrate food. It is found in all fruits and vegetables. An intake of 300 g would provide 50 percent of an average daily requirement of energy. Providing energy is the principal function of the carbohydrates in our food. Many fruits and some vegetables also contain significant amounts of the simple sugars glucose and fructose, as well as the disaccharide sucrose, ordinary sugar, which contains both glucose and fructose.

When starch is digested by the enzymes in the saliva and gastric juice, it combines with water and breaks down to form the small molecules of glucose, which pass through the walls of the intestines into the bloodstream and are transported to the cells all over the body. There they are burned to provide the energy that we need to operate our biochemical mechanisms, to do work, and to keep warm. The glucose that is present in foods also enters the bloodstream and is handled in the same way. Human beings and their predecessors have been accustomed to metabolizing about 300 g of glucose (mostly from starchy foods) every day for millions of years.

The situation with fructose is different from that with glucose. Human beings have always ingested some fructose, in the fruits and honey that were part of their diet. Until about two hundred years ago the average daily intake of fructose was quite small, only about 8 g. Then, as ordinary sugar (sucrose) from sugar beets and sugarcane began to be generally available the daily intake of fructose rose tenfold, to about 75 g per day.

The reason for this great increase in the intake of fructose is that when sucrose is ingested it reacts with water to form equal amounts of glucose and fructose. Each 100 g of sucrose gives 53 g of glucose and 53 g of fructose; that is why it is referred to as a disaccharide. In the United States we eat about 100 pounds of sugar (sucrose) per year. This is 125 g per day, corresponding, when it is digested, to 66 g of fructose per day. With about 8 g from fruits and honey, the average daily intake becomes 74 g per day.

Our bodies have been accustomed to metabolizing only 8 g of fructose per day. It is accordingly not surprising that the nearly tenfold overload causes problems. There is little doubt that this great intake of fructose, to which human beings have been subjected only during the last century, is the cause of many of our ills, as will be discussed in Chapter 6.

Water is the fourth major nutrient. It is required for life in the amount of about one liter (l) per day, partially to produce urine to carry off the harmful substances that have been extracted from the blood by the filtering processes that operate in the two million filtering units (nephrons) in the kidneys. A larger intake of water, preferably about 3 liters (more than 3 quarts) per day, is needed for the best of health. A good habit is to drink a glass of water every hour. Soft drinks provide water, but they are undesirable because of the sugar or the sugar substitutes that they contain. Carbonated water, orange juice, and other fruit juices are good sources of water, as is also beer, in limited amount.

One reason for a high intake of water is that it leads to a high volume of urine; this reduces the burden on the kidneys, which excrete a dilute urine with less work than they do a concentrated urine. That is especially important for persons with impaired kidney function.

Another reason is that with a high intake of water there is less chance that crystals of one kind or another will form out of the body fluids. Gout results from the formation of crystals of sodium urate in the joints and tendons, and pseudo-gout from the similar crystallization of calcium pyrophosphate dihydrate. Urinary calculi (kidney stones) involve the formation of masses of crystals held in a protein matrix. The crystals are calcium and magnesium phosphates and urates or, less commonly, cystine. About 1 percent of people have a tendency to form these stones. The formation can be averted by keeping the water intake high, never allowing the urine volume to drop.

The various classes of foods—meats, fish, fruits and vegetables, grains and nuts, dairy products—all have value in providing protein, fat, carbohydrates, minerals, vitamins, and other valuable micronutrients, such as gamma-aminobenzoic acid, choline, lecithin, and the ubiquinones. The amounts of these important constituents are different in different foods, and it is wise to have a varied diet, one that appeals to you, and to supplement it with the important vitamins and minerals in order to get them in the optimum amounts.

The servings of meat and fish must be kept small in order to keep the total protein intake down to the recommended amount, 0.8 g per kilogram body weight.

Ovolactovegetarians, who accept eggs and milk but not meat and fish, can keep in good health by taking supplementary vitamins and minerals. Strict vegetarians need to select their vegetable foods with care to insure that they have the proper intake of those vegetables that provide the essential amino acids that are present in only small amounts in most vegetable foods.

The intake of fat should be limited, but enough should be eaten to provide the essential fats.

Fruits, vegetables, grains, and nuts should be eaten in a satisfying variety and amount. Fruits and vegetables provide some protein and fat, large amounts of carbohydrates, and also vitamins, minerals, and other micronutrients. A high intake was needed in past centuries in order to provide the minimum amounts of these micronutrients, as well as carbohydrate for energy. In the new era of modern nutrition the optimum intakes of vitamins, more than can conveniently be provided by fruits and vegetables, are available in supplements, as discussed throughout this book. It is wise, nonetheless, to supplement the vitamin supplements with a good intake of fruits and vegetables.

Seeds and nuts are low in vitamins and high in protein and fat as well as carbohydrate and total energy. For example, a 1-ounce snack of almonds provides 180 kilocalories (kcal) of food energy, 5 g of protein, 16 g of fat, and 6 g of carbohydrate. A similar snack of peanuts provides 170 kcal of energy, 7 g of protein, 14 g of fat, and 5 g of carbohydrate.

The amount of carbohydrate eaten should be kept down to the amount that permits the ingested fat to be burned rather than deposited in the body. You may have to limit your consumption of alcohol and of nuts and other snacks, as well as the size of your meals. The intake of sucrose (white sugar, brown sugar, raw sugar, honey, candy, sweet desserts) should be kept low. Corn syrup consists of glucose, and it is an acceptable sweetener unless sucrose has been added to make it sweeter—check the label. The obesity and atherosclerosis, the two most common nutritional afflictions arising from bad habits with respect to the macronutrients, that follow upon violation of these simple rules are discussed in Chapter 6.

# 5

## *Foods as the Source of Heat and Energy*

One of the characteristics of human beings is that they are able to do work. They also are able to keep warm in a cold environment. A source of energy is required for doing work and keeping warm.

Many of the substances in our food that enter the bloodstream—the fats and the amino acids as well as the carbohydrates—are burned in the cells of our tissues and organs to provide the energy for various biochemical reactions, including those in our muscles that permit us to do physical work and those that generate the heat energy to keep us warm. This process of burning is the enzyme-catalyzed combination of the fuel molecules with oxygen molecules that are distributed through the body by the blood. The hydrogen atoms burn to water, $H_2O$, and the carbon atoms to carbon dioxide, $CO_2$, which is carried to the lungs and exhaled. The nitrogen atoms form urea, $H_4N_2CO$, which is excreted in the urine.

The average amount of food energy required by men is 2000 to 3500 kilocalories (kcal) per day and for women 1600 to 2400. Young people require more and old people less. The quantity 2500 kcal is the average daily amount.

This amount of energy could heat a bathtub full of water (increasing the temperature of 25 gallons of water from 50°F to 100°F). If it could all be used to do work, it could lift a weight of 1400 pounds to the top of a mile-high mountain. With these calculations in mind, we can understand that we need more food in the winter than in the summer, in cold climates than in warm climates, and that heavy physical work or strenuous exercise increases the need for food.

The concept of food energy was discovered in 1842 by a young German physician, Julius Robert Mayer (1814-1878). He was the ship's surgeon on a Dutch ship sailing to Java when he wondered why the sailors, who were doing just as much work every day, ate much less food in the Indian Ocean than in the North Sea, and why the hard-working sailors ate more than the officers. He concluded that the food a person ingests provides a certain amount of energy, which can be used either for heat or for work.

At the same time the English physicist James Prescott Joule was making experiments (reported in 1843) to determine the relation between work and heat. These two thoughtful persons discovered the very important physical law called the conservation of energy.

The energy values of a food can be determined by burning a weighed amount of the food and measuring the amount of heat given off. It is convenient to give the values for a standard amount, 100 grams (g, or 3 1/2 ounces) of the food. The energy values are 900 kcal per 100 g of fat, 415 kcal per 100 g of starch, and about 430 kcal per 100 g of protein. The values for the sugars are a little smaller than for starch: 395 kcal per 100 g for sucrose, lactose (milk sugar), and maltose (malt sugar, a disaccharide made from starch by action of an enzyme), and 375 kcal per 100 g for glucose and fructose.

In the table below there are given values of the fractions of the energy provided by fat, protein, and carbohydrate in several diets—the average American diet, the diet recommended by the U.S. Senate Select Committee on Nutrition and Human Needs, and an intermediate diet. The third diet contains more fat and less carbohydrate than that of the Senate Committee. Part of the reason for recommending the intermediate amount of fat is that we need the essential fats, and we obtain these essential fats almost entirely in the food that we eat.

A diet with 10 percent of the energy provided by protein and giving 2500 kcal requires 58 g of protein. To keep the protein intake down to this level requires that the intake of meat and fish be limited. Half a pound of beefsteak provides more than 58 g of protein, allowing for no other protein

| Energy distribution of some diets. | | | |
|---|---|---|---|
| | *Present U.S. diet* | *Dietary goal*[1] | *Intermediate diet* |
| Fat | 42% | 30% | 40% (1000 kcal/day) |
| Protein | 12% | 12% | 10% (250 kcal/day) |
| Carbohydrate | 46% | 58% | 50% (1250 kcal/day) |
| Starch | 20% | 38% | 30% |
| Naturally occurring sugars | 6% | 10% | 10% |
| Sucrose | 20% | 10% | 10% |
| TOTAL | 100% | 100% | 100% (2500 kcal/day) |

[1]*Dietary Goals for the United States.* Senate Select Committee on Nutrition and Human Needs. U.S. Government Printing Office, Washington, D.C. (1976).

foods. One egg provides 6 g; one glass of milk 8 g; one slice of bread 3 g; one serving of baked beans 8 g; one serving of potatoes, green beans, or other vegetable 2 to 6 g; a serving of breakfast cereal 4 to 8 g. Lamb, pork, and fish contain 15 to 20 percent protein, beef about 30 percent. The intake of meat and fish should be kept to about a quarter of a pound per day. Probably the greatest benefit of all offered by the recommended diet comes from decreasing the intake of sucrose, ordinary sugar, as is discussed in the next chapter.

Much interest in the value of meat in the diet was created over half a century ago by observations made by the Arctic explorer Vilhjalmur Stefansson. He was born in Manitoba, Canada, of Icelandic parents, in 1879, and when he was only a year or two old he (and his parents) lived mainly on fish for a year, because of a famine in the area. After graduating from the University of Iowa, studying anthropology for three years at Harvard, and making two archaeological trips to Iceland, he began his Arctic research in 1905. He lived with the Eskimos for a year, learning their language and culture, and he concluded that it was possible to remain in reasonably good health on the Eskimo diet of meat alone, eaten as the Eskimos eat it.

By 1926 he had lived a total of nine years on a meat-only diet, during eleven and a half years spent in the Arctic. The longest period that he ate no food other than meat was nine months. A study of him made in 1922, when he was forty-three, showed him to be in the state of health expected for his age (Lieb, 1926); for example, his blood pressure was 115/55. He died at the age of eighty-two.

Because of Stefansson's claim that it was possible to be healthy on a diet of meat only, a carefully planned experiment was carried out with Stefansson and another Arctic explorer, beginning in 1927. For one year the two men ate nothing but meat (beef, lamb, veal, pork, chicken, both fat and lean portions, and also at times liver, kidney, brain, bacon, and bone marrow). Stefansson also ate some eggs, butter, and fish, when he had trouble obtaining meat while traveling. The meat was usually boiled or stewed, but they ate some raw marrow. They drank no milk. They were in a hospital under observation for the first six months and then resumed their usual activities but adhered to their diet. They reported that they had no craving for other foods. They complained, however, that the boiled mutton was not so good as the musk ox, caribou, or mountain sheep described in

Stefansson's autobiography, *Discover* (1962). They were carefully studied throughout the year, with the conclusion that they were in as good health at the end of the year as at the beginning.

The diet contained about 230 g of fat, 120 g of protein, and only 5 to 10 g of carbohydrate per day. The high intake of animal fat did not seem to harm them (Torrey and Montu, 1931).

Their tolerance for glucose was low at the end of the year but became normal within two weeks on a mixed diet.

It is remarkable that they did not develop vitamin-deficiency diseases on the exclusively meat diet. Presumably fresh meat contains a minimum supply of vitamin C and other vitamins. Stefansson (1918) reported that three of the seventeen members of the Canadian Arctic Expedition became scorbutic during the winter of 1916-1917. These three had been eating some foods in a cache that had been left by an earlier expedition. They developed scurvy, whereas the others, who ate only fresh meat, did not.

I do not conclude that a meat diet is the best, even though fresh meat may alone provide the minimum amounts of all nutrients, with the fat providing most of the energy. Vitamin supplements and a mixed diet, with a limited intake of sugar, lead to the best health.

Stefansson's experience has its relevance to public anxiety about fat in the diet. That anxiety was awakened in 1955, when President Dwight David Eisenhower suffered a coronary occlusion. The president's cardiologist, Paul Dudley White of the Harvard Medical School, took the occasion to instruct the public about the role of cholesterol in atherosclerosis and to advise reduction in the intake of fat-containing foods. Stefansson was moved to challenge White with his own good health on a high-fat diet and his observations of the health of the Eskimos he knew so well. He concluded with the rhetorical question: "We eat carbohydrates, fat, and protein. We make gunpowder from saltpeter, sulfur, and charcoal. How can we say which one makes the explosion?" White withdrew his doctrinaire stricture and wrote a chastened introduction to a new edition of Stefansson's account of his dietary adventures published under the title *The Fat of the Land.*

The energy content of alcohol is discussed in the following chapter.

# 6

## *Two Eating Problems*

It is from the numerous deficiency diseases, caused by lack of essential elements in the diet, that the students of nutrition first learned about the micronutrients and the various ways in which they serve the healthy organism. Today, in the well-off and well-fed industrial countries of the world, the science of nutrition is learning to contend with afflictions that attend overabundance rather than deficiency of the macronutrients. Efforts to manage the two most common of these afflictions, *obesity* and *atherosclerosis,* generate more controversy, if that is possible, than that which attends discussion of the micronutrients, especially the vitamins.

Obesity is the condition of being grossly overweight, excessively fat, much beyond the normal weight for the person's height and build. It constitutes a serious problem for many people.

The normal weights for women between 5 feet and 6 feet tall are 116 to 155 pounds, with leeway of about 10 or 15 pounds each way, depending on build. For men between 5 feet 4 inches and 6 feet 4 inches the values are 135 to 185 pounds, with leeway of 15 to 20 pounds. Overweight by 25 percent is accompanied by some inconvenience, by 40 percent by increased incidence of illness, and by shortening of life expectancy by four years. Overweight by 50 percent causes much inconvenience, a more than doubled incidence of illness, and a ten-year decrease in life expectancy (Pauling, 1958).

In past centuries and millennia the deposition of fat in the human body has served an important purpose. The supply of food was often irregular. When plentiful food was at hand, as when a mastodon was killed, people ate as much as they could. The protein (excess amino acids) and carbohydrates (glucose) were burned in the body cells to provide the needed energy, and the fat was stored in deposits under the skin and elsewhere in the body, in order that it might be burned later, to prevent death by starvation when food became scarce.

We may conclude that the way to prevent the excessive deposition of fat is to restrict the intake of all food—protein, carbohydrate, and fat—to the quantity required every day for heat and work. There is little gain from restricting just one kind of food. Even if fat is restricted, there is still some fat in the diet, and if there is enough carbohydrate to provide the energy needs, this fat will be deposited and will lead to obesity.

No crash diet or fad diet can solve the obesity problem, because these diets are so disagreeable and such a continuing nuisance that the obese person soon gives up. A successful treatment is one that will be adhered to, year after year. To achieve such continued compliance the diet should appeal to the appetite. It is not the kind of food that controls the body weight, but it is instead the total food energy, in relation to size, build, and amount of exercise. The food should be the kind that pleases the person, but the amounts eaten must be limited.

This point has been emphasized by Brian Leibovitz in his 1984 book, in which he criticizes various fad diets for control of weight and improvement of health. Representative of his comments are his statements about the Pritikin diet. On the jacket of Nathan Pritikin's book *The Pritikin Promise: 28 Days to a Longer, Healthier Life* there is the following exhortation:

> Follow my safe 28-day diet and exercise program and I promise
> you:
> You'll feel really alive every day;
> You'll reduce risk of heart disease, diabetes, high blood pressure,
> breast and colon cancer;
> You'll lose weight without hunger.

Leibovitz comments:

> The Pritikin program is a low-protein, low-fat, and high-
> carbohydrate regimen, and to its credit it emphasizes the
> importance of unrefined foods. Oil, butter, salt, sugar, and
> red meats are not allowed on the Pritikin plan. Since neither
> butter nor oils are allowed, foods must be broiled or steamed.
> The Pritikin diet, while basically sound, suffers from two
> major drawbacks, however. To begin, it is unnecessarily
> Spartan. Although there are some good reasons to cut down
> on excessive consumption of meat, diary products, oil, butter,
> salt, and sugar, . . . it is not necessary to eliminate them
> entirely from the diet. In my experience, because it is so strict,
> many who try the Pritikin diet have trouble staying on it.

The moral is: do not be extreme; for example, do not adopt a single-food diet, such as the Zen Macrobiotic diet, which involves eliminating foods until only brown rice is eaten. Adhering to such a diet can result in death. Instead, adopt eating habits that are sensible and also satisfying to you, so that you can adhere to them year after year.

A common tragic outcome of faddism in dieting and the anxiety caused by the difficulty of observing fad diets is the anorexia nervosa that seizes adolescent girls. It is estimated that between 5 and 20 percent of adolescents (95 percent female) with anorexia nervosa die of protein, energy, and vitamin starvation. Often the young person has a voracious appetite, but a large meal is followed by induced vomiting (called bulimia). This disease, which is not associated with poverty or scarcity of food, seems to be psychological, the result of a fear of becoming overweight. Anorexia nervosa is a serious disease. The patient requires expert treatment, including psychotherapy.

Many actions can be taken to improve one's health without interfering seriously with the enjoyment of life. A sensible control of the diet is one such action. Another is the regular use of dietary supplements, which is the theme of this book.

One point that must not be forgotten in weight control is that alcohol is a food. Potable alcohol, ethanol ($C_2H_5OH$), has a rather high heat of combustion, 700 kilocalories (kcal) per 100 grams, closer to that of fat (900) than of carbohydrate (400). One jigger (1.5 ounces) of strong liquor (80 to 100 proof) provides 100 to 120 kcal. One pint of beer provides 160 kcal. One glass of wine provides 100 to 150 kcal. Accordingly a moderate drinker, imbibing two or three drinks a day, may receive 300 to 400 kcal of food energy from the alcohol, and a heavy drinker may receive 1000 to 1500 kcal, as much as one half of the daily energy requirement.

One result is that heavy drinkers get fat. Moreover, even moderate drinkers have an added tendency toward obesity. To lose weight you must cut down on your intake not only of protein, carbohydrate, and fat, but also of alcohol.

Another effect of a high intake of alcohol is that the drinker doesn't eat very much and may begin to suffer from a deficient intake of vitamins and minerals, unless he or she takes vitamin-mineral supplements. In a study of randomly selected residents in San Mateo County, California, H. D. Chope and L. Breslow found that moderate drinkers are healthier than teetotallers but that heavy drinkers, who consume more than four drinks per day, are less healthy (Chope and Breslow, 1955). Part of their poor health may be the result of vitamin-mineral malnutrition.

Especially in this country, there are few people who have not heard that the diseases of the heart and circulatory system, the number one cause of death, have been associated with fat in the bloodstream. With this knowledge in mind, almost everyone accepts the further proposition, advanced by many physicians and most nutritionists, that high concentration of fat in the bloodstream is caused by high intake of fat in the diet.

John Yudkin, professor of physiology in Queen Elizabeth College of London University (1945-1954), professor of nutrition and dietetics (1954-1971), and now emeritus professor of nutrition, has a different view of the matter. He has presented his view in a series of scientific papers and in the book *Sugar: Chemical, Biological, and Nutritional Aspects of Sucrose,* edited by Yudkin, Edelman, and Hough (1971). He has summarized his findings for the lay public in his book *Sweet and Dangerous* (1972).

Yudkin traced the widely held theory about fat to a paper by Ancel Keys, of the University of Minnesota. "In 1953," wrote Yudkin, Keys "drew attention to the fact that in six different countries there was a highly suggestive relationship between the intake of fat and their death rates from coronary disease. This was certainly one of the most important contributions made to the study of heart disease. It has been responsible for an avalanche of reports by other research workers throughout the world; it has changed the diets of hundreds of thousands of people; and has made huge sums of money for producers of foods that are incorporated into these special diets."

Against the general public acceptance of the proposition that coronary heart disease is caused by a high intake of animal fat (saturated fat) and the eating of foods containing cholesterol, Yudkin himself has shown that for the same countries the correlation of coronary disease with intake of sugar is much better than that with intake of fat. He found that persons who develop coronary disease have been ingesting more sucrose, ordinary sugar, than those who have not developed the disease, and he remarks that "no one has ever shown any difference in fat consumption between people with and people without coronary diseases, but this has in no way deterred Dr. Keys and his followers." Yudkin's observation has been confirmed by a large-scale, long-term epidemiological study of the population of

Framingham, Massachusetts, conducted under the auspices of the National Institutes of Health, which showed no correlation between the intake of fat and the incidence of heart disease. Nevertheless, perhaps in part because of the now huge economic interest in the link between fats in the food and cholesterol and the blood, the naive one-to-one correspondence persists in physicians' advice and in the public mind. The idea is dying hard, as we shall see in Chapter 17.

Coronary heart disease, which occurred very rarely seventy-five years ago, is today one of the principal causes of death. In 1957 Yudkin reported a study of the death rate from coronary disease in fifteen countries in relation to the average intake of sugar. The annual coronary death rate per 100,000 persons increases steadily from 60 for an intake of 20 pounds of sugar per year to 300 for 120 pounds per year, and then more sharply to about 750 for 150 pounds per year. In 1964 and 1967 Yudkin and his coworkers reported the results of two studies of the average intake of sucrose (during the period of some years before they had developed the disease) of sixty-five male patients in London with myocardial infarction or peripheral arterial disease, and also of fifty-eight male control subjects, of whom some were healthy and some were patients hospitalized with other diseases. The patients with heart disease were 45 to 65 years old, with average 56.1, and the control subjects were in the same age range, with average 55.1.

The mean sugar intake of the men who developed cardiovascular disease was 140 pounds per year, and that of the controls was 80 pounds per year. This difference has very high statistical significance, the calculated confidence level being greater than 99.999 percent. We are led to the conclusion that men with a large intake of sucrose have a far greater chance of developing heart disease in the age range forty-five to sixty-five than those with a small intake of sucrose. A second study gave essentially the same results.

Yudkin's work has been criticized on the ground that his method of determining the intake of sucrose, by questioning the patient, within three weeks after his hospitalization, about his normal eating habits, was unreliable. He carried out an investigation to check this point and concluded that this method is as reliable as the much more elaborate method usually used by nutritionists.

Coronary disease, including angina pectoris, which because of its striking symptoms would surely not have been ignored by the physicians of earlier centuries, seems to be a disease of modern times. It has been reported in the medical literature only during the last hundred years. The increasing incidence of the disease closely parallels the increasing consumption of sugar. It is not at all correlated with the consumption of animal fat (saturated fat) or of total fat.

Yudkin quotes several studies that indicate strongly that sucrose, and not animal fat, is the villain in the heart-disease story. Dr. A. M. Cohen in Jerusalem found that Yemenite Jews who had been in Israel only ten years or less had very little coronary disease, whereas those who had been in Israel twenty-five years had a high incidence of the disease. In the Yemen their diet had been high in animal fat and low in sugar, and in Israel they had adopted the usual high-sugar diet of the country. This observation shows clearly that a diet high in saturated fat does not necessarily lead to a high incidence of coronary disease, and it supports Yudkin's conclusion that a high-sucrose diet does lead to coronary disease.

Moreover, the East African Masai and Samburu tribes live mostly on milk and meat and accordingly have a high consumption of animal fat;

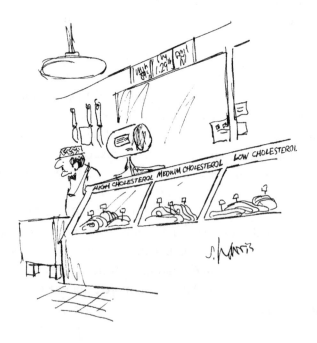

nevertheless, they have very little heart disease. In the past the black population in South Africa as a whole had almost no coronary disease; during the last ten years their consumption of sugar has increased greatly and the incidence of coronary disease is rising rapidly.

The epidemiological evidence that there is a correlation between the amount of cholesterol in the blood, if not in the diet, and the incidence of heart disease is convincing. When the level of cholesterol is decreased, the incidence of coronary disease decreases. The procedure that has been recommended to decrease the level of cholesterol is to cut down the intake of eggs, meat, and other foods that contain cholesterol. The cholesterol ingested in food does not, however, go directly into the bloodstream. It may be that another procedure is even better than reducing the intake of cholesterol. This procedure is to change our intake of nutrients that are known to be involved in the synthesis and destruction of cholesterol in our bodies. Yudkin has convincingly put the sugar sucrose in this category.

As explained in Chapter 4, the metabolism of sucrose yields in its first step equal quantities of glucose and fructose. Glucose proceeds directly into the metabolic steps that yield its energy to the biochemical machinery of the cells of the body. Fructose metabolism goes in part by a different route such that it produces acetate, which is a precursor of the cholesterol that we synthesize in our liver cells.

It has been shown in a trustworthy clinical study that the ingestion of sucrose leads to an increase in the cholesterol concentration in the blood. This important study was reported by Milton Winitz and his associates in 1964 and 1970. These investigators studied eighteen subjects who were kept in a locked institution, without access to other food, during the whole period of the study (about six months). After a preliminary period with ordinary food, they were placed on a chemically well-defined small-molecule diet (seventeen amino acids, a little fat, vitamins, essential minerals, and glucose as the only carbohydrate). The only significant physiological change that was found was in the concentration of cholesterol in the blood serum, which decreased rapidly for each of the eighteen subjects. The average concentration in the initial period, on ordinary food, was 227 milligrams per deciliter. After two weeks on the glucose diet it had dropped to 173, and after another two weeks to 160. The diet was then changed by replacing one quarter of the glucose by sucrose, with all of the other dietary constituents kept the same. Within one week the

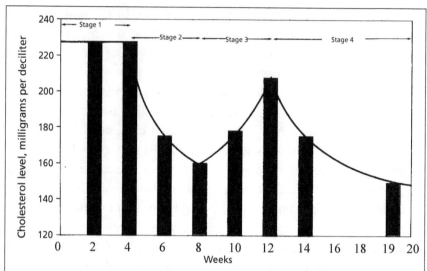

Cholesterol in the blood. In a locked ward eighteen male experimental subjects received at first ordinary food and then a rigorously specified diet in which protein requirements were met by amino acids, the bulk requirement by essential fats, and the carbohydrate requirement by glucose. Four stages in the experiment are charted here. STAGE I: For the first four weeks the subjects ate ordinary food. STAGE 2: From the fourth to the eighth week, their diet contained only glucose as carbohydrate. STAGE 3: From the eighth week to the twelfth week, their source of carbohydrate was mixed: 75 percent glucose and 25 sucrose. STAGE 4: After the twelfth week, their diet returned to glucose (as in stage 2). Note that their blood cholesterol decreased significantly each time the sucrose was eliminated.

average cholesterol concentration had risen from 160 to 178, and after two more weeks to 208. The sucrose was then replaced by glucose. Within one week the average cholesterol concentration had dropped to 175, and it continued dropping, leveling off at 150, 77 less than the initial value (see the illustration above).

This important experiment, in which the only change made was to replace some of the glucose in the diet with sucrose and then return to the sucrose-free diet, shows conclusively that an increased intake of sucrose leads to an increased level of blood cholesterol. Because of the relation between bloodstream cholesterol and heart disease, this experiment ties the consumption of sucrose directly to increased incidence of heart disease. Moreover, the sucrose-cholesterol effect has its biochemical basis established in the fact that fructose, formed in the digestion of sucrose, undergoes reactions in the body leading to acetate, which is then in part converted to cholesterol. This clinical trial conducted by Winitz and his collaborators strongly supports the conclusion reached by Yudkin that sugar (sucrose) is dangerous as well as sweet.

The ordinary diet, with 20 percent of the food energy from sucrose, corresponds to an average intake of 125 g per day, 100 pounds per year. To cut this intake in half greatly improves the health, decreasing the chance of developing heart disease and other diseases, lowering the blood cholesterol, and strengthening the body's natural defense mechanisms.

You can decrease your intake of sucrose by half very easily by developing some good habits.

1. Keep away from the sugar bowl. Do not add sugar to your tea or coffee. A rounded teaspoonful of sugar weighs 9 g. Each time that you refrain from adding it to your cup of coffee or tea you decrease your intake of sucrose by that amount.
2. Do not eat prepared breakfast cereals (frosted cereals) with added sugar. Some of these cereals are 50 percent sugar. When you eat a 2-ounce serving you eat 28 g of sucrose. Eat sugar-free cereals, and add only a small amount of sugar.
3. Do not eat sweet desserts regularly. As Yudkin has pointed out, this does not mean that when you are a guest you should refuse to eat the dessert your hostess has prepared.
4. Do not drink soft drinks (carbonated beverages), except club soda (carbonated water). The usual 6-ounce bottle or can of a cola drink contains 17 g of sucrose. If you were to drink four of them per day and eat the ordinary American diet, your sucrose intake would be 155 pounds per year, and, according to Yudkin, you would be fifteen times as likely to die of heart disease at an early age as if you restricted your intake to 50 pounds per year by following these rules.

A glass of ginger ale contains 14 g of sucrose, a glass of cream soda 17 g, a glass of fruit-flavored soda (citrus, cherry, grape, strawberry, Tom Collins mix, other) 20 g, a glass of root beer 18 g, a glass of tonic water (quinine water) 14 g.

I do not recommend the diet sodas, in which the sucrose is replaced by artificial sweeteners, because I am worried about the possible toxicity of these nonorthomolecular substances. The soft drink that I recommend for every person except those on a low-sodium diet is club soda, which contains no sucrose. I also recommend water.

If you keep your intake of sugar down, vitamin C can supply the rest of your insurance against high cholesterol concentration in your bloodstream. As I explain in Chapter 17, where we return to the subject of heart disease, vitamin C is involved in the biochemistry of the synthesis and destruction of cholesterol in our bodies.

# II
## *THE NEW NUTRITION*

# 7

## *How Vitamins Were Discovered*

Scurvy, beriberi, pellagra, pernicious anemia, and rickets are diseases that over past millennia caused a tremendous amount of suffering and millions of deaths. We know today that each of these diseases is the result of a deficiency in the amount of an important kind of molecule in the organs and tissues of the body. Scurvy results from an insufficient supply of vitamin C; beriberi, from an insufficient supply of vitamin $B_1$ (thiamine); pellagra, from an insufficient supply of vitamin $B_3$ (niacin). Pernicious anemia results from an insufficient amount of vitamin $B_{12}$ (cobalamin) in the blood, caused by the failure of the patient to synthesize a substance that carries the vitamin across the intestinal wall. Rickets (defective bone growth) is caused by a lack of vitamin D in the diet or by insufficient exposure of the skin to sunlight. This knowledge, which has been obtained only during the last one hundred years, has led to nearly complete control of the diseases in the developed countries and to great improvement in the general health of their populations.

Scurvy has been known for centuries, but it was not until 1911 that its cause was clearly recognized to be a dietary deficiency. Until the 1880s the disease was common among sailors on board ships taking long voyages. It also frequently broke out among soldiers in an army on campaign, in communities in times of scarcity of food, in cities under siege, and in prisons and workhouses. Scurvy plagued the California gold miners 140 years ago and the Alaskan gold miners 90 years ago.

The onset of scurvy is marked by a failure of strength, by depression, restlessness, and rapid exhaustion on making an effort. The skin becomes sallow or dusky. The patient complains of pain in the muscles. He is mentally depressed. Later his face looks haggard. His gums ulcerate, his teeth drop out, and his breath is fetid. Hemorrhages of large size penetrate the muscles and other tissues, giving him the appearance of being extensively bruised. The later stages of the disease are marked by profound exhaustion, diarrhea, and pulmonary and kidney troubles, leading to death.

The ravages of scurvy among the early sea voyagers were terrible. On a long voyage the sailors lived largely on biscuits, salt beef, and salt pork, which contain very little vitamin C. Between 9 July 1497 and 30 May 1498, the Portuguese navigator Vasco da Gama made the voyage of discovery of the sea route around Africa to India, sailing from Lisbon to Calicut. During this voyage 100 of his crew of 160 died of scurvy. In the year 1577 a Spanish galleon was found adrift in the Sargasso Sea, with everyone on board dead of scurvy. Late in 1740 the British admiral George Anson set out with a squadron of six ships manned by 961 sailors. By June 1741, when he reached the island of Juan Fernandez, the number of sailors had decreased to 335, more than half of his men having died of scurvy. The conqueror of Mexico, Hernando Cortes, discovered Baja California in 1536 but had to turn back before discovering California itself because his sailors were dying of scurvy.

The idea that scurvy could be prevented by a proper diet developed only slowly. In 1536 the French explorer Jacques Cartier discovered the St. Lawrence River and sailed upstream to the site of the present city of Quebec, where he and his men spent the winter. Twenty-five of the men died of scurvy, and many others were very sick. A friendly Indian advised them to drink tea made of the leaves and bark of the arbor vitae tree, *Thuja occidentalis.* The treatment was beneficial. The leaves or needles of this tree were later shown to contain about 50 milligrams of vitamin C per 100 grams.

The sixteenth-century English admiral Sir John Hawkins found that on a very long voyage the crew suffered from scurvy in proportion to the length of time they were restricted to dry foods. They recovered rapidly as soon as they had access to a supply of succulent plants, including citrus fruits.

Since fresh fruits and vegetables are obviously the most difficult of all supplies to maintain on shipboard, efforts were made to find a substitute capable of marine transport.

In 1747, while in the British naval service, the Scottish physician James Lind carried out a now-famous experiment with twelve patients severely ill with scurvy. He placed them all on the same diet, except for one item, one or another of the reputed remedies that he was testing. To each of two patients he gave two oranges and one lemon per day; to two others, cider;

to the others, dilute sulfuric acid, or vinegar, or sea water, or a mixture of drugs. At the end of six days the two who had received the citrus fruits were well, whereas the other ten remained ill. Lind carried out further studies, which he later described in his book *A Treatise on Scurvy* (1753).

The experiences of the great English explorer Captain James Cook in controlling scurvy are particularly striking. Cook was the son of a day laborer on a farm in Yorkshire. As a boy he showed unusual ability, and at eighteen he was apprenticed to a ship owner, who encouraged him in his study of mathematics and navigation. After he joined the navy he advanced rapidly and became one of the world's greatest explorers.

The story of his dealing with scurvy among his crews on his Pacific voyages during the period 1768 to 1780 has been told by Kodicek and Young in *Notes and Records of the Royal Society of London* (1969). These authors quote the following song by the sailor T. Perry, a member of the crew of Cook's flagship *H.M.S. Resolution:*

> We were all hearty seamen, no colds did we fear
> And we have from all sickness entirely kept clear
> Thanks be to the Captain, he has proved so good
> Amongst all the Islands to give us fresh food.

This song, written two hundred years ago, indicates that Cook's sailors believed that something in the fresh food provided them with protection against colds, as well as against other diseases.

Captain Cook made use of many antiscorbutic agents. Whenever the ships reached shore he ordered the sailors to gather fruits, vegetables, berries, and green plants. In South America, Australia, and Alaska the leaves of spruce trees were gathered and made into an infusion called spruce beer. Nettletops and wild leeks were boiled with wheat and served at breakfast. Cook began one voyage with a supply of 7,860 pounds of sauerkraut, enough to provide 2 pounds per week for a period of a year for each of the seventy men on board his first flagship, the *Endeavour.* (Saukerkraut contains a good amount of vitamin C, about 30 milligrams [mg] per 100 grams.) The result of his care was that, despite some illness, not a single member of his crew died of scurvy during his three Pacific voyages, carried out at a time when scurvy was still ravaging the crews of most vessels on such protracted expeditions. Cook's scientific contributions were recognized by his election as a Fellow of the Royal Society of London, which awarded him the Copley Medal for his work on the prevention of scurvy.

Although the most intelligent travelers since the time of Hawkins had expressed their opinion that the juice of citrus fruits—principally oranges, lemons, and limes—was a good substitute for fresh fruit and vegetables in preventing scurvy, acceptance by the public was slow. Such juice was expensive and troublesome to carry, so skippers and ship owners found it expedient to be skeptical. In the controversy some attempts to find a solution involved using orange, lemon, and lime juice that had been boiled down to a syrup. But they were unsuccessful. We know today that most of the ascorbic acid in the juice was destroyed by this process. Controversy over the value of fresh citrus juice continued. Finally, however, in 1795, forty-eight years after Lind had carried out his striking experiment, the British Admiralty ordered that a daily ration of fresh lime juice (not boiled to a syrup) be given to the sailors. Scurvy soon disappeared from the British Navy. From this salutary practice the British sailor came to be known as a "Lime-juicer," or "Limey."

The spirit of free enterprise remained dominant in the British Board of Trade, however, and scurvy continued to ravage the British merchant marine for seventy years longer. Not until 1865 did the Board of Trade pass a similar lime-juice regulation for the merchant marine.

At the present time scurvy, complicated by other deficiency diseases, is found in populations that are ravaged by starvation and severe malnutrition, usually as a result of poverty. In the United States scurvy is also occasionally observed in people who are not poverty-stricken: among infants six to eighteen months old who are fed a formula without vitamin supplement and such persons as middle-aged or elderly bachelors or widowers who for convenience and through ignorance ingest a diet deficient in the essential nutrients.

E. Cheraskin, W. M. Ringsdorf, Jr., and E. L. Sisley in their book *The Vitamin C Connection* (1983) recount the story of a forty-eight-year-old woman in California who came to the hospital because of pain, indigestion, and swelling of the abdomen. Over a period of four years she had six surgical operations. Each time the abdomen was found to be full of blood. In the effort to prevent the recurrent bleeding, her ovaries, uterus, appendix, spleen, and part of the small intestine were removed. Finally, after four years, a doctor asked her what she ate and found that her diet contained essentially no fruits or vegetables and that she took no supplementary vitamins. She was getting a little vitamin C in her food, enough to keep her from dying of scurvy but not enough to keep her blood vessels strong enough to prevent internal bleeding. Her blood-level of vitamin C was only 0.06 mg per deciliter. When she was put on 1000 mg of vitamin C per day she regained normal health, qualified, however, by the surgery she had endured (Cooke and Milligan, 1977).

Not many people in the United States develop this sort of incipient scurvy. I believe, however, for reasons discussed throughout this book, that most of the American people suffer from a mild or even rather serious prescorbutic condition and also from deficiencies in other essential nutrients. The regular intake of supplements of vitamin C and other vitamins and minerals, in addition to a good diet and other health practices, can lead to a better life for almost every person.

The article on scurvy in the eleventh edition of the *Encyclopedia Britannica* (1911) states that the incidence of scurvy depends upon the nature of the food and that it is disputed whether the cause is the absence of certain constituents in the food or the presence of some actual poison.

The study of another vitamin-deficiency disease, beriberi, was then in a similar state. Beriberi was prevalent in eastern Asia, where rice is the staple food, and also in the Pacific islands and South America. It involves paralysis and numbness, starting from the legs and leading to cardiac and respiratory disorders and to death. In the Dutch East Indies, about one hundred years ago, soldiers, sailors, prisoners, mine workers, plantation workers, and persons admitted to a hospital for minor ailments were dying of the disease by the thousands. Young men in seemingly good health sometimes died suddenly, in terrible distress through inability to breathe.

In 1886 a young Dutch physician, Christiaan Eijkman, was asked by the Dutch government to study the disease. For three years he made little progress. Then he noticed that the chickens in the laboratory chickenhouse were dying of a paralytic disease closely resembling beriberi. His studies of the chickens' disease were suddenly brought to an end, when the chickens that had not yet died recovered and no new cases developed. He found, on investigating the circumstances, that the man in charge of the chickens had been feeding them, from 17 June to 27 November, on polished rice (with the husks removed) prepared in the military hospital kitchen for the hospital patients. Then a new cook took charge of the kitchen; he refused, as Eijkman was to report in his address accepting the Nobel Prize for physiology and medicine in 1929, to "allow military rice to be taken for civilian chickens." The disease had broken out among the chickens on 10 July and disappeared during the last days of November.

It was immediately confirmed that a diet of polished rice causes death of chickens in three or four weeks, whereas they remain in good health when fed unpolished rice. A study of 300,000 prisoners in 101 prisons in the Dutch East Indies was then made, and it was found that the incidence of beriberi was three hundred times as great in the prisons where polished rice was used as a staple diet as in those where unpolished rice was used.

Eijkman found that he could isolate an extract from the bran of the rice that had protective power against beriberi. At first he had thought that some substance in the bran acted as an antidote for a toxin assumed to be present in polished rice, but by 1907 he and his collaborator, Gerrit Grijns, had concluded that the bran contains a nutrient substance that is required for good health.

In the meantime a number of investigators had been studying the nutritional value of foods. It was shown that for good health certain minerals are needed (compounds of sodium, potassium, iron, copper, and other metals), as well as proteins, carbohydrates, and fats. The Swiss biochemist Lunin found in 1881 that mice died when they were fed a mixture of purified protein, carbohydrate, fat, and minerals, whereas those fed the same diet with the addition of some milk survived. He concluded that "a natural food such as milk must therefore contain besides these known principal ingredients small quantities of unknown substances essential to life." Similar observations were made in the same laboratory (in Basel) ten years later by another Swiss biochemist, Socin, who found that small amounts of either egg yolk or milk, in addition to the purified diet, sufficed to keep the mice in good health. In 1905 the Dutch physiologist Pekelharing found that very small amounts of the unknown essential substances in milk were enough to keep the animals in good health. Between 1905 and 1912 the English biochemist F. Gowland Hopkins carried on similar studies with rats. His results were announced in 1911 and published in detail in 1912. Hopkins shared the 1929 Nobel Prize with Eijkman.

In 1911 Casimir Funk, a Polish biochemist then working in the Lister Institute in London, published his theory of "vitamines," based upon his review of the existing knowledge about diseases associated with faulty nutrition. He suggested that four such substances are present in natural foods and that they serve to provide protection against four diseases—beriberi, scurvy, pellagra, and rickets. Funk coined the word *vitamine* from the Latin word *vita* ("life") and the chemical term *amine,* a member of a class of compounds of nitrogen, which includes, of course, the amino acids. Later, when it was found that some of these essential substances do not contain nitrogen, the word was changed to vitamin.

In the meantime the American investigator E. V. McCollum had been studying nutritional factors at the University of Wisconsin. He and his coworkers reported in 1913 the need for two "necessary" food factors, one soluble in fats and one in water. In 1915 he named them "fat-soluble A" and "water-soluble B." This was the start of the modern nomenclature of the vitamins. The vitamin that prevents scurvy was then named water-soluble C, and the one that prevents rickets was named fat-soluble D. When "water-soluble B" was found to contain not only the protective agent against beriberi but also several others, they were given the names $B_1$, $B_2$, and so on to $B_{17}$. Some of these substances have been found not to be vitamins, their requirement for life and health being uncertain, but the names $B_1$, $B_2$, $B_3$, $B_6$, and $B_{12}$ are still used.

During the following years a number of efforts were made to isolate pure vitamin C from lemon juice and other foods. The pure vitamin was finally obtained in 1928, by Albert Szent-Györgyi. He was working on another problem and at first did not know that his new substance was vitamin C. He named the substance hexuronic acid. Szent-Györgyi was given the Nobel Prize for physiology and medicine for 1937 in recognition of his discoveries concerning the biological oxidation processes, with especial reference to vitamin C and to the role of fumaric acid in these processes.

Szent-Györgyi was born in Budapest in 1893. He studied medicine in Budapest and immediately began his career as an investigator in the fields of physiology and biochemistry. While he was working in the Netherlands in 1922 he began a study of the oxidation reactions that cause a brown pigmentation to appear in certain fruits, such as apples and bananas, as they decay. In the course of these studies he found that cabbages contain a reducing agent (an agent that can combine with oxygen) that prevents the formation of the brown pigment, and that the adrenal glands of animals contain the same reducing agent or a similar one. Because of his interest in physiological oxidation-reduction reactions he began to try to isolate this reducing agent from the plant tissues and from adrenal glands.

In 1927 Szent-Györgyi received the fellowship from the Rockefeller Foundation, permitting him to spend a year in the laboratory of F. Gowland Hopkins in Cambridge, England. Here he succeeded in isolating the substance from plant tissues and from the adrenal glands of animals. He then spent a year at the Mayo Clinic, Rochester, Minnesota, where he succeeded in obtaining 25 grams (g) of the substance, which he had called hexuronic acid. In 1930 he returned to Hungary, where he found that Hungarian paprika contains large amounts of the substance. He and his collaborators, and also the American investigators Waugh and King, showed in 1932 that Szent-Györgyi's substance was vitamin C. Szent-Györgyi himself had found that the chemical formula of the substance is $C_6H_8O_6$. He gave some of the crystalline material to the English sugar chemist W. M. Haworth, who determined its structural formula, establishing the atom-to-atom connections in the molecule (to be discussed in more detail in Chapter 9). Szent-Györgyi and Haworth then changed its name to ascorbic acid, meaning the acidic substance that prevents and cures scurvy.

Haworth demonstrated also the two chemical reactions by which the sugar dextrose or glucose, a carbohydrate with the formula $C_6H_{12}O_6$, is made to give up four hydrogen atoms to be transformed to $C_6H_8O_6$, with two molecules of water as byproduct. Essentially the same reactions are conducted by the living cells that manufacture vitamin C and by the chemical reactors that make the identical "synthetic" vitamin C. The very simplicity of the molecule and its manufacture from glucose, the principal fuel sustaining life in tissue cells, suggest the importance of vitamin C and explain its ubiquity in the tissues of the body.

Two twentieth-century American chemists, Robert R. Williams and Roger J. Williams, have made important contributions to our knowledge about the B vitamins. Their parents were missionaries, and they were born in India. R. R. Williams worked for many years as director of chemical research for Bell Telephone Laboratories in New York City on problems such as improving the electrical insulation on submarine cables. He set up a laboratory in his home and devoted his spare time to trying to isolate the substance in rice hulls that protects against beriberi. After years of work he and his collaborators, R. R. Waterman (his son-in-law) and E. R. Buchman, succeeded in isolating the substance, which they named thiamine, in determining its chemical constitution, and in devising ways of synthesizing it, making it available at a low price for improving the health of people all over the world.

R. J. Williams, when he was professor of chemistry at Oregon State University in 1933, discovered another B vitamin, which he named pantothenic acid. Later, at the University of Texas, he studied a factor in extracts from yeast and liver that had been reported in 1931 and 1938 by other investigators to be effective in controlling anemia in animals. In 1941 he and his students had decided that it was a vitamin, which they named folic acid.

In 1916 the American physician J. Goldberger reported that the disease pellagra, which was causing great suffering and many deaths among the poor people in the southern United States, could be prevented by improved nutrition (milk and eggs) and in no other way. Then in 1937 the American biochemist C. A. Elvehjem and his students at the University of Wisconsin showed that niacin or niacinamide cured a similar disease, blacktongue, in dogs, and in the same year these substances, vitamin $B_3$, were shown to cure pellagra in human beings.

There are interesting stories that might be recounted about the other vitamins. For example, after some red crystals of a cobalt compound that has an astounding protective effect against pernicious anemia had been isolated, the greatest organic chemists in the world were unable to determine the chemical constitution of the substance. Today called vitamin $B_{12}$, it is a complex molecule containing 183 atoms of carbon, hydrogen, nitrogen, oxygen, phosphorus, and cobalt. Its structure was ultimately resolved by an X-ray crystallographer, Dorothy Hodgkin, at Oxford University. For this work she was given the Nobel Prize for chemistry in 1964. While there is more to tell about the history of how vitamins were discovered, let us turn now to their role in the physiology of good health.

# 8

## *Vitamins and Evolution*

We are accustomed to thinking of human beings as the highest of all species of living organisms. In one sense they are: they have achieved effective control over a large part of the earth and have even begun to extend their realm as far as the moon and Mars. But in their biochemical capabilities they are inferior to many other organisms, including even unicellular organisms, such as bacteria, yeasts, and molds.

The red bread mold *(Neurospora),* for example, is able to carry out in its cells a great many chemical reactions that human beings are unable to carry out. The red bread mold can live on a very simple medium, consisting of water, inorganic salts, an inorganic source of nitrogen, such as ammonium nitrate, a suitable source of carbon, such as sucrose, and a single vitamin, biotin. All other substances required by the red bread mold are synthesized by it, using its internal biochemical mechanisms. The red bread mold does not need to have any amino acids in its diet, because it is able to synthesize all of them and also to synthesize all of the vitamins except biotin.

The red bread mold owes its survival, over hundreds of millions of years, to its great biochemical capabilities. If, like humans, it were unable to synthesize the various amino acids and vitamins, it would not have survived, because it could not have solved the problem of obtaining an adequate diet.

From time to time a gene in the red bread mold undergoes a mutation, such as to cause the cell to lose the ability to manufacture one of the amino acids or vitaminlike substances essential to its life. This mutated spore gives rise to a deficient strain of red bread mold, which could stay healthy only with an addition to the diet that suffices for the original type of the mold. The scientists G. W. Beadle and E. L. Tatum carried on extensive studies of mutated strains of the red bread mold, when they were working in Stanford University, beginning about 1938. They were able to keep the mutant strains alive in the laboratory by providing each strain with the additional food that it needed for good health, as shown by a normal rate of growth.

It was mentioned in Chapter 7 that the substance thiamine (vitamin $B_1$) is needed by human beings to keep them from dying of beriberi, and that chickens fed on a diet that contains none of this food also die of a neurological disease resembling beriberi. It has been found, in fact, that thiamine is needed as an essential food for all other animal species that have been studied, including the domestic pigeon, the laboratory rat, the guinea pig, the pig, the cow, the domestic cat, and the monkey. We may surmise that the need of all of these animal species for thiamine as an essential food, which they must ingest in order not to develop a disease resembling beriberi in human beings, resulted from an event that took place more than five hundred million years ago.

Let us consider the epoch, early in the history of life on earth, when the early animal species from which present-day birds and mammals have evolved populated a part of the earth. We assume that the animals of this species nourished themselves by eating plants, possibly together with other food. All plants contain thiamine. Accordingly the animals would have in their bodies the thiamine that they had ingested with the foodstuffs that they had eaten, as well as the thiamine that they themselves synthesized by use of their own synthetic mechanism. Now let us assume that a mutant animal appeared in the population, an animal that, as the result of the impact of a cosmic ray on a gene or of the action of some other mutagenic agent, had lost the biochemical machinery that still permitted the other members of the species to manufacture thiamine from other substances. The amount of thiamine provided by the ingestion of food would suffice to keep the mutant well nourished, essentially as well nourished as the unmutated animals. The mutant would have an advantage over the unmutated animals, in that it would be liberated from the burden of the machinery for manufacturing its own thiamine. As a result, the mutant would be able to have more offspring than the other animals in the population. By reproduction the mutated animal would pass its advantageous genetic change along to some of its offspring, and they too would have more than the average number of offspring. Thus in the course of time this advantage, the advantage of not having to do the work of manufacturing thiamine or to carry within itself the machinery for this manufacture, could permit the mutant type to replace the original type.

To recapitulate: Many different kinds of molecules must be present in the body of an animal in order that the animal be in good health. Some of these molecules can be synthesized by the animal; others must be ingested as foods. If the substance is available as a food, it is advantageous to the animal species to rid itself of the burden of the machinery for synthesizing it.

It is believed that, over the millennia, the ancestors of human beings were enabled, over and over again, by the availability of certain substances as foods, including the essential amino acids and the vitamins, to simplify their own biochemical lives by shuffling off the machinery that their ancestors had needed for synthesizing these substances. Evolutionary processes of this sort gradually, over millions of years, led to the appearance of new species, including man.

Some interesting experiments concern competition between strains of organisms that require a certain substance as food and those that do not require the substance, because they have the ability to synthesize it themselves. These experiments were carried out at the University of California, Los Angeles, by Zamenhof and Eichhorn, who published their findings in 1967. They studied a bacterium, *Bacillus subtilis,* by comparing a strain that had the power of manufacturing the amino acid tryptophan and a mutant strain that had lost the ability to manufacture it. If the same numbers of cells of the two strains were put in a medium that did not contain any tryptophan the strain that could manufacture tryptophan survived, whereas the other strain died out. If, however, some cells of the two strains were put together in a medium containing a good supply of tryptophan, the scales were turned. The mutant strain, which had lost the ability to manufacture the amino acid, survived, and the original strain, with the ability to manufacture the amino acid, died out. The two strains of bacteria differed only in a single mutation, the loss of the ability to manufacture tryptophan. We are hence led to conclude that the burden of using the machinery for tryptophan synthesis was disadvantageous to the strain possessing this ability and hampered it in its competition with the mutant strain, to such an extent as to cause it to fail in this competition. The number of generations (cell divisions) required for takeover in this series of experiments (starting with an equal number of cells, to a million times as many cells of the victorious strain) was about fifty, which would correspond to only about fifteen hundred years for humans (thirty years per generation).

We may say that Zamenhof and Eichhorn carried out a small-scale experiment about the process of the evolution of species. This experiment, and several others that they also carried out, showed that it can be advantageous to be free of the internal machinery for synthesizing a vital substance, if the vital substance can be obtained instead as a food from the immediate environment.

Most of the vitamins required by humans for good health are also required by animals of other species. Vitamin A is an essential nutrient for all vertebrates for vision, maintenance of skin tissue, and normal development of bones. Riboflavin (vitamin $B_2$), pantothenic acid, pyridoxine (vitamin $B_6$), nicotinic acid (niacin), and cyanocobalamin (vitamin $B_{12}$) are required for good health by the cow, pig, rat, chicken, and other animals. It is likely that the loss of the ability to synthesize these essential substances, like the loss of the ability to synthesize thiamine, occurred rather early in the history of animal life on earth, when the primitive animals began living largely on plants, which contain a supply of these nutrients.

Irwin Stone pointed out in 1965 that, whereas most species of animals can synthesize ascorbic acid, humans and other primates that have been tested, including the rhesus monkey, the Formosan long-tail monkey, and the ringtail or brown capuchin monkey, are unable to synthesize the substance and require it as a supplementary vitamin. He concluded that the loss of the ability to synthesize ascorbic acid probably occurred in the common ancestor of the primates. A rough estimate of the time at which this mutational change occurred is twenty-five million years ago (Zuckerkandl and Pauling, 1962).

The guinea pig and an Indian fruit-eating bat are the only other mammals known to require ascorbic acid as a vitamin. The red-vented bulbul and some other Indian birds (of the order Passeriformes) also require ascorbic acid. The overwhelming majority of mammals, birds, amphibians, and reptiles have the ability to synthesize the substance in their tissues, usually in the liver or the kidney.† The loss of the ability by the guinea pig, the fruit-eating bat, the red-vented bulbul, and other passeriform birds probably resulted from independent mutations in populations of these species of animals living in an environment that provided an ample supply of ascorbic acid in the available foodstuffs.

We may ask why ascorbic acid is not required as a vitamin in the food of the cow, pig, horse, rat, chicken, and many other species of animals that do require the other vitamins needed by humans. Ascorbic acid is present in green plants, along with these other vitamins. When green plants became the steady diet of the common ancestor of humans and other mammals, hundreds of millions of years ago, why did not this ancestor undergo the mutation of eliminating the mechanism for synthesizing ascorbic acid, as well as those for synthesizing thiamine, pantothenic acid, pyridoxine, and other vitamins?

I think the answer is that for optimum health more ascorbic acid was needed than could be provided under ordinary conditions by the usually available green plants. Part of the extra amount is needed by animals because ascorbic acid is required for the synthesis of collagen, as will be explained in Chapter 9. This protein is present in large amounts in the bodies of animals but not in plants.

Let us consider the common precursor of the primates, at a time about twenty-five million years ago. This animal and his ancestors had for hundreds of millions of years continued to synthesize ascorbic acid from the glucose in the foods that they had ingested. Let us assume that a population of this species of animals was living, at that time, in an area that provided an ample supply of food with an unusually large content of ascorbic acid, permitting the animals to obtain from their diet approximately the amount of ascorbic acid needed for optimum health. A cosmic ray or some other mutagenic agent then caused a mutation to occur, such that the enzyme in the liver that catalyzes the conversion of L-gulonolactone to ascorbic acid was no longer present in the liver. Some of the progeny of this mutant animal would have inherited the loss of the ability to synthesize ascorbic acid. These mutant animals would, in the environment that provided an ample supply of ascorbic acid, have an advantage over the ascorbic-acid-producing animals, in that the mutants had been relieved of the burden of constructing and operating the machinery for producing ascorbic acid. Under these conditions the mutant would gradually replace the earlier strain.

A mutation that involves the loss of the ability to synthesize an enzyme occurs often. Such a mutation requires only that the gene be damaged in some way or be deleted. (The reverse mutation, leading to the ability to produce the enzyme, is difficult, and would occur only extremely rarely.) Once the ability to synthesize ascorbic acid has been lost by a species of animals, that species depends for its existence on the availability of ascorbic acid as a food.

The fact that most species of animals have not lost the ability to manufacture their own ascorbic acid shows that the supply of ascorbic acid available generally in foodstuffs is not sufficient to provide the optimum amount of this substance. Only in an unusual environment, in which the available food provided unusually large amounts of ascorbic acid, have circumstances permitted a species of animal to abandon its own powers of synthesis of this important substance. These unusual circumstances occurred for the precursor of humans and other primates, for the guinea pig, for the Indian fruit-eating bat, and for the precursor of the red-vented bulbul and some other species of passeriform birds, but they have not occurred, through the hundreds of millions of years of evolution, for the precursors of most other animals. Thus the consideration of evolutionary processes, as presented in the foregoing analysis, indicates that the ordinarily available foodstuffs might well provide nearly the optimum amounts of thiamine, riboflavin, niacin, vitamin A, and other vitamins that are required as essential nutrients by all mammalian species, but be deficient in ascorbic acid. For this food, essential for humans but synthesized by many other species of animals, the optimum rate of intake is indicated to be larger than the rate associated with the ingestion of the ordinarily available diet.

Thus, while the loss of the capacity to synthesize vitamin C conferred some evolutionary advantage on the primates and other lines, this genetic deletion also exposed them to some risk. Dr. Claus W. Jungeblut, a pioneer as early as the 1930s on the use of vitamin C for the therapy of infectious disease, advanced an interesting argument, new to me, in a letter to me on 10 February 1971: ". . . One might even go a step further here by asking why the *guinea pig,* of all common laboratory animals, shares with man certain physiological characteristics that include susceptibility not only to scurvy but also to anaphylactic shock, diphtheritic intoxication, pulmonary tuberculosis, a poliomyelitis-like neurotropic virus infection, and last but not least a form of viral leukemia that is indistinguishable from its human counterpart. None of the vitamin-C-synthesizing laboratory animals (rabbits, mice, rats, hamsters, etc.) answer positively to this call."

I have checked the amounts of various vitamins present in 110 raw, natural plant foods, as given in the tables in the metabolism handbook published by the Federation of American Societies for Experimental Biology (Altman and Dittmer, 1968). When the amounts of vitamins corresponding to one day's food for an adult (the amount that provides 2500 kilocalories [kcal] of energy) are calculated, it is found that for most vitamins this amount is about three times the daily allowance recommended by the Food and Nutrition Board. For ascorbic acid, however, the average amount in the daily ration of the 110 plant foodstuffs is 2.3 grams (g), about forty times the amount recommended as the daily allowance for a person with a caloric requirement of 2500 kcal per day (see table on facing page).

It is almost certain that some evolutionarily effective mutations have occurred in humans and their immediate predecessors rather recently (within the last few million years) such as to permit life to continue on an intake of ascorbic acid less than that provided by raw plant foods containing a high content of ascorbic acid. These mutations might involve an increased ability of the kidney tubules to pump ascorbic acid back into the blood from the glomerular filtrate (dilute urine, being concentrated on passage through the tubules) and an increased ability of certain cells to extract ascorbic acid from the blood plasma. The adrenal glands have been found to be richly supplied with ascorbic acid, extracting it from the blood and employing it in the synthesis of adrenalin, the all-important mobilizer of the body in response to stress; the supply of ascorbic acid in the adrenals may be available to the rest of the body by return to the bloodstream when the supply from nutrition runs low. On general principles we can conclude, however, that these mechanisms require energy and are a burden to the organism. The optimum rate of intake of ascorbic acid might still be within the range given above, 2.3 g per day or more, or might be somewhat less; and, of course, there is always the factor of biochemical individuality, discussed in Chapter 10.

It is not unreasonable to think that over the last millions of years the human body has adjusted somewhat to the food that was available and was eaten, so that the amounts of various nutrients in the food might be an

**Water-soluble content (mg) of 110 raw natural plant foods (referred to amount giving 2500 kcal of food energy).**

| | Thiamine | Riboflavin | Nicotinic acid | Ascorbic acid |
|---|---|---|---|---|
| Nuts and grains (11) | 3.2 | 1.5 | 27 | 0 |
| Fruit, low-C (21) | 1.9 | 2.0 | 19 | 600 |
| Beans and peas (15) | 7.5 | 4.7 | 34 | 1000 |
| Berries, low-C (8) | 1.7 | 2.0 | 15 | 1200 |
| Vegetables, low-C (25) | 5.0 | 5.9 | 39 | 1200 |
| **Average for 110 foods** | 5.0 | 5.4 | 41 | 2300 |
| Intermediate-C foods (16) | 7.8 | 9.8 | 77 | 3400 |
| Collards | 10.8 | 17 | 92 | 5000 |
| Chives | 7.1 | 11.6 | 45 | 5000 |
| Cabbage | 6.2 | 5.0 | 32 | 5100 |
| Brussels sprouts | 5.6 | 8.9 | 50 | 5700 |
| Cauliflower | 10.0 | 9.3 | 65 | 7200 |
| Mustard greens | 8.9 | 18 | 65 | 7800 |
| Kale | | | | 8200 |
| Broccoli spears | 7.8 | 18 | 70 | 8800 |
| Black currants | 2.3 | 2.3 | 14 | 9300 |
| Parsley | 6.8 | 15 | 68 | 9800 |
| Hot red chili peppers | 3.8 | 7.7 | 112 | 14200 |
| Sweet green peppers | 9.1 | 9.1 | 57 | 14600 |
| Hot green chili peppers | 6.1 | 4.1 | 115 | 15900 |
| Sweet red peppers | 6.5 | 6.5 | 40 | 16500 |

*Nuts and grains:* almonds, filberts, macadamia nuts, peanuts, barley, brown rice, whole grain rice, sesame seeds, sunflower seeds, wild rice, wheat.

*Fruit (low in vitamin C, less than 2500 mg):* apples, apricots, avocados, bananas, cherries (sour red, sweet), coconut, dates, figs, grapefruit, grapes, kumquats, mangoes, nectarines, peaches, pears, pineapple, plums, crabapples, honeydew melon, watermelon.

*Beans and peas:* broad peas (immature seeds, mature seeds), cowpeas (immature seeds, mature seeds), lima beans (immature seeds, mature seeds), mung beans (seeds, sprouts), peas (edible pod, green mature seeds), snapbeans (green, yellow), soybeans (immature seeds, mature seeds, sprouts).

*Berries (low-C, less than 2500 mg):* blackberries, blueberries, cranberries, loganberries, raspberries, currants, gooseberries, tangerines.

*Vegetables (low-C, less than 2500 mg):* bamboo shoots, beets, carrots, celeriac root, celery, corn, cucumber, dandelion greens, eggplant, garlic cloves, horseradish, lettuce, okra, onions (young, mature), parsnips, potatoes, pumpkins, rhubarb, rutabagas, squash (summer, winter), sweet potatoes, green tomatoes, yams.

*Intermediate-C foods (2500-4900 mg):* artichokes, asparagus, beet greens, cantaloupe, chicory greens, Chinese cabbage, fennel, lemons, limes, oranges, radishes, spinach, strawberries, swiss chard, ripe tomatoes, zucchini.

indication of the optimum intakes of these nutrients. During the past few years paleontologists, anthropologists, and other scientists have obtained a great amount of information about the foods eaten by primitive human beings during the period from forty thousand years ago to the development of agriculture ten thousand years ago. Studies have also been made of the few hunter-gatherer societies that have survived until recently or until the present time. A review of the subject of paleolithic nutrition was published in 1985 by Dr. S. Boyd Eaton and Dr. Melvin Konner of the School of Medicine and the Department of Anthropology of Emory University, Atlanta, Georgia. This article has provided much of the basis for the following paragraphs.

Five million years ago fruits and other vegetable foods were the main dietary constituents of the primates. It was about then that the lines leading to present-day humans and apes diverged. The ancestors of human beings began eating increasing amounts of meat. Modern man (*Homo sapiens*) developed about forty-five thousand years ago. His diet was about 50 percent vegetable material and 50 percent meat, including fish, shellfish, small animals, and large animals.

As agriculture developed, about ten thousand years ago, which greatly increased the use of grains as food, the amount of vegetables in the diet became as great as 90 percent, with a drastic decline in the amount of meat. European humans thirty thousand years ago, with a high intake of meat, were about 6 inches taller than their descendants after the development of agriculture. Eaton and Konner state that "The same pattern was repeated later in the New World: the Paleo-indians were big-game hunters 10,000 years ago, but their descendants, in the period just before European contact, practiced intensive food production, ate little meat, were considerably shorter, and had skeletal manifestations of suboptimal nutrition, which apparently reflect both the direct effects of protein-calorie deficiency and the synergistic interaction between malnutrition and infection. Since the Industrial Revolution, the animal-protein content of Western diets has become more nearly adequate, as indicated by increased average height: we are now nearly as tall as were the first biologically modern human beings. However, our diets still differ markedly from theirs, and these differences lie at the heart of what has been termed 'affluent malnutrition.' "

Eaton and Konner point out that the quality of modern meat is different from that of Paleolithic meat. Domesticated animals are fatter than wild animals. Meat now often contains 25 to 30 percent fat, whereas game contains only about 4 percent fat. The vegetable foods are also different. Hunter-gatherers eat roots, beans, nuts, tubers, fruits, flowers, and edible gums but only small amounts of cereal grains, such as wheat, oats, and rice, which constitute a large part of our modern diet.

Eaton and Konner point out that the late Paleolithic diet compares with the present American average diet in the following ways: more protein, less fat; the same amount of carbohydrate (but more starch, less sucrose); the same amount of cholesterol (about 600 milligrams [mg] per day); more fiber (36 g vs. 20 g per day); much less sodium; more potassium and more calcium; much more vitamin C (400 mg per day vs. 88 mg per day). They conclude that "The diet of our remote ancestors may be a reference standard for modern human nutrition and a model for defense against certain 'diseases of civilization.' "

# 9

## Vitamins in the Body

It was the vitamin-deficiency diseases, as we saw in Chapter 7, that led to the discovery of the vitamins. The sharp definition and the severity of the symptoms of these diseases testify to the fact that each of the vitamins plays a decisive role in one or more of the vital processes in the cells and tissues of the body. So specific and immediate is the efficacy of a given vitamin in its action upon the deficiency disease with which it is identified that one might take it to be a "wonder drug." One needs to be reminded that vitamins are foods. They catalyzed the evolution of our species. They remain essential to our existence and our health.

A striking characteristic of human beings and other living organisms is that they carry out thousands of different chemical reactions between substances that under ordinary conditions would not react with one another. Every day we burn about a pound of fuel, carbohydrate (mainly glucose) and fat to provide body heat and energy. This combination takes place at body temperature, 98.6°F. But we know that these substances—starch, sugar, butter, etc.—do not burn at ordinary temperatures. It may even be hard to make them burn at a much higher temperature. For example, if you take a cube of sugar (sucrose) and hold the flame of a burning match to one corner, you will find that some of the sugar will melt, but it will not catch fire.

How is it possible for living organisms to make carbohydrates and fats react with oxygen (burn) at body temperature? The answer is that they make use of auxiliary substances that have the power to speed up chemical reactions without any change in themselves. These substances are called catalysts; they are said to catalyze the reactions.

If you put a very small amount of cigarette ash (if you know someone who still smokes) on the corner of a cube of sugar and touch a match flame to it, the sugar will catch fire and will continue to burn until the cube is consumed. The burning takes place on the surface of the ash particles, which themselves remain unchanged, so that a little bit of ash can catalyze the combustion of a large amount of sugar.

The catalysts in the human body are called enzymes (named after the Greek word for yeast); yeast contains enzymes that accelerate the process of fermentation, the conversion of glucose into alcohol by reaction with oxygen. They are proteins, with large molecules, often containing ten thousand or twenty thousand atoms. They are highly specific in their enzymatic activity, often able to speed up only a single biochemical reaction or a few similar ones. There may be as many as fifty thousand different kinds of enzymes in the body of a single human being.

Some enzymes are pure protein, just a folded chain of amino-acid residues. Others consist of a protein molecule with something added, an addition required to give it the ability to catalyze its specific chemical reaction. This added part is called a coenzyme.

Both metals and vitamins (or substances made from vitamins, such as thiamine diphosphate, made by combining thiamine, vitamin $B_1$, and phosphoric acid) serve as coenzymes in many enzyme systems in the human body. For example, the molecule of alcohol dehydrogenase, which catalyzes the oxidation of alcohol to acetate in the liver, contains two atoms of zinc, which are required for its enzymatic activity. One enzyme, cysteamine oxidase, contains an atom of iron, an atom of copper, and an atom of zinc. The reason that a trace element such as molybdenum is required in extremely small amounts is that it serves as a coenzyme, permitting the active enzyme to work over and over again in catalyzing a chemical reaction that is essential for health. In the same way only a small daily intake of a vitamin may be required (a few millionths of a gram of $B_{12}$), but through its catalytic activity it produces a far larger amount of some vital substance.

Most of the vitamins are known to serve as coenzymes in a number of enzyme systems. Pantothenic acid, for example, is a part of coenzyme A, which combines with the protein apoenzymes (see page 99) to give active enzymes required for many reactions. One of these reactions is the conversion in the brain of choline to acetylcholine, one of the messengers involved in brain activity. Nicotinamide, one form of vitamin $B_3$, is an essential part of two important coenzymes, diphosphopyridine nucleotide and triphosphopyridine nucleotide. There is some evidence that these coenzymes are involved in two hundred enzyme systems, and in fact the number may be much greater. Vitamin $B_6$, usually as pyridoxal phosphate, is required as a coenzyme for more than one hundred known enzyme systems, and the other vitamins, with vitamin C an exception, also serve as coenzymes.

Often the apoenzyme available in the body is only partially converted to active enzyme. The amount of active enzyme can be increased by increasing the intake of the vitamin that serves as coenzyme. This effect is an important part of the rationale behind the modern science of nutrition, with its emphasis on optimum intakes.

The devastating symptoms of scurvy, expressed in the wasting and disintegration of the tissues of the body, suggested a large and ubiquitous presence in the body for the factor in nutrition we know today as vitamin C. Fortunately the disease yielded to the simple therapy of supplying a small ration of the foods that contain the vitamin. The therapy worked its cure long before the vitamin was identified and still longer before its biochemical role began to be as well understood as at is today. While much remains to be learned, more is known about the function of vitamin C than of any other vitamin. For that reason, as well as for its well-established supreme importance, we shall here consider at closer range what vitamin C—also called ascorbic acid—is, what it does in the body, and how it works.

Ascorbic acid is a white, crystalline powder, which dissolves readily in water. Its solution has an acidic taste, resembling that of orange juice. It is a weak acid, somewhat stronger than acetic acid found in vinegar, but weaker than citric acid (in lemons and grapefruit), lactic acid (in sour milk and sauerkraut), and tartaric acid (in grapes). In body fluids, which are usually neither acidic nor basic, ascorbic acid is completely dissociated into an ascorbate ion and a hydrogen ion. The hydrogen ion combines with basic groups of proteins or with a bicarbonate ($HCO_3$) ion. It is the ascorbate ion that participates in the many physiological reactions that require vitamin C, especially the scurvy-preventing synthesis of the critically important protein collagen.

Vitamin C may also be taken as the salts of ascorbic acid, in particular sodium ascorbate and calcium ascorbate. These molecules dissolve in the body fluids to produce ascorbate ions, which have the same properties and physiological action as the ascorbate ion from ascorbic acid. Vitamin C may thus be taken by mouth, in solution or in tablet form, as ascorbic acid, as sodium ascorbate, or as calcium ascorbate. Only the latter two, the salts, can be taken by intravenous injection, however, because the acid solution damages the veins or tissues.

The ways in which ascorbic acid functions in the human body relate first to the fact that it engages on both sides of the universal oxidation-reduction reaction that subtracts or adds hydrogen atoms to a molecule. It is readily oxidized to dehydroascorbic acid by the surrender, to oxidizing agents, of the two hydrogen atoms (designated by the symbol H) shown attached to the two oxygen atoms (O) at the top of the structural diagrams of the two molecules displayed below:

Ascorbic Acid                Dehydroascorbic Acid

(For the structure of ascorbic acid in three-dimensional space, see the illustration on page 72.)

This action is readily reversible, for dehydroascorbic acid acts as a strong oxidizing agent, and by picking up two hydrogen atoms is reduced to ascorbic acid. It is likely that the reducing power of ascorbic acid and the oxidizing power of dehydroascorbic acid are responsible for some of the physiological properties of the substance.

The synthesis of collagen, for which vitamin C is essential, proceeds in the body as one of its major manufacturing enterprises. A person who is dying of scurvy stops making this substance, and his body falls apart—his joints fail, because he can no longer keep the cartilage and tendons strong, his blood vessels break open, his gums ulcerate and his teeth fall out, his immune system deteriorates, and he dies (Cameron, 1976).

Collagen is a protein, one of the thousands of different kinds of proteins in the human body. Most proteins occur in only small amounts; the various enzymes, for example, are so powerful in their ability to cause specific chemical reactions to take place rapidly that only a gram or two or even a few milligrams may be needed in the body. There are a few exceptions. In the red cells of the blood there is a great amount of hemoglobin, amounting to 1 percent of a person's weight. Hemoglobin, however,

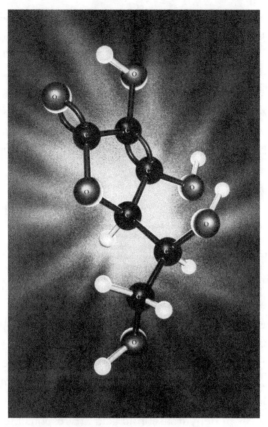

*Molecular structure of vitamin C. Ascorbic acid has a distinctive shape or
configuration in three-dimensional space, shown here in the conventional
ball (atoms) and stick (atomic bonds) model, that underlies its function in the
biochemistry of the body. Four carbon atoms (indicated by the letter C) and an
oxygen atom (O) form a central pentagonal ring, shown tilted at an angle to the
plane of the page. The four bonds on each carbon atom—which give organic
molecules their endless structural diversity—bind each of them to four other atoms
or to three others with a double bond binding one of the three. The bottom carbon in
the ring holds a large side group, which extends upward above the plane of the page.
Attached to the two carbons in this side group are two hydroxyl groups, an oxygen
atom with an attached hydrogen. Vitamin C is needed for the vital hydroxylation
reactions that introduce hydroxyl groups into many other molecules, notably the
adrenal hormone and the collagen molecule that forms connective tissue (see the
illustration on page 75). The shape of the vitamin-C molecule fits it, hand and glove
style, to the shape of the enzymes with which it works in these reactions.*

does not get the prize. There is even more collagen in the skin, bones, teeth, blood vessels, eye, heart, and, in fact, essentially all parts of the body. Collagen as strong white fibers, stronger than steel wire of the same weight, and as yellow elastic networks (called elastin), usually together with macropolysaccharides, constitutes the connective tissue that holds our bodies together.

When bones, skin, cartilage, and other parts of the animal body are boiled in water for a long time, the molecules are hydrolyzed (react with water molecules) to form smaller molecules, called gelatin. Gelatin is a reasonably good food, but it lacks the essential amino acids phenylalanine and tryptophan. Soup stock is a gelatin solution, and aspic and, of course, gelatin desserts are based on gelatin.

Like other proteins, collagen consists of polypeptide chains; the long chains of this fibrous molecule contain about one thousand amino-acid residues, about sixteen thousand atoms. It differs from almost all other proteins in being substantially composed of but two amino acids, glycine and hydroxyproline. Collagen is a kind of supermolecule, however, in its three-dimensional architecture. The polypeptide chains of the two amino acids, alternating with one another and punctuated by the presence of certain other amino acids, are coiled in a left-handed helix. Three of these helical strands are twisted around one another, like the strands of a rope, in a right-handed superhelix, to compose the complete molecule.

Understandably, the synthesis of this structure proceeds in steps. While it has been known for half a century that vitamin C is essential to the manufacture of collagen, the process is only now yielding to inquiry. It appears that vitamin C is involved at every step.

First a three-stranded structure is assembled, with the amino acids glycine and proline as its principal components. This is not yet collagen but its precursor, procollagen. A recent study shows that vitamin C must have an important role in its synthesis. Prolonged exposure of cultures of human connective-tissue cells to ascorbate induced an eightfold increase in the synthesis of collagen with no increase in the rate of synthesis of other proteins (Murad et al., 1981, 1983). Since the production of procollagen must precede the production of collagen, vitamin C must have a role in this step—the formation of the polypeptide chains of procollagen—along with its better understood role in the conversion of procollagen to collagen.

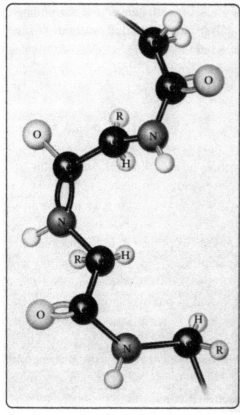

*Structure of collagen. The collagen molecule is stronger than steel wire of the same weight. One of the most abundant proteins, it supplies the body's connective tissue, the natural plastic of which the body is largely made. Vitamin C plays essential roles in its synthesis, apparently at every stage (see facing page).*

*Collagen owes its properties not only to its chemical composition but also to the physical arrangement of its component atoms in three-dimensional space. The atoms—of carbon, hydrogen, oxygen, and nitrogen—are organized in three polypeptide chains. Each of these chains is coiled in a left-handed helix, and the three chains are twisted around one another, as the strands of a rope, to form a right-handed superhelix, one full turn of which is shown schematically at left on facing page.*

*The illustration on this page shows the arrangement of atoms in one full turn of the left-handed helix of the polypeptide chain (in the small box on page 75) in the conventional ball (atoms) and stick (atomic bonds) model. A polypeptide chain is assembled by the head-to-toe linkage of amino acids by peptide bonds. These bonds tie the nitrogen atom (N) in one amino acid to a carbon atom (C) in another.*

*In the three peptide groups in the full turn of the helix shown here, note the double bond that ties the carbon to the nitrogen in the middle peptide group. This is the peptide bond; it could as well be shown binding the carbon to the oxygen (O), as it is in the peptide groups at the top and bottom of the turn. The resonating of the bond between these two alignments holds the six atoms of the peptide group in a plane. (The six atoms, from the top, are a carbon festooned with two hydrogens [H] or with one hydrogen and a side group [R], which are outside the plane, the carbon, the oxygen bonded to the carbon, the nitrogen, the hydrogen bonded to the nitrogen, and a second festooned carbon.) By contrast, the single bond that links the nitrogen to the festooned carbon that is shared with the neighboring peptide group permits the planar peptide groups to rotate about a common axis and form the helix.*

*Some 1000 peptide groups composed of 16,000 atoms make up the thin fiber of the collagen molecule, 2800 angstroms (1 angstrom [Å] is one hundred-millionth of a centimeter) long and only 72 angstroms thick. The long collagen molecules link up to form still longer strands. These strands, with the collagen molecules overlapping by a quarter of their length (700 angstroms), line up and cross-link to form the collagen fibril at the far right on facing page. The periodic striations in the collagen fibril (see electromicrograph on facing page) reflect the linkage and cross-linkage of the overlapping molecules of collagen in the fibril.*

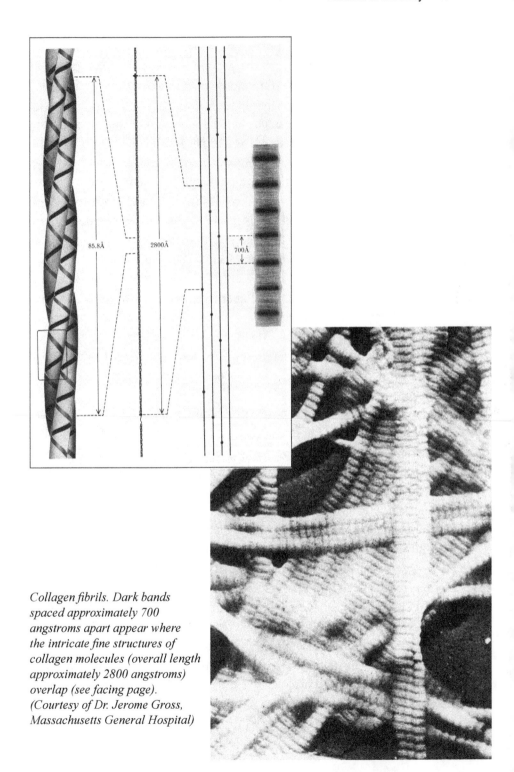

*Collagen fibrils. Dark bands
spaced approximately 700
angstroms apart appear where
the intricate fine structures of
collagen molecules (overall length
approximately 2800 angstroms)
overlap (see facing page).
(Courtesy of Dr. Jerome Gross,
Massachusetts General Hospital)*

That conversion involves a reaction that substitutes a hydroxyl group, OH, for a hydrogen atom, H, in the proline residues at certain points in the polypeptide chains, converting those residues to hydroxyproline. This hydroxylation reaction secures the chains in the triple helix of collagen. The hydroxylation, next, of the residues of the amino acid lysine, transforming them to hydroxylysine, is then needed to permit the cross-linking of the triple helices into the fibers and networks of the tissues.

These hydroxylation reactions are catalyzed by two different enzymes: prolyl-4-hydroxylase and lysyl-hydroxylase. Vitamin C also serves with them in inducing these reactions. It has recently been shown by Myllylä and his colleagues that, in this service, one molecule of vitamin C is destroyed for each H replaced by an OH (Myllylä et al., 1984).

We have come upon two big reasons why we require for good health much larger amounts of vitamin C than are present in the plants we use as food. First, there is the body's continuing need for the synthesis of large amounts of collagen for growth and for replacement of the collagen degraded by daily wear and tear. Second, vitamin C, in the critical reactions that assemble collagen in the tissues, does not serve merely as a catalyst but is destroyed.

The function of vitamin C involves another aspect of the molecule: its architecture in the three dimensions of space. Vitamin C is a chiral substance: its molecules have handedness. (The word *chiral* is derived from the Greek work *cheir,* which means "hand.") Ascorbic acid is often called L-ascorbic acid, to identify the molecules as left-handed (L for *levo,* "left") rather than right-handed (D for *dextro,* "right"). Like a single hand, the molecule of L-ascorbic acid is not identical with its mirror image.

Chirality may almost be said to be characteristic of life. It is true that some inorganic substances are chiral: the mineral quartz, for example, forms right-handed and left-handed crystals, as do some other minerals, but living organisms have exploited chirality to a far greater extent than has the inorganic part of nature. The organic molecules that life processes build around the carbon atom derive their chirality from a property of carbon atoms. On its four bonds carbon may gather four different kinds of atoms or groups; such molecules must be either right-handed or left-handed and, like hands, differ from their mirror image.

Our principal macronutrients are carbohydrates, fats, and proteins. All of the carbohydrates are chiral. This fact is illustrated in some of their names. Glucose is also called dextrose; its molecules may be considered to be right-handed. Our principal food starch, which is a sort of polymer (a condensation product of glucose, with elimination of water), may also be said to be right-handed. Starch is digested to form glucose by enzymes that are themselves chiral—these enzymes can digest ordinary right-handed starch (D-starch), but not left-handed starch. Fructose (fruit sugar) is also called levulose; it may be said to be a left-handed sugar. Its left-handedness accounts for the fact that it is not all burned for its energy content, as glucose is, but serves in part as a raw material for the synthesis of cholesterol.

Most of the fats are not chiral, but some related substances (lipids) are. An example is vitamin E: D-alpha-tocopherol and L-alpha-tocopherol have different vitamin-E activity.

Proteins are chiral. These extremely important macromolecules (a human being may synthesize fifty thousand different kinds of protein molecules to do different jobs in the body) consist of long chains of amino-acid residues, all of which are chiral, except those of the simplest amino acid, glycine. It is a remarkable fact that all of the more than twenty amino acids that make up the proteins in human beings, in other animals, and in plants have the same handedness: they are all L-amino acids, except for glycine, which is identical with its mirror image.

We can understand now why living organisms are made of only one kind of amino acids. The principal ways in which the chains of amino-acid residues are folded in stable proteins are known, and we can see that these structures are stable when they are made of one kind, either the D kind or the L kind, but they cannot be made with D and L mixed.

The earth might just as well be populated with living organisms made with D-amino acids as with those made with L-amino acids. A man who was suddenly converted into an exact mirror image of himself would not at first know that anything had changed; he could drink water, inhale air and use the oxygen molecules in it for combustion, exhale carbon dioxide, and carry on other bodily functions just as well as ever—so long as he did not eat any ordinary food. If he were to eat ordinary plant or animal food, he would find that he could not digest it. (In Lewis Carroll's *Through the Looking Glass* Alice said, "Perhaps looking-glass milk isn't good to drink." We know now that she was right in her surmise.)

This mirror-image man could be kept alive only on a diet containing synthetic D-amino acids, made in the chemical laboratory. He could not have any children, unless he would find a wife who had been subjected to the same process of reflection into a mirror image of her original self. Also he would die of scurvy, even if he had plenty of ordinary vitamin C, because vitamin C is itself a chiral molecule, L-ascorbic acid.

Ascorbic acid has accordingly four stereoisomers—four molecules with identical atomic constituents linked to one another in the same order but arrayed differently in three-dimensional space. We may therefore call the three-dimensional molecule LL and the others LD, DL, and DD. LL is the ordinary vitamin C, L-ascorbic acid. DD is its exact mirror image, with properties exactly the same as those of L-ascorbic acid (unless they involve chirality)—the same melting point and the same solubility in water—but one rotates the plane of polarized light in a clockwise way and the other in the opposite way (but through exactly the same angle). But the DD substance, which is called D-xyloascorbic acid, has no vitamin-C activity. The substances LD and DL, which are mirror images of each other, also provide no protection against scurvy.

This fact shows that the action of vitamin C does not depend simply on its activity as a reducing or oxidizing agent, which it has in common with its stereoisomers. Instead it depends upon the shape of its molecules, which presumably fit into a complementary cavity in the hydroxylation enzymes with which it works in the synthesis of collagen and thereby forms a reactive complex. Further study is needed to determine the structure of these enzymes and of others that can form such complexes with vitamin C. There are probably many different kinds, because vitamin C carries on so many different functions in our bodies.

The hydroxylation reaction, which vitamin C promotes in the synthesis of collagen, has a role in many other physiological processes. A substance called carnitine, for example, helps to supply the fuel that energizes the contraction of muscle fiber. Its synthesis from the amino acid lysine takes place through five successive reactions, each catalyzed by a specific enzyme. The second and fifth involve hydroxylation, for which vitamin C is needed.

In the adrenal glands, hydroxylation reactions mediated by vitamin C, present in large amounts, similarly convert the amino acid tyrosine first to dopa, then to dopamine and at last to noradrenaline in the manufacture of the all-important hormone adrenaline, which floods the body in moments of stress and activates the muscles for flight or fight. In this critical cycle the ascorbic acid is reconstituted from semidehydroascorbate by a special electron-transport mechanism, and so the vitamin is not destroyed.

This review of the function of vitamin C in the biochemistry of the body explains why we require large intakes of this vitamin, larger than those of other vitamins and larger than is supplied by the usual quantities of vegetables and fruits consumed in the diet. Setting aside the factor of biochemical individuality, to be discussed in the next chapter, for a moment, we may ask what is the optimum daily supplementary intake of vitamin C.

Plants need only small amounts of this vitamin. They do not manufacture collagen to make their structures strong; they use a carbohydrate, cellulose, for this purpose. I have checked the amounts of various vitamins present in 110 raw, natural plant foods, as given in the tables in the metabolism handbook published by the Federation of American Societies for Experimental Biology (Altman and Dittmer, 1968). When the amounts of vitamins corresponding to one day's food for an adult (the amount that provides 2500 kilocalories [kcal] of energy) are calculated, it is found that for most vitamins this amount is about three times the Recommended Daily Allowance (RDA) of the Food and Nutrition Board. For ascorbic acid, however, the average amount in the daily ration of the 110 plant foodstuffs is 2300 milligrams (mg), about forty times the amount recommended as the daily allowance for a person with a requirement of 2500 kcal per day (see the table in Chapter 8). This calculation suggests that the RDA ought to prescribe at least forty times its stingy 60 mg of vitamin C.†

The average ascorbic-acid content of the fourteen plant foodstuffs richest in this vitamin is 9.4 grams (g) per 2500 kcal. Peppers (hot or sweet, green or red) and black currants are richest of all the foods in the table, with 15 g per 2500 kcal.

The foregoing argument represents an extension and refinement of arguments advanced by the biochemists G. H. Bourne and Irwin Stone. In 1949 Bourne pointed out that the food ingested by the gorilla consists largely of fresh vegetation, in quantity such as to give the gorilla about 4500 mg of ascorbic acid per day, and that before the development of agriculture humans existed largely on green plants, supplemented with some meat. He concluded that "it may be possible, therefore, that when we are arguing whether 10 to 20 mg of vitamin C a day is an adequate intake we may be very wide of the mark. Perhaps we should be arguing whether 1000 or 2000 mg a day is the correct amount." Stone (1967) quoted this argument and supplemented it by consideration of the rate of manufacture of ascorbic acid by the rat. The rat under normal conditions is reported to synthesize ascorbic acid at a rate between 26 mg per day per kilogram of body weight (Burns, Mosbach, and Schulenberg, 1954) and 58 mg per day per kilogram of body weight (Salomon and Stubbs, 1961). If the assumption is made that the same rate of production would be proper for a human being, a person weighing 70 kilograms (kg, 154 pounds) should ingest between 1800 and 4100 mg per day under ordinary circumstances.

Other animals, including the goat, cow, sheep, mouse, squirrel, gerbil, rabbit, cat, and dog, also manufacture ascorbic acid at a high rate, averaging about 10,000 mg per day for 70 kilograms (kg) (154 pounds) of their body weights (Chatterjee et al., 1975a). It is hard to believe that these animals would make this large amount of ascorbic acid if it were not beneficial to them, and it is also hard to believe that humans are so much different from other animals that they can keep in the best of health with only two-hundredths of the amounts that animals use. If the need for ascorbic acid in our diet were really as small as the RDA published by the Food and Nutrition Board, then the mutation that deprived the primates of the capacity to synthesize their own vitamin C would surely have occurred six hundred million years ago, and dogs, cows, pigs, horses, and other animals would be obtaining ascorbic acid from their food, instead of manufacturing it in their liver cells. I conclude, therefore, that 2300 mg per day is less than the optimum rate of intake of ascorbic acid for an adult human being.

In general, the dietary requirements of humans have been found to be closely similar to those of other primates, and studies of vitamin C in these primates should yield valuable information about the optimum human intake of this vitamin. Monkeys are used in large numbers in medical research. As I mentioned in Chapter 1, much effort has been devoted by the Subcommittee on Laboratory Animal Nutrition to finding the intakes of various nutrients that puts them in the best of health. These careful studies have led to the formulation of several, rather similar recommended diets for laboratory monkeys. The amount of ascorbic acid in these diets lies in the range of 1.75 g per day to 3.50 g per day, scaled up to 70 kg of body weight; the 1.75 g per day scaled from the prescription for rhesus monkeys (Rinehart and Greenberg, 1956) and 3.50 g per day from that for squirrel monkeys (Portman et al., 1967). These monkeys weigh only a few kilograms, but there is little doubt that the need for ascorbic acid is proportional to body weight, for the amounts manufactured by animals that have the ability to make this substance are found to be rather closely proportional to body weight over a tremendous range, from a 20-g mouse to a 70-kg goat. From these studies with monkeys we may conclude that the requirement of vitamin C by humans might lie in the range of 1.75 g to 3.5 g per day.

Additional evidence has been provided by a study of the optimum intake of ascorbic acid by guinea pigs. Yew (1973) found that observations of growth rates both before and after surgical stress; recovery times after anesthesia; and the times needed for scab formation, wound healing, and the production of hydroxyproline and hydroxylysine during wound healing all support the conclusion that young guinea pigs ordinarily need about 5.0 mg per 100 g of body weight per day and that under stress the needs are even higher. For humans the corresponding intake is 3.5 g per day under ordinary conditions, a larger amount under stress.

Why have not similar studies been carried out with human beings? Part of the answer is that it is much harder to study humans than animals. Another part is that many physicians and nutritionists seem to have accepted the idea that vitamin C has no value for human beings except to prevent scurvy and that it would be a waste of effort to attempt to determine the optimum intake. Still another aspect of this matter is that these authorities persist in ignoring the many studies that have been carried out demonstrating that an intake of several grams per day leads to improved health.

I conclude that the optimum daily intake of ascorbic acid for most adult human beings lies in the range 2.3 g to 10 g. The amount of individual biochemical variability (Chapter 10) is such that for a large population the range may be as great as from 250 mg to 20 g or more per day.

These amounts are much larger than the RDA of vitamin C published of the Food and Nutrition Board, as previously noted. The recommendation of this board, said to be designed for the maintenance of good nutrition of practically all healthy people in the United States, is 35 mg per day for infants, 45 mg per day for children, increasing to 60 mg per day for adults (80 for pregnant women and 100 for lactating women). In making its recommendation the board stated that the minimum daily intake of ascorbic acid needed to prevent scurvy is about 10 mg, and that the somewhat larger amounts recommended should provide a generous increment for individual variability and a surplus to compensate for potential losses in food. The idea that beneficial effects would result from a larger intake of ascorbic acid was rejected, on the basis of reports that physical and psychomotor performances of men had not been improved by supplements of between 70 mg and 300 mg of ascorbic acid per day, and that the occurrence of bleeding gums in military personnel was not affected by supplements of 100 mg or 200 mg per day for periods of three weeks. There are, however, many published reports about beneficial effects of vitamin C ingested in larger amounts.

Ascorbic acid is not a dangerous substance. It is described in the medical literature as "virtually nontoxic." Guinea pigs that were given, orally or by intravenous infusion (of sodium ascorbate, the sodium salt of ascorbic acid), 0.5 percent of their body weight per day for a period of days showed no symptoms of toxicity (Demole, 1934). This amount corresponds for a human being to about 350 g (three quarters of a pound) per day. Many dogs and cats have been given large doses for control of distemper, influenza, rhinotracheitis, cystitis, and other diseases, with beneficial results and no signs of toxicity (Belfield and Stone, 1975; Belfield, 1981, 1983). The amount used was 1 g per pound of body weight per day, injected intravenously (in two doses, morning and afternoon), corresponding to about 150 g per day for an adult human being. Human beings themselves have taken 10 to 20 g of vitamin C every day for twenty-five years with no development of kidney stones or other side effects (Klenner, 1971; Stone, 1967). Patients with glaucoma have been treated with about 35 g of vitamin C (0.5 g per kg body weight) each day for more than seven months (Virno et al., 1967; Bietti, 1967). The only side effect reported was looseness of the bowels during the first three to four days. Patients with viral diseases or schizophrenia have received as much as 100 g per day with no symptoms of toxicity (Klenner, 1971; Herjanic and Moss-Herjanic, 1967). One cancer patient has taken 130 g per day for nine years, with benefit. A large amount (several grams) of ascorbic acid taken without other food may cause an upset stomach and looseness of the bowels in some people, but more serious side effects have not been reported.

Ascorbic acid may be described as no more toxic than ordinary sugar (sucrose), and far less toxic than ordinary salt (sodium chloride). There is no reported case of the death of any person from eating too much ascorbic acid, nor, indeed, of serious illness from this cause.

It might be possible to ingest from the food we eat the amount of vitamin C that I recommend as optimum. This would require, however, a cuisine loaded with peppers (hot or sweet, green or red) and black currants. Other plant foods afford less than the 350 mg of vitamin C per 100 g measured in these foods. Orange juice, lemon juice, lime juice, grapefruit juice, tomato juice, mustard greens, spinach, and brussel sprouts contain a good quantity of ascorbic acid, from 25 mg to 100 mg per 100 g. Green peas and green beans, sweet corn, asparagus, pineapple, tomatoes, gooseberries, cranberries, cucumbers, and lettuce contain from 10 mg to 25 mg per 100 g. Somewhat smaller amounts—less than 10 mg per 100 g—are found in eggs, milk, carrots, beets, and cooked meat. (See the table on page 65.)

The ascorbic acid in foodstuffs is easily destroyed by cooking at high temperatures, especially in the presence of copper and to some extent of other metals. Cooked foods usually retain only about half of the ascorbic acid present in the raw foods. The loss of the vitamin can be kept to a minimum by cooking for a short period of time, with a minimum amount of water and with the water not discarded, because it has extracted some of the vitamin from the food.

A good ordinary diet, including green vegetables and orange or tomato juice, may provide 100 mg of ascorbic acid per day. Many people, however, do not obtain even this rather small amount. A 1971-1972 study by the Health Resources Administration of the U.S. Department of Health, Education, and Welfare of 10,126 people aged one to seventy-four in ten representative geographical areas of the country found that half of the people received less than 57.9 mg of vitamin C per day and about one-third of the people received less than the RDA of 60 mg per day for an adult

(Abraham et al., 1976). Only 30 percent had a daily intake greater than 100 mg, and only 17 percent greater than 150 mg. The average intake of people below the poverty level is 78 percent of that of the whole population, and 57 percent of them receive less than the RDA.

Fortunately, this important dietary requirement may be met in any amount desired—from the optimum daily intake to the larger therapeutic amounts which we shall consider later in this book—by ingesting supplemental quantities of the pure substance, crystalline ascorbic acid, or one of its salts.

# 10

## *Biochemical Individuality*

The genetic mutation that deleted the capacity to manufacture vitamin C in the primate line presents one vivid example of the countless genetic variations from which natural selection produced the diversity of biological organisms we know in the world today. Such biochemical insight permits us to see evolution, as it were, from the inside. It gives a quantitative measure of the wealth of differences among individuals within a single species upon which natural selection acts in choosing the "fittest." It shows each of us human beings to possess a biochemical individuality that is scarcely expressed in (but only partly accounts for) the differences we observe in one another.

Let us consider some genetic characteristic, such as the weight of the liver relative to the total weight of the human being or the concentration of a certain enzyme in the red cells of the blood. It is found that, when a sample of a hundred human beings is studied, this characteristic varies over a wide range. The variation often is approximately that given by the standard, bell-shaped probability function. It is customary to say that the "normal" range of values of the characteristic is that range within which 95 percent of the values lie and that the remaining 5 percent of the values, representing the extremes, are abnormal. If we assume that five hundred characteristics are independently inherited, then we can calculate that there is only a small chance, 4 percent, that one person in the whole population, of the world would be normal with respect to each of these five hundred characteristics.

It is estimated, however, that a human being has a complement of one hundred thousand genes, each of which serves some function, such as controlling the synthesis of an enzyme. The number of characteristics that can be variable, because of a difference in the nature of a particular gene, is presumably somewhere near one hundred thousand rather than only five hundred; and accordingly we reach the conclusion that no single human being on earth is normal (within the range that includes 95 percent of all human beings) with respect to all characteristics. This calculation is, of course, oversimplified. It helps emphasize, however, that human beings differ from one another and that each human being must be treated as an individual, biologically as well as morally.

The species *Homo sapiens* is more heterogeneous, with respect to genetic character, than most other animal species. Nevertheless, heterogeneity has been found also for laboratory animals such as guinea pigs. It was recognized long ago that guinea pigs fed the same scurvy-producing diet, containing less than 5 milligrams (mg) of ascorbic acid per day per kilogram of body weight, differed in the severity of the scurvy that they developed and in the rapidity with which they developed it. A striking experiment was carried out in 1967 by Williams and Deason. These investigators obtained some male weanling guinea pigs from an animal dealer. After a week of observation during which the guinea pigs were on a good diet, including fresh vegetables, they were placed on a diet free of ascorbic acid or with known amounts added. They were divided into eight groups, each of ten to fifteen guinea pigs, with one of the groups receiving no ascorbic acid and the other groups receiving varying amounts through a pipette into the mouth. About 80 percent of the animals receiving no ascorbic acid or only 0.5 mg per kilogram per day developed signs of scurvy, whereas only about 25 percent of those receiving between 1 mg and 4 mg per kilogram per day, and none of those receiving 8 mg per day or more, developed these signs. These results agree with the customary statement that about 5 mg per kilogram per day of ascorbic acid is required to prevent scurvy in guinea pigs.

It was observed, however, on the one hand, that two animals receiving only 1 mg per kilogram per day remained healthy and gained weight over the entire period of the experiment (eight weeks). One of them showed a total gain in weight larger than that for any animal receiving two, four, eight, or sixteen times as much ascorbic acid.

On the other hand, seven of the guinea pigs receiving 8, 16, or 32 mg per kilogram per day were unhealthy and showed very small growth during the first ten days on the diet. They were then provided with a larger amount of the vitamin, five of them with 64 mg per kilogram per day and two of them with 128 mg per kilogram per day. These animals showed a remarkable response: whereas they had grown only 12 grams (g), on the average, in a period of ten days on the smaller amounts of ascorbic acid, their growth during the ten-day period after beginning to receive the larger amounts was, on the average, 72 g. The indicated conclusion is that these animals, seven of the thirty that were given between 8 mg and 32 mg per kilogram per day, required more vitamin C for good health than the others. Williams and Deason (1967) reached the conclusion that there is at least a twentyfold range in the vitamin-C needs of individual guinea pigs in a population of a hundred. They pointed out that the population of human beings is presumably not more uniform than that of the guinea pigs used in their experiments and that accordingly the individual variation in the vitamin-C needs of humans is probably just as great.

I have accepted their conclusion, and similar conclusions reached by other investigators, in suggesting that the optimum rate of intake of ascorbic acid by human beings may extend over a wide range, perhaps the eightyfold range from 250 mg per day to 20 g per day or an even wider range.

Vitamin C has been under investigation, reported in thousands of scientific papers, ever since it was discovered fifty years ago. The reader of this book might well be justified in asking first, why the range of values of the optimum intake of this important substance was not reliably determined long ago and, second, why no one can tell him or her what amount to take to be in the best of health. Part of the answer to the first question is that only a very small amount of the vitamin, perhaps 10 mg per day, is enough to keep most people from developing scurvy, and physicians and nutritionists accepted the idea that no larger amount is needed. Even though some physicians had observed forty or fifty years ago that amounts a hundred or a thousand times larger have value in controlling various diseases, as described elsewhere in this book, the medical profession and most scientists ignored the evidence.

Another part of the answer to this first question is that studies that would yield the answer can be carried out only with great effort and at great expense. It is much easier to investigate some powerful drug that has an immediate beneficial effect on the patient (although it is harder to check the possible long-term damage that the powerful drug may do to some fraction of the people for whom it is prescribed). Several excellently planned and executed epidemiological studies involving nutritional and other factors in relation to the incidence of disease and the chance of death at various ages have been carried out. In some of these studies the nature of the ingested food has been tabulated, and the amounts of vitamin C and other vitamins in the diet have been calculated using tables giving the vitamin contents of various foods. Some of these studies show that the incidence of disease and the chance of death at each age are less for people with a larger intake of vitamin C (and also for some other vitamins) than for those with a smaller intake. In these studies, however, the intakes of vitamin C are small, usually, for example, 0 mg to 50 mg per day for the low-intake group and between 50 mg and 100 mg for the high-intake group.

In their San Mateo County, California, study, Lester Breslow and his colleagues in 1948 interviewed 577 randomly selected residents of the county who were fifty years old or older. They obtained much information about their state of health and about environmental, behavioral, and nutritional factors that might affect it. After seven years they examined the death records and compared the age-corrected death rates for the subpopulations related to the different factors. Of all of these factors, the intake of vitamin C was found to have the greatest correlation with the age-corrected death rate, even greater than that for cigarette smoking (Chope and Breslow, 1955).

Whereas cigarette smokers have at each age twice the chance of dying that a nonsmoker has, the persons with a lower intake of vitamin C (calculated from the content of vitamin C in the food that they ate) had a chance of dying 2.5 times greater than the persons with a higher intake of the vitamin. The amount of illness was also correspondingly greater. This difference means that the length of the period of good health and of life was ten years greater for the persons with the higher intake than for those with the lower intake of vitamin C. The dividing line was 50 mg per day, approximately equal to the recommended dietary allowance. The average intake of the low-intake group was 24 mg per day and that of the high-intake group was 127 mg per day.* It is interesting that drinking a large glass of orange juice each day (about 90 mg of ascorbic acid in 6 ounces

---

*These averages are calculated on the assumption that the distribution of intakes for each of the two groups is the same as that for the corresponding groups (age over sixty) in the First Health and Nutrition Examination Survey, 1971-72 (Abraham, Lowenstein, and Johnson, 1976).

of juice) or taking a 100-mg tablet each day would put a person in the high-intake group.

Part of the improvement in health in the high-intake group may be attributed to other substances in the foods that provided the extra vitamin C. There is no doubt that orange juice, lettuce and other vegetables, and fruits contain important nutrients in addition to vitamin C. But the effect of a higher intake of vitamin A in improving the health was found in the San Mateo study to be only half as great as that of vitamin C, and the effect of niacin, one of the B vitamins, was only one-quarter as great. The foods with a high content of vitamin A and niacin, although they have value in improving the health, are not so valuable as those with a high content of vitamin C.

When vitamin C is taken by mouth, most of it is absorbed into the blood through mucous membranes of the mouth and the upper part of the small intestine. If the amount taken is rather small, up to 250 mg, about 80 percent is absorbed into the blood. With larger doses the amount absorbed is less, about 50 percent for a dose of 2 g and still smaller for larger doses (Kubler and Gehler, 1970).† Accordingly it is more economical to ingest vitamin C in smaller doses, such as 1 g every three hours, than to take a single, much larger dose once a day. Also, a quantity of sodium ascorbate injected into the bloodstream is more effective in the treatment of disease than the same amount taken by mouth.

For a small daily intake of ascorbic acid, up to about 150 mg, the concentration in the blood plasma is nearly proportional to the intake: this concentration is about 5 mg per liter for a daily intake of 50 mg, 10 mg per liter for 100 mg, and 15 mg per liter for 150 mg. Above an intake of 150 mg per day the concentration in the blood increases much less with increasing intake, reaching about 30 mg per liter for an intake of 10 g per day (ascorbic acid plus dehydroascorbic acid; Harris, Robinson, and Pauling, 1973).

The reason for this change when the intake exceeds about 150 mg per day is that a larger amount of the vitamin then begins to be excreted in the urine. One of the functions of the kidney is to clear the blood of unwanted and harmful molecules, the molecules of toxic substances that have got into the blood through the food or impure air or of waste products such as urea, the compound of nitrogen that is formed when old protein molecules in the body are degraded. Every twenty minutes the entire volume of the blood passes by a set of molecular filters in the two million glomeruli of the kidney. In the glomeruli the capillaries through which the blood is flowing have small holes in them. These holes, the pores of the glomerular filter, are small enough that the protein molecules in the blood, such as the antibodies (globulins) that protect us against disease, cannot pass through them, but water molecules and other small molecules, such as those of blood sugar (glucose) and ascorbic acid, can pass through. The blood pressure operates to push part of the water of the blood, together with its burden of small molecules, through these pores into a surrounding capsule.* The glomerular filtrate, with its dilute urine, is produced in amounts of about 180 liters (l) per day, thirty-six times the volume of the blood itself. We cannot stand to lose so much water, and fortunately there is a mechanism to concentrate the urine to the usual volume of one or two l a day. As the glomerular filtrate moves along through tubules toward the vessels that carry the urine to the bladder, molecular pumps in the walls of the tubules transfer most of the water back into the bloodstream.** The blood sugar is valuable as a fuel for the body, and it would not be good to lose it. Accordingly, there are special tubular pumps to pump the glucose molecules back into the blood. There are also special pumps for other important molecules, including those of vitamin C.

This is fortunate, because if the process of tubular reabsorption of vitamin C did not operate, even a big dose of the vitamin would be nearly completely excreted in an hour or two. In fact, a person who ingests 100 mg per day excretes only about 10 mg in the urine. As discussed in Chapter 7, the necessity of conserving our supply of ascorbic acid arose when our ancestors lost the ability to synthesize it and we were required to depend on what we could obtain in our food. We have developed the mechanism of tubular reabsorption to such an extent that it works nearly perfectly (pumping 99.5 percent of the ascorbate in the glomerular filtrate back into the bloodstream) until it reaches the limit of its pumping capacity. This

---

•A seriously ill person or a person in shock may have such low blood pressure that he cannot produce any urine.

**The process of concentrating the urine is regulated by the antidiuretic hormone, which is secreted by the pituitary gland. Some people develop a rather rare illness, diabetes insipidus, involving an insufficient output of this hormone; their urine volume may reach 40 liters per day, requiring them to drink an equal amount of water.

limit is reached when the concentration in the blood plasma equals about 14 mg per liter, corresponding to a daily intake of about 140 mg.

On the one hand, when the discovery was made that at higher intakes than 140 mg per day a greatly increased amount of vitamin C is excreted in the urine, the idea developed that at 140 mg per day the tissues of the body are saturated with the vitamin and are beginning to reject any additional amount. Although this idea is false, it continues to be advanced in the medical and nutritional literature, and the intake of 140 mg per day, corresponding to the so-called tissue saturation, is considered to be an upper limit to the amount of vitamin C required for "ordinary good health."

An argument similar to those developed in Chapter 9, on the other hand, leads us to the conclusion that this intake, at which the tubular pumps reach their capacity, is a *lower* limit to the optimum intake (Pauling, 1974c). Let us compare a tubular pump for ascorbic acid that pumps until the concentration of ascorbic acid in the blood is 14 mg per liter with one that operates only until the concentration is 13 mg per liter. The second pump is 7 percent smaller than the first and requires 7 percent less energy, which is provided by the food that we burn as fuel, for its operation. The smaller pump would accordingly be less of a burden to us than the larger one. Then why should we have developed the larger pump? The answer surely is that we need the larger pump to conserve the extra 7 percent of vitamin C. Hence the limit to which tubular reabsorption has been developed represents a lower limit to the optimum intake of vitamin C. This lower limit is more than twice the Recommended Daily Allowance (RDA) set by the Food and Nutrition Board.

If a large amount of vitamin C is taken, 62 percent of the amount that enters the bloodstream is excreted in the urine, so that only about 38 percent remains in the body to carry on its valuable functions. It is, however, good to have vitamin C in the urine. It protects against urinary infections and also against cancer of the bladder, as will be shown in Chapter 19.

Moreover, that fraction of a large dose of vitamin C taken by mouth that remains in the intestines has value. DeCosse and his coworkers studied the effect of 3 g per day of ascorbic acid in controlling the growth of adenomatous polyps of the rectum in people who have inherited the tendency to develop them (1975). This polyposis is serious because the polyps usually develop into a malignant cancer. In a group of eight patients, the polyps regressed completely in two and partially in three.

The appearance of vitamin C in the urine has been used by nutritional authorities as an argument against a high intake. Dr. Fredrick J. Stare in his book *Eating for Good Health* (1969) states that 60 mg or 70 mg per day is enough: "An extra amount of the vitamin cannot be stored in the body and is simply excreted. You don't need vitamin-C pills under normal circumstances." These statements are repeated by him in his latest book, *Panic in the Pantry* (Whelan and Stare, 1975). The statements are not true.

The observations that have been made on the concentration of ascorbate in the blood plasma corresponding to the capacity of the mechanism of tubular reabsorption in different people give some information about biochemical individuality with respect to vitamin C. In one study, with nineteen subjects, the capacity varied between 10 mg and 20 mg per liter (Friedman, Sherry, and Ralli, 1940). Similar variation has been found by other investigators.

Ascorbic acid is present in the various body fluids and organs, especially the leukocytes and the blood. Its concentration in the brain is also high. When a person with an insufficient supply of ascorbic acid ingests a quantity of it, it moves very rapidly from the blood serum into the leukocytes, other cells, and organs such as the spleen. The amount remaining in the blood serum may be so small, less than the capacity of the mechanism of tubular reabsorption, that very little is eliminated in the urine.

A test was developed long ago (Harris and Ray, 1935) to show the avidity with which the tissues remove ascorbic acid from the blood serum. This test, called a loading test, involves giving the subject a certain amount of vitamin C by mouth or by injection, collecting the urine for the following six hours, and analyzing it for ascorbic acid. If an oral dose of about 1 g is given, most people whose blood serum is not depleted of the vitamin eliminate about 20 to 25 percent of it in the urine in six hours.

A person who eliminates a smaller fraction of the ingested ascorbic acid may do so either because he or she has been living on a diet containing an insufficient quantity of the vitamin, such that the tissues are depleted, or because some biochemical abnormality of his or her body operates to remove ascorbate from the blood serum very rapidly, perhaps by

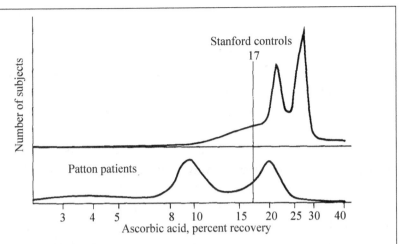

*Vitamin C and schizophrenia. In a 1973 study, forty-four patients hospitalized with acute schizophrenia and forty-four Stanford University students took a 1.76-gram dose of ascorbic acid (vitamin C) by mouth. Researchers measured the fraction of the dose excreted in the urine over the next six hours. Many of the students (upper curve) eliminated about 25 percent of the ascorbic acid, a somewhat smaller group eliminated about 20 percent, and some of the students eliminated a still smaller amount. The lower curve, for the schizophrenic patients, seems to show three similar groups, with the two peaks shifted to the left, indicating elimination of smaller amounts of ascorbic acid, and with a larger fraction of the patients eliminating only a small amount of the vitamin. The 17 percent line divides low excretors from high excretors.*

converting it rapidly into other substances. It was reported by VanderKamp in 1966 that patients with chronic schizophrenia required a loading dose of ascorbic acid about ten times greater than that required by other persons to cause the appearance of a certain amount in the urine. This observation was verified by Herjanic and Moss-Herjanic (1967).

The results of another loading test are shown in the illustration above (Pauling and others, Chapter 2 in Hawkins and Pauling, 1973). In this study forty-four patients recently hospitalized with acute schizophrenia and forty-four other subjects were given 1.76 grams of ascorbic acid by mouth, and the fraction excreted in the urine in six hours was measured. There was a twentyfold individual variation in this fraction, from 2 percent to 40 percent, with the schizophrenic patients excreting only about 60 percent as much as the others. This variation is probably partly nutritional and partly genetic in origin. The distribution functions suggest that there are three kinds of human beings with respect to their handling of ascorbic acid, the low excretors, the medium excretors, and the high excretors. This idea has not, however, been thoroughly tested as yet.

Some of the subjects in this study were given 1.76 g of ascorbic acid every day for eight days, and the fraction excreted in the six hours after the last dose was determined. Of sixteen low excretors (less than 17 percent excreted), eight had moved out of the low-excretor class, whereas the excretion of the other eight remained low. This observation suggests that these persons have an abnormal way of handling their ingested vitamin C. They might require much larger intake to be in good health.

Several serious genetic diseases, such as phenylketonuria, galactosemia, and methylmalonicaciduria, are discussed in Chapter 11. Of the many such diseases now known, some can be controlled by a large intake of an appropriate vitamin. It is harder to recognize a mild genetic disease than a serious one, but the mild genetic diseases may in the aggregate cause more suffering than the serious ones, because so many more people suffer from them. It is likely that many of the low excretors of ascorbic acid shown in the illustration on the previous page have a genetic detect such that a low intake of vitamin C is more damaging to them than to other people. For them a larger intake of the vitamin may be essential if they are to avoid a short and miserable life. At the present time it is very difficult to determine the nutritional needs of an individual person except by trial of various intakes, but we may hope that reliable clinical tests that show the individual needs will be developed before long.

# III

## *ORTHOMOLECULAR MEDICINE*

# 11

## *Orthomolecular Medicine Defined*

I believe that in general the treatment of disease by the use of substances, such as ascorbic acid, that are normally present in the human body and are required for life is to be preferred to treatment by the use of powerful synthetic substances or plant products, which may, and usually do, have undesirable side effects. Such substances as vitamin C and most of the other vitamins are remarkable for their low toxicity and absence of side effects when taken in amounts larger than those usually available in the diet. I have coined the term *orthomolecular medicine* for the preservation of good health and the treatment of disease by varying the concentrations in the human body of substances that are normally present in the body and are required for health (Pauling, 1968b). Dr. Bernard Rimland (1979) has emphasized my point by suggesting that conventional medicine, which uses drugs, be called toximolecular medicine.

Death by starvation, kwashiorkor, beriberi, scurvy, or any other deficiency disease can be averted by providing an adequate daily intake of carbohydrates, essential fats, proteins (including the essential amino acids), essential minerals, and thiamine, ascorbic acid, and other vitamins. To achieve the best of health, the rate of intake of essential foods should be such as to establish and maintain the optimum concentrations of essential molecules, such as those of ascorbic acid.

An example of orthomolecular medicine is the treatment of diabetes mellitus by the injection of insulin. Diabetes mellitus is a hereditary disease, usually caused by a recessive gene. The hereditary defect results in a deficient production by the pancreas of the hormone insulin. The primary action of insulin is to cause an increase in the rate of extraction of glucose from the blood into the cells, where it can be metabolized. In the absence of insulin the concentration of glucose in the blood of the patient becomes much greater than normal, resulting in manifestations of the disease.

Insulin extracted from cattle pancreas or pig pancreas differs only slightly in its molecular structure from human insulin, and it has essentially the same physiological activity. The injection of cattle insulin or pig insulin in a human is essentially the provision of the normal concentration of insulin in the body of the patient; it permits the metabolism of glucose to take place at the normal rate and thus serves to counteract the abnormality resulting from the genetic defect. Insulin therapy is accordingly an example of orthomolecular therapy. Its major disadvantage is that the insulin can only be introduced into the bloodstream by injection.

Another example of orthomolecular treatment of this disease, if it is not serious, is by adjusting the diet, regulating the intake of sugar, especially, in such a way as to keep the glucose concentration in the blood within the normal limits. A third example is increasing intake of vitamin C to decrease the need for insulin. Dice and Daniel (1973) reported from the study of one diabetic subject that for each gram of L-ascorbic acid taken by mouth the amount of insulin required could be reduced by two units.

A fourth way to control diabetes, by using so-called oral insulin, a drug taken by mouth, does not constitute an example of orthomolecular medicine, because oral insulin is a synthetic drug, foreign to the human body, which may have undesirable side effects.

Another disease that is treated by orthomolecular methods is phenylketonuria. It results from a genetic defect that leads to a decreased amount or effectiveness of an enzyme in the liver that in normal persons catalyzes the oxidation of one amino acid, phenylalanine, to another, tyrosine. Ordinary proteins contain several percent of phenylalanine, providing a much larger amount of this amino acid than a person needs. The concentration of phenylalanine in the blood and other body fluids of the patient becomes abnormally high, if he or she is on a normal diet, causing mental deficiency, severe eczema, and other manifestations. The disease can be controlled by a diet, beginning in infancy, that contains a smaller amount of phenylalanine than is present in ordinary foods. In this way the concentration of phenylalanine in the blood and other body fluids is kept to approximately the normal level, and the manifestations of the disease do not appear.

A somewhat similar disease, which can also be controlled by orthomolecular methods, is galactosemia. It involves the failure to manufacture an enzyme that carries out the metabolism of galactose, which is a part of milk sugar (lactose). The disease manifests itself in mental retardation, cataracts, cirrhosis of the liver and spleen, and nutritional failure. These manifestations are averted by placing the infant on a diet free of milk sugar, with the result that the concentration of galactose in the blood does not exceed the normal limit.

A conceivable sort of orthomolecular therapy for phenylketonuria or other hereditary diseases involving a defective gene would be to introduce the gene (molecules of deoxyribonucleic acid, or DNA), separated from the tissues of another person, into the cells of the person suffering from the disease. For example, some molecules of the gene that directs the synthesis of the enzyme that catalyzes the oxidation of phenylalanine to tyrosine could be separated from liver cells of a normal human being and introduced into the liver cells of a person with phenylketonuria. This sort of change in the genetic character of an organism has been carried out for microorganisms but not yet for human beings, and it is not likely that it will become an important way of controlling genetic defects until many decades have passed.

Another possible method of orthomolecular therapy for phenylketonuria, resembling the use of insulin in controlling diabetes, would be the injection of the active enzyme. There are two reasons why this treatment has not been developed. First, although it is known that the enzyme is present in the liver of animals, including humans, it has not yet been isolated in purified form. Second, the natural mechanism of immunity, which involves the action of antibodies against proteins foreign to the species, would operate to destroy the enzyme prepared from the liver of animals of another species. This mechanism in general prevents the use of enzymes or other proteins from animals other than humans in the treatment of diseases of human beings.

There is still another possible type of orthomolecular therapy. The molecules of many enzymes consist of two parts: the pure protein part, called the apoenzyme, and a nonprotein part, called the coenzyme. The active enzyme, called the holoenzyme, is the apoenzyme with the coenzyme attached to it. Often the coenzyme is a vitamin molecule or a closely related molecule. It is known, for example, that a number of different enzymes in the human body, catalyzing different chemical reactions, have thiamine diphosphate, a derivative of thiamine (vitamin $B_1$), as coenzyme.

In some cases of genetic disease the enzyme is not absent but is present with diminished activity. One way in which the defective gene can operate is to produce an apoenzyme with abnormal structure, such that it does not combine readily with the coenzyme to form the active enzyme. Under ordinary physiological conditions, with the normal concentration of coenzyme, perhaps only 1 percent of the abnormal apoenzyme has combined with the coenzyme. According to the principles of chemical equilibrium, a larger amount of the abnormal apoenzyme could be made to combine with the coenzyme by increasing the concentration of the coenzyme in the body fluids. If the concentration were to be increased one hundred times, most of the apoenzyme molecules might combine with the coenzyme, to give essentially the normal amount of active enzyme.

There is accordingly the possibility that the disease could be kept under control by the ingestion by the patient of a very large amount of the vitamin that serves as a coenzyme. This sort of orthomolecular therapy, involving only a substance normally present in the human body (the vitamin), is, in my opinion, the preferable therapy.

An example of a disease that sometimes is controlled in this way is the disease methylmalonicaciduria. Patients with this disease are deficient in the active enzyme that catalyzes the conversion of a simple substance, methylmalonic acid, to succinic acid. It is known that cyanocobalamin (vitamin $B_{12}$) serves as the coenzyme for this reaction. It is found that the provision of very large amounts of vitamin $B_{12}$, giving concentrations about a thousand times the normal concentration, causes the reaction to proceed at the normal rate for many patients.

The use of very large amounts of vitamins in the control of disease, called megavitamin therapy, is an important procedure in orthomolecular medicine. It is my opinion that in the course of time it will be found possible to control hundreds of diseases by megavitamin therapy. For example, Abram Hoffer and Humphry Osmond demonstrated, as was mentioned in Chapter 3, that many patients with schizophrenia are benefitted by megavitamin therapy (Hoffer, 1962; Hoffer and Osmond, 1966). Their treatment includes the administration of nicotinic acid (niacin) or nicotinamide (niacinamide) in amounts of 3 grams (g) to 18 g per day, together with 3 g to 18 g per day of ascorbic acid, and good amounts of other vitamins (Hawkins and Pauling, 1973; Pauling, 1974b).

It is usually thought that a drug that is claimed to be a cure for many different diseases cannot have any value against any one of them. Yet there is evidence, summarized in this book, that a large intake of vitamin C helps to control a great many diseases: not only the common cold and the flu, but also other viral and bacterial diseases, such as hepatitis, and also quite unrelated diseases, including schizophrenia, cardiovascular disease, and cancer. There is a reason for this difference between vitamin C and ordinary drugs. On the one hand, most drugs are powerful substances that interact in a specific way with one kind of molecule or tissue or agent of disease in the body so as to help to control a particular disease. The substance may, however, interact in a harmful way with other parts of the body, thus producing the side effects that make drugs dangerous.

Vitamin C, on the other hand, is a normal constituent of the body, required for life. It is invoked in essentially all of the biochemical reactions that take place in the body and in all of the body's protective mechanisms. With the ordinary intake of vitamin C these reactions and mechanisms do not operate efficiently; the person ingesting only the 60-milligram (mg) Recommended Dietary Allowance (RDA) is in what might be called ordinary poor health—what the physicians and nutritionists call "ordinary good health." The optimum intake of vitamin C, together with other health measures, can provide really good health, with increased protection against all diseases. That increase in protection is secured, as we shall see in Chapter 12, by strengthening the immune system, a process in which vitamin C plays a crucial role. The optimum intake is necessarily large. When that lesson is learned and practiced, the protection provided by vitamin C may well be the most important of all methods of orthomolecular medicine. While less is known about the other vitamins, there is no doubt that, used in the proper amounts, they also can be of great value.

In the chapters that follow, we shall consider the ways in which supplemental intake of the vitamins can prevent many diseases, sustain the body's resistance to the stress and damage of illness, and provide effective therapy in a manner preferable to that by drugs and, when necessary, in association with drugs and other conventional methods of treatment.†

If no mention is made of some disease, readers should not conclude that improved nutrition is not helpful. For many diseases and medical problems there are reports about the apparent effectiveness of a high intake of one vitamin or the use of some other orthomolecular substance. Reports of this sort are usually not published in the standard medical journals, but they may be found, for example, in *Prevention* magazine. The reports may not be reliable; the writer may have reached the unjustified conclusion that the improvement in health that occurred when he or she increased the intake of a vitamin was caused by that increase, when in fact it was just a coincidence. If the same report is made many times, however, it may be given some credence, even though medical investigators have, because of their lack of interest in vitamins, failed to carry out any definitive studies.

It is especially important to try improved nutrition in the effort to control "incurable" diseases, as was pointed out by Cheraskin and Ringsdorf (1971), who gave multiple sclerosis as one of their examples. A recommendation to try a drug when there is not strong evidence for its probable effectiveness should not be made, of course, because drugs are dangerous. It is fortunate that vitamins are so lacking in toxicity and harmful side effects that this caveat does not apply to them.

I remember a young physician who came to my home thirteen years ago and said, "Dr. Pauling, you saved my life. I was dying of chronic hepatitis, but I heard about high-dose vitamin C, and it has cured me."

Since then good studies of the value of vitamin C in the prevention and treatment of hepatitis have been made (Chapter 14), but there are other diseases for which such studies have not yet been carried out. One of these is amyotrophic lateral sclerosis (ALS), brought to public attention as the disease of which the famous Yankee baseball player Lou Gehrig died. In August 1985 I received a letter from a physician who described himself in the following way: "I am a medical 'miracle.' I've suffered from ALS for over eight years, with loss of function pretty well localized, and no spreading. I take between 12 and 20 grams of ascorbic acid every day, avoid fats and greases, and take at least 200 mg of a full B complex every day."

The acceptance of orthomolecular medicine would surely help somewhat to solve one of the great present-day problems, the high cost of health care. In 1965 the total public and private spending on health care in the United States was $40 billion; in twenty years it has increased tenfold, to $400 billion (Report of the Department of Health and Human Services, 1985). The increasing cost of medical care, amplified by inflation, accounted for 76 percent of this increase and population growth for 11 percent. The cost of health care was 6 percent of the gross national product in 1965 and 11 percent in 1985. This increase reflects both the rapid rise in charges for medical services (after corrections for inflation) and the increasing availability of expensive high-technology methods of diagnosis and treatment. A recent discussion (Atkins et al., 1985) of high-tech cardiology mentioned some of the new technologies now in use: telemetry units for monitoring arrhythmias, diagnostic cardiac catheterization, invasive electrophysiologic assessments, permanent artificial pacemakers, electrocardiography and Doppler studies for assessing cardiac function, nuclear imaging, open-heart surgery, and heart transplantation. The discussion went on to new technologies soon to be applied: magnetic resonance imaging; high-speed computerized tomography scanning of the heart; and implantable "cardioverters" that automatically correct potentially lethal arrhythmias. Additional technologies include implantable defibrillators in high-risk patients to restore the cardiac beat after arrest, artificial heart implantation, and laser angioscopy to visualize atherosclerotic coronary plaques directly and to guide the "recanalizing" of obstructive narrowing.

Among the problems associated with this development are the very high cost and the pressures from both patients and physicians to make sometimes inappropriate use of the techniques. Dr. George A. Beller, of the University of Virginia, listed ten forces that operate against cost containment in cardiology: First, physicians are motivated to provide the highest quality of care possible, regardless of cost. Second, most physicians are still on a fee-for-service basis. Third, physicians are paid the highest premium for performing technologically sophisticated procedures. Fourth, physicians are likely to try to convince hospital administrators to acquire the latest innovations. Fifth, the administrators are under pressure to increase the hospital's share of patients in the face of competition and therefore view it desirable to acquire these technologies. Sixth, patients are attracted to hospitals offering the latest equipment, services, and modern technologies. Seventh, suppliers of high-tech goods and services have an interest in continued growth. Eighth, some physicians feel pressured to order tests that they know are probably unnecessary because a consultant has written them as suggestions in the patient's chart. If the patient does not do well, failure to follow the consultant's advice could be considered negligent in court. The fear of a malpractice suit is certainly an inhibiting factor in cost containment. Ninth, it is often difficult to distinguish tests that are undertaken for clinical research from tests that are necessary for clinical management. Tenth, the need for an ultimate diagnosis has been a prevailing factor in cardiologic practice.

Beller also pointed out that another force is our society's special sympathy for those who are suffering. He quoted Gregory Pence of the University of Alabama as saying, "Medical costs are uncontrollable because we lack moral agreement about how to deny medical services. Deciding how to say 'no,' and to say it with honesty and integrity, is perhaps the most profound, most difficult moral question our society will face in the coming years."

These are difficult problems. I believe that orthomolecular medicine can contribute to their solution. Vitamins are much less expensive than drugs. The amount of suffering caused to the patient by the treatment should be taken into consideration—a high intake of vitamins improves the state of well-being of the patient and helps to control the unpleasant side effects of some conventional therapies. Finally, if the aim of medical care is not merely to cure sickness but to promote health, then it should be foremost in the physician's mind that improved nutrition can help the patient significantly in reaching the goal of a good and satisfying life.

# 12

## *The Immune System*

Our bodies are protected from onslaughts from both without and within by our natural protective mechanisms. The most important of these is the immune system. By keeping that system operating as effectively as possible we can make a significant contribution to our own good health.

When vitamins were first isolated and investigated half a century ago it was observed that a deficiency in any one of several of them resulted in impairment of the immune system, such as a decrease in the number of leukocytes in the blood and in a decreased resistance to infection. The vitamins required for good immunity are vitamin A, vitamin $B_{12}$, pantothenic acid, folic acid, and vitamin C. These are also the vitamins that seem to strengthen the immune system when they are taken in amounts larger than those usually recommended. The effect on the immune system is greatest for vitamin C. I shall discuss the evidence in this chapter.

When we were discussing the immune system in relation to cancer in our book *Cancer and Vitamin C* (Cameron and Pauling, 1979), Dr. Ewan Cameron and I wrote that the immunological defense system has the difficult task of distinguishing foe from friend by first recognizing "nonself" (the invading vectors of disease, such as bacteria or malignant cells) as distinct from "self" (the normal cells). Recognition depends upon the evaluation of differences in molecular structure. For the viral and bacterial vectors of disease these differences are striking, and their recognition is relatively easily accomplished, whereas for the cancer cells the differences are slight, and the immune mechanisms must be highly competent in order to be effective. As pictured by Lewis Thomas, former president of the Memorial Sloan-Kettering Cancer Center, the immune system functions as a police force, constantly patrolling the body and checking the cells, keeping an eye open for cells that have become malignant, and, when they have been recognized, destroying them.

There is much evidence that vitamin C is essential for the efficient working of the immune system. The mechanisms of the immune system involve certain molecules, mainly protein molecules that are present in solution in the body fluids, as well as certain cells. Vitamin C is involved both in the synthesis of many of these molecules and in the production and proper functioning of the cells.

Antibodies (also called immunoglobulins) are rather large protein molecules, each molecule consisting of about fifteen thousand or twenty-five thousand atoms. A human being is able to make about a million different kinds of antibody molecules. Each kind is able to recognize a particular group of atoms, called a haptenic group or hapten, carried in its antigen, a foreign molecule. Most people do not make antibodies that can combine with their own haptens. Those unfortunate people who do so suffer from a special sort of disease, an "autoimmune" disease; it is possible that lupus erythematosis and glomerular nephritis may be such diseases.

The haptenic groups in an antigen stimulate the cells in the body that manufacture the corresponding specific antibodies to divide and to form a clone of a large number of cells. These new cells liberate the specific antibodies into the blood, where they can combine with the antigenic molecules or cells and mark them for destruction.

It has been found that an increased intake of vitamin C leads to the manufacture of more antibody molecules. Increase in antibodies of types IgG and IgM was reported by Vallance (1977). He studied subjects who for nearly a year were isolated in a British research station in Antarctica, out of contact with any sources of new infection, which, by stimulating immunoglobulin production, would have introduced a disturbing factor. Prinz and his coworkers gave 1 gram (g) of vitamin C to twenty-five healthy male university students and a placebo to twenty similar subjects. After seventy-five days they found that for the vitamin-C subjects there was a significant increase in the serum levels of the immunoglobulins IgA, IgG, and IgM (Prinz et al., 1977). A similar dependence of the production of antibodies on the intake of vitamin C has also been observed in guinea pigs, which share our dependence on outside sources for a supply of this vitamin (Prinz et al., 1980).

IgA is the form of antibody that is present in the largest amount (together with some IgM) in nasal secretions; it is largely responsible for the antiviral action of these secretions. All three forms are present in blood and interstitial fluid, IgM in the largest amount.

Bacterial cells and malignant cells that have been identified as foreign by the molecules of specific antibodies adhering to them have to be prepared for destruction by combination with some other protein molecules, the components of complement, that are present in the bloodstream. There is some evidence that vitamin C is involved in the synthesis of the Cl-esterase component of complement and that the amount of this important substance increases with increase in the intake of this vitamin. Without this important component of complement the whole complement cascade is inoperable and the "nonself" cells would not be destroyed. There is no doubt that vitamin C is required also in humans for the synthesis of Cl-esterase, because this component of complement contains protein molecules that are similar to the molecules of collagen that are known to require vitamin C for their synthesis.

After the foreign cells or malignant cells have been identified and marked for destruction they are attacked and destroyed by the phagocytic (cell-eating) cells that patrol the body. These phagocytic cells are white cells, leucocytes, in the blood and other body fluids. Leucocytes are found in large numbers in the pus formed in suppurating abscesses or sores, where they have been fighting an infection.

Leucocytes that are made in the lymph glands are lymphocytes. They are conveyed in the lymph (a suspension of the cells in a clear yellowish fluid resembling blood plasma) through the lymphatic vessels to the bloodstream. The lymphocytes seem to be the most important of the phagocytic cells in the battles against cancer and other diseases. A malignant tumor is often observed to be infiltrated with lymphocytes, and a high degree of lymphocyte infiltration is now accepted as a reliable indicator of a favorable outcome of the disease. Moreover, it has been demonstrated that guinea pigs maintained on very low intakes of vitamin C tolerate skin grafts from other guinea pigs, and that this tolerance is related to their abnormally low lymphocyte ascorbate levels (Kalden and Guthy, 1972). When the guinea pigs are given large amounts of vitamin C the skin grafts are promptly rejected, showing that the immune systems are again functioning.

These observations and the well-known fact that leucocytes are phagocytically effective only if they contain a rather large amount of ascorbate led Dr. Ewan Cameron and me to suggest in 1974 that a high intake of vitamin C would permit the lymphocyte part of the defense mechanisms against cancer to function at high efficiency. This prediction has now been confirmed. Working in the National Cancer Institute, Yonemoto and his coworkers (Yonemoto, Chretien, and Fehniger, 1976; Yonemoto, 1979) studied five healthy young men and women, eighteen to thirty years old, who initially were receiving the ordinary low intake of vitamin C. They took samples of blood, separated the lymphocytes, and measured their rate of blastogenesis (production of new lymphocyte cells by budding) when stimulated by an antigenic foreign substance, phytohemagglutinin. Then they gave each subject 5 g of vitamin C on each of three successive days. The rate of formation of new lymphocytes, as measured by the same test of the separated cells, had nearly doubled (an increase of 83 percent) in a few days. and it remained high for another week. A dose of 10 g per day for three days caused this rate to triple, and a dose of 18 g per day caused it to reach four times the original value. This study leaves little doubt that a high intake of vitamin C by cancer patients increases the effectiveness of the body's protective mechanism involving lymphocytes and leads to a more favorable prognosis for the patient suffering from cancer or an infectious disease. More extensive studies of this sort are needed to determine the intake of vitamin C, both orally and intravenously, that leads to the maximum rate of blastogenesis of lymphocytes. The indication from the work of Yonemoto and his coworkers is that the optimum oral intake may be greater than 18 g per day.

Many investigators have reported that an increase in the intake of vitamin C by either normal subjects or patients with certain diseases leads to increased motility of leucocytes and their more rapid movement to the site of an infection (Anderson, 1981, 1982; Panush et al., 1982). There is further evidence that when they arrive, vitamin C increases their capacity for phagocytosis. This is the process in which leucocytes surround and destroy bacterial cells or malignant cells that have been identified as foreign and marked for destruction; the individual leucocyte surrounds and engulfs the foreign cell. Vitamin C is required for this process. It was discovered long ago that leucocytes are not phagocytically effective if they do not contain enough ascorbate (Cottingham and Mills, 1943). A recent study (Hume and Weyers, 1973) has shown that persons on an ordinary Scottish diet and in good health had a little more ascorbate in their leucocytes than the amount needed for phagocytic activity but the amount dropped to half this value on the first day after they had contracted colds, and it stayed low for several days, rendering them susceptible to secondary bacterial infections. An intake of 250 milligrams (mg) of ascorbic acid per day was not enough to keep the amount of ascorbate in the leucocytes up to the level required for effective phagocytosis, but 1 g per day plus 6 g per day beginning at the onset of the cold was found to be enough to keep this important protective mechanism operating.

I conclude from this study that the prophylactic intake of ascorbic acid, the dose taken regularly to preserve good health and provide protection against disease, almost certainly should be more than 250 mg per day for most people. Other considerations led me to suggest the range 250 mg to 4000 mg, or even 10,000 mg, for recommended daily intake for most people (Pauling, 1974c). Such an intake should decrease the chance of contracting the common cold or influenza and, if a viral infection is contracted, should prevent a secondary bacterial infection from developing.

Irwin Stone (1972) has described vitamin C in relation to bacterial diseases in the following words:

1. It is bactericidal or bacteriostatic and will kill or prevent the growth of the pathogenic organisms.*
2. It detoxicates and renders harmless the bacterial toxins and poisons.
3. It controls and maintains phagocytosis.
4. It is harmless and nontoxic and can be administered in the large doses needed to accomplish the above effects without danger to the patient.

Another, more recently recognized, agent in the immune system is the interferons. These are proteins with antiviral activity, which are produced by cells infected by a virus and possibly also by malignant cells. Spreading to neighboring cells, the interferons change them in such a way as to enable them to resist infection. There is some evidence that interferons help in the effort by the human body to control a developing cold or other infection or cancer. Different kinds of interferon are synthesized by different animal species. Human beings make about twenty different kinds of interferon molecules, with somewhat different activities, in different cells in the body. Interferon has attracted lively interest because very few drugs have any effectiveness against viral infections and cancer.

*Evidence for this statement will be considered in Chapter 14.

Since interferons are proteins, animal interferons act as antigens in human beings and cannot be injected without sensitizing the person in such a way that further injections would cause serious allergic reactions. Human interferons, made from human leucocytes in cell culture, are now available, but at a rather high price. Studies have indicated that injections of these substances have some value in treating cancer and infectious diseases (Borden, 1984).

The suggestion that an increased intake of vitamin C would lead to the production of larger amounts of the interferons (Pauling, 1970a) has been verified. Until more evidence becomes available about the value of injections of human interferon, we may be wise to follow the advice of Cameron: "Take more vitamin C and make your own interferon!"

The prostaglandins are small molecules (lipids, related to fats) that play a potent, central role in the functioning of the human body. Acting as hormones, they are involved in regulation of the heart beat, the flow of blood, the damage done to cells by drugs, and the responses of the immune system. Their isolation and characterization have occurred mainly since 1960, with many discoveries made since 1970. The formula of prostaglandin PGE1 is $C_{20}H_{34}O_5$, and the other prostaglandins have the same or closely similar formulas.

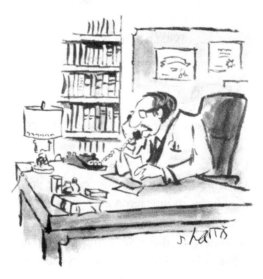

"TAKE SOME INTERFERON, AND CALL ME IN THE MORNING."

Whenever any tissue is disturbed or damaged it releases prostaglandins (Vane, 1971). The prostaglandins, especially PGE2 and PGF2-alpha, are involved with other substances in producing inflammation of the tissues—redness, swelling, pain, tenderness, and heat—resulting from increased flow of blood and the movement of leucocytes and other cells and substances to the region in response to the hormones. As we shall see in the comparison of drugs and vitamins in Chapter 26, the function of the prostaglandins in inflammation is controlled to some extent by aspirin. In 1978 Horrobin reported that vitamin C inhibits the synthesis of PGE2 and PGF2-alpha, and in this way the vitamin also exerts a considerable anti-inflammatory action. He reported, however, that whereas aspirin inhibits the synthesis of PGE1, vitamin C increases the amount synthesized (Horrobin, Oka, and Manku, 1979). The prostaglandin PGE1 is involved in the formation of lymphocytes and plays a major part in the regulation of immune responses. Accordingly the effect of vitamin C in stimulating the production of PGE1 is an additional way in which the intake of the optimum amount of vitamin C strengthens the immune system and contributes to the maintenance of better health.

# 13

## *The Common Cold*

Most people catch several colds each year, usually in the fall, winter, and spring. When you catch a cold, after you have been exposed to cold viruses being spread by some other person, you may sneeze, feel a chill and scratchiness of the throat, develop a runny nose or stopped-up nose, and show other signs of the viral infection. Later, as the cold develops, you may feel rather miserable for two or three days. At this time it is usually wise to stay at home and rest in bed—for your own well-being and to spare your family and your colleagues the risk of exposure to your cold. After a week or ten days you have usually recovered.

Having a cold two or three times a year is not pleasant. What is worse, the cold may be attended by serious complications—bronchitis, sinus infection, infection of the middle ear, infection of the mastoid bone (mastoiditis), meningitis, bronchopneumonia or lobar pneumonia, or exacerbation of some other disease, such as arthritis or kidney disease or heart disease.

The common cold (acute coryza) is an inflammation of the upper respiratory tract caused by infection with a virus.* This infection alters the physiology of the mucous membrane of the nose, the perinasal sinuses, and the throat. The common cold occurs more often than all other diseases combined. This infection does not occur, however, in small isolated communities; exposure to the virus, carried by persons from the outside, is needed. Thus, the Norwegian island of Spitsbergen used to be isolated during seven months of the year. The 507 residents of the principal town of the island, Longyearbyen, were nearly free of colds through the cold winter, with only four colds recorded in three months. Then within two weeks after the arrival of the first ship some 200 of the residents had become ill with colds (Paul and Freese, 1933).

---

*A discussion of the many viruses that can cause the common cold is given in the book *The Common Cold,* by Sir Christopher Andrewes, 1965.

Development of a cold after exposure to the virus is determined to some extent by the state of health of the person and by environmental factors. Fatigue, chilling of the body, wearing of wet clothing and wet shoes, and the presence of irritating substances in the air are traditionally cited as preludes to a cold. Experimental studies indicate, however, that these factors are not so important as is generally believed (Andrewes, 1965; Debré and Celers, 1970, page 539).

The period of incubation, between exposure and the manifestation of symptoms, is usually two or three days. The first symptoms are the familiar ones cited in the first paragraph of this chapter. Headache, general malaise (an indefinite feeling of uneasiness or discomfort), and chills (a sensation of coldness attended with convulsive shaking of the body, pinched face, pale skin, and blue lips) often attend the progress of the cold. A slight increase in temperature, usually to not over 101°F (38.3°C), may occur. The mucous membranes of the nose and pharynx are swollen. One nostril or both nostrils may be blocked by the thickened secretions. The skin around the nostrils may become sore, and cold sores (caused by the virus *Herpes simplex*) may develop on the lips.

The customary treatment for the common cold includes resting in bed, drinking fruit juice or water, ingesting a simple and nutritious diet, preventing irritants such as tobacco smoke from entering the respiratory tract, and alleviating the symptoms to some extent by the use of aspirin, phenacetin, antihistamines, and other drugs (see Chapter 26). After some days the tissues of the nose and throat, weakened by the virus infection, are often invaded by bacteria. This secondary infection may cause the nasal secretions to become purulent (to contain pus). Also, the secondary infection may spread to the sinuses, the middle ears, the tonsils, the pharynx, the larynx, the trachea, the bronchi, and the lungs. As mentioned above, mastoiditis, pneumonia, meningitis, and other serious infections may follow. Control of the common cold thus would lead to a decrease in the incidence of more serious diseases.

Not everyone is susceptible to infection with the common cold. Most investigators have noted that an appreciable proportion of the population, 6 to 10 percent, never have colds. This fact provides justification for hope that a significant decrease in the number of colds can be achieved through increase in the resistance of individuals to viral infection. It is likely that the ability of 6 to 10 percent of the population to avoid colds is the result of their natural powers of resistance. Like other physiological properties, the resistance of individuals to viral infection probably can be represented by a distribution curve that has approximately the normal bell shape. The 6 to 10 percent of the population that are resistant to colds presumably correspond to the tail end of the curve, those people with the largest natural powers of resisting viral infections. If in some way the natural resistance of the whole population could be shifted upward, a larger percentage of the population would lie in the range corresponding to complete resistance to the infection and would never have colds. This argument indicates strongly that a study of the factors involved in the natural resistance to viral infection, such as nutritional factors, could lead to a significant decrease in the susceptibility of the population as a whole to the common cold. Considering, along with this possibility, that the common cold disappears in isolated communities like Spitsbergen, I am moved to declare again my belief that the nuisance and menace of the common cold might be stamped out entirely.

I have made a rough estimate of the significance of the common cold, measured in dollars. Let us assume that the average loss of time because of serious illness with the common cold is seven days per person per year. The person suffering from a cold or series of colds during the year might stay away from work, or might have a decreased effectiveness, or might be sufficiently ill and miserable to feel that the seven days are wasted. In any event, a measure of the damage done by the common cold might be roughly taken as the person's loss of productivity and income for the seven days during the year when he or she is most seriously ill. The personal income of the people of the United States is about $3,000 billion per year (1985). The income per week is this quantity divided by fifty-two. We may accordingly be justified in saying that the damage done by the common cold to the people of the United States each year can be described roughly as corresponding to a monetary loss of $60 billion per year.*

This corresponds to a loss in income or its equivalent in well-being of about $250 per year per person. It is easy to understand why the people of the United States spend hundreds of millions of dollars per year on cold medicines, despite their limited effectiveness.

*A smaller estimate, $5 billion per year, was given by Fabricant and Conklin in their book *The Dangerous Cold,* 1965. The increase is the result of population growth and monetary inflation.

It has been known for more than twenty years that most people can keep from having colds, or, if a cold develops, can suppress most of its disagreeable manifestations, by the proper use of vitamin C. There is no need for you to be made miserable by the common cold.

In the medical literature, nonetheless, it continues to be said that no clearly effective method of treatment of the common cold has been developed. The various drugs that are prescribed or recommended have some value in making the patient more comfortable, by giving relief from some of the more distressing symptoms, but they have little effect on the duration of the cold. The fact that doctors have not had a good way of preventing and treating the common cold has been the subject of many jokes. The doctor says to the patient, "You have a cold. I don't know how to treat it, but if it develops into pneumonia, come to see me because I can cure pneumonia." There is another joke that appeared after the first edition of my book *Vitamin C and the Common Cold* was published in 1970. The doctor says to the patient, "You are suffering from an overdose of vitamin C, so I shall give you an injection of cold viruses to counteract it."

A great many people have reported to me that their lives were changed by reading my book. Whereas during previous years they had suffered from many colds, their increased intake of vitamin C had been effective in providing complete protection against this disease. Other people, however, reported that following my recommendations did not keep them from developing colds that were just about as serious as those that they had caught earlier. The continued study of this problem has led me to conclude that human beings, with their biochemical individuality, differ quite a bit from one another in the amount of vitamin C required to provide protection against the common cold. For some people the achievement of really good health and protection against cold viruses requires the intake of a far larger amount of vitamin C than was recommended in my book. I now believe that every person can protect himself or herself against the common cold, or, if a cold begins to develop, can make its symptoms far less serious than they would be otherwise, by taking the amount of vitamin C that is appropriate to him or her.

If you have established your optimum nutritional intake of vitamin C, you will find yourself going through the common-cold season without a cold. This statement may, in fact, be put the other way around. If you go through the season cold-free, you have probably found your optimum nutritional intake of vitamin C.

Your heightened resistance may nonetheless be overridden. When you feel the first symptoms of a cold coming on, you should increase your intake of vitamin C at once to the therapeutic level. In my own experience, this means taking 1 gram (g) or more of vitamin C per hour throughout the waking hours of the day. Cold symptoms are usually suppressed at once, and they remain so if the therapeutic dose is maintained for the duration of what would otherwise have been the cold. The one discomfort in this regimen may be a looseness of the bowels in the first few days.

My simple prescription remains, of course, heresy to orthodox nutritionists and most practitioners of medicine. I was on a television show, with David Frost, some years ago with the nutrition authority Dr. Fredrick J. Stare, *Mademoiselle's* "Big Name in nutrition," as my fellow guest. Stare and I made somewhat different statements about vitamin C and its value, and the hour-long program came nearly to its end. Finally, Stare said, "I know that Dr. Pauling's method of preventing the common cold is no good, because I tried it, and it didn't work." I started to ask a question about how he had tried it, but Frost said, "Gentlemen, I am sorry that our time is up, and I thank you for having been on the program." Then, as we were walking away, Stare turned to me and said "Of course, I didn't use the astronomical amount that *you* recommend."

This story has some bearing on the question of why physicians on the whole have not been recommending the use of vitamin C to their patients to help prevent the common cold and other diseases. Although physicians, as part of their training, are taught that the dosage of a drug that is prescribed for the patient must be very carefully determined and controlled, they seem to have difficulty in remembering that the same principle applies to the vitamins. Stare probably could have prevented his cold from developing if he had taken the "astronomical amount" that I recommend.

I believe that every cold or other illness that a person suffers from damages his or her body in a permanent way to some extent, and shortens his or her life expectancy. Using vitamin C to prevent colds may slow down the aging process. This is part of the contribution that results from following the regimen that I urge in this book for the prolongation of life and especially of the period of well-being, during which life is really enjoyed.

The answer to the apparent contradiction between the opinions expressed by authorities in nutrition and my own experience is a simple one. Vitamin C has only rather small value in providing protection against the common cold when it is taken in small amounts, but it has great value when it is taken in large amounts. Most of the studies referred to in the editorial article in the August 1967 issue of *Nutrition Reviews,* mentioned in Chapter 3, involved giving small amounts of ascorbic acid to the subjects, usually 200 milligrams (mg) per day. But even these studies indicate that such small amounts have some protective value, not very great, against the common cold. The amount of protection increases with increase in the amount of ingested vitamin C and becomes nearly complete with 10 g to 40 g per day taken at the immediate onset of the cold.

The study of vitamin C in relation to the common cold began only a few years after the vitamin was identified as ascorbic acid. Dr. Roger Korbsch of St. Elisabeth Hospital, Oberhausen, Germany, was one of the first to publish an account of such a study, in 1938. The fact that ascorbic acid has been reported to be effective against several diseases, including gastritis and stomach ulcers, suggested that he try it in treating acute rhinitis and colds. In 1936 he found that oral doses of up to 1 g per day were of value against rhinorrhea, acute rhinitis, and secondary rhinitis and accompanying manifestations of illness, such as headache. He then found that the injection of 250 or 500 mg of sodium ascorbate on the first day of a common cold almost always led to the immediate disappearance of all the signs and symptoms of the cold, with a similar injection sometimes needed on the second day. He stated that ascorbic acid is far superior to other cold medicines, such as aminopyrine, and is without danger, in that there is no evidence that there are serious side effects, even with large doses.

A trial was then made in Germany (Ertel, 1941) in which 357 million daily doses of vitamin C were distributed among 3.7 million pregnant women, nursing mothers, suckling infants, and schoolchildren. Ertel reported that the recipients of the vitamin C enjoyed better health, in several different respects, than the corresponding control populations. The only quantitative information given by him is that with one group of schoolchildren for which good statistical data were collected the amount of illness with respiratory infections was 20 percent less than the year before.

In 1942 Glazebrook and Thomson reported the results of a study carried out in an institution where there were about 1500 students, whose ages ranged from fifteen to twenty years. The food was poorly prepared, being kept hot for two hours or more before serving, and the total intake of ascorbic acid was determined to be only about 5 to 15 mg per student per day. Some of the students (335) were given additional ascorbic acid, 200 mg per day, for a period of six months, and the others (1100) were kept as controls. The incidence of colds and tonsillitis was 14 percent less among the students given ascorbic acid than among the controls. The number of serious cases of colds or tonsillitis requiring admission to sick quarters was 25 percent less for the students receiving ascorbic acid than for the controls. This difference has high statistical significance (only 1 percent probability in a uniform population). The average number of days of hospitalization per student because of infection (common cold, tonsillitis, acute rheumatism, pneumonia) was 2.5 days for the students receiving ascorbic acid and 5.0 days for the controls. There were 17 cases of pneumonia and 16 cases of acute rheumatism among the 1100 controls, and no case of either disease among the 335 students receiving ascorbic acid. The probability of such a great difference in two samples of a uniform population is so small (less than 0.3 percent) as to indicate very strongly that vitamin C has value in providing protection against these serious infectious diseases, as well as against the common cold and tonsillitis.

A study made famous by detractors of my prescription of vitamin C is that of Cowan, Diehl and Baker, which I cited in Chapter 3. The main result of the study is that the students who received the placebo lost an average of 1.6 days from school because of colds, and those who received vitamin C in only a small dose, 200 mg per day, lost only an average of 1.1 days, 31 percent less. The probability that this difference would occur in a uniform population is only 0.1 percent, so that it is highly likely that this decrease in the amount of illness was caused by the ascorbic acid.

In such a test, the best experiments are those in which the subjects are divided into two groups, in a random way, with the substance being tested (ascorbic acid) administered to the subjects in one group, and a placebo (an inactive material resembling the preparation to be tested: for example, a capsule containing citric acid might be used as a placebo for ascorbic acid) administered to those of the other group. In a blind experiment the subjects do not know whether or not they are receiving the placebo. Sometimes a double-blind study is made, in which the investigators evaluating the effects of the preparation and the placebo do not know which of the subjects received the preparation and which received the placebo until the study is completed, this information being kept by some other person.

The results of the first carefully controlled, double-blind study with a larger daily amount, 1000 mg, of ascorbic acid were reported in 1961 by Dr. G. Ritzel. a physician with the medical service of the school district of the city of Basel, Switzerland. He carried out the study at a ski resort with 279 boys during two periods of five to seven days. The conditions were such that the incidence of colds during these short periods was large enough (approximately 20 percent) to permit results with statistical significance to be obtained. The subjects were of the same age (fifteen to seventeen) and had similar nutrition during the period of study. In accordance with the double-blind protocol, neither the participants nor the physicians had any knowledge about the distribution of the 1000-mg ascorbic-acid tablets and the placebo tablets. The tablets were distributed every morning and were taken by the subjects under observation in such a way that the possibility of interchange of tablets was eliminated. The subjects were examined daily for symptoms of colds and other infections. The records were largely on the basis of subjective symptoms, partially supported by objective observations (measurement of body temperature, inspection of the respiratory organs, auscultation of the lungs, and so on). Persons who showed cold symptoms on the first day were excluded from the investigation.

After the completion of the investigation a completely independent group of professional people carried out the statistical evaluation of the observations with the identity of the recipients of the ascorbic acid and the placebo tablets concealed by identification numbers. The group receiving ascorbic acid showed only 39 percent as many days of illness per person as the group receiving the placebo; the number of individual symptoms per person was only 36 percent as great for the ascorbic-acid group as for the placebo group. The statistical evaluation showed that these differences are statistically significant at better than the 99 percent level of confidence. We see that in Ritzel's study the vitamin-C subjects had only about one-third as much illness as the placebo subjects.

In another ski-camp study, with forty-six students as subjects, Bessel-Lorck (1959) found that those students who received 1 g of vitamin C per day had only about half as much illness as those who received no vitamin C.

After the publication of my *Vitamin C and the Common Cold,* several excellent double-blind studies were carried out. The first one, in Toronto, Canada (Anderson, Reid, and Beaton, 1972) involved 407 subjects receiving ascorbic acid (1 g per day plus 3 g per day for three days at the onset of any illness) and 411 subjects receiving a closely matching placebo. The duration of the study was four months. The number of days confined to house per subject was 30 percent less for the ascorbic-acid group than for the placebo group, and the number of days off work per subject was 33 percent less. The authors mention that these differences have high statistical significance (99.9 percent level of confidence).

Another study, under quite different conditions, involved 112 soldiers undergoing operational training in northern Canada (Sabiston and Radomski, 1974). Half of the subjects received 1 g of ascorbic acid per day during the four weeks of the study, and the other half received a placebo. The average number of days of illness was 68 percent less for the ascorbic-acid subjects than for the placebo subjects.

The average amount of protection against the common cold found in these four studies in which 1 g or 2 g was given per day is 48 percent; that is, on the average, the subjects who received vitamin C had only about one-half as much illness as those who received the inactive tablet.

Since identical twins have, in principle, identical immune systems, they commend themselves for studies of this kind. Two unfortunately flawed studies comparing one twin on placebo and the other on vitamin C have been reported. Carr and his colleagues conducted a hundred-day double-blind study of ninety-five pairs of identical twins in Australia, fourteen to sixty-four years old, average twenty-five years, in which one of each pair took a 1000-mg tablet of vitamin C each day and the other took a well-matched placebo, with all subjects also taking a vitamin tablet containing 70 mg of vitamin C. The results of this study were published in three separate articles (Carr, Einstein, et al., 1981a, 1981b; Martin, Carr, et al., 1982). Of the ninety-five pairs of twins, however, fifty-one pairs were living together. For these pairs there was little difference in the amount of illness between the twin with the high intake of C and the twin with the low intake. I think that the probable explanation is that the twins living together were not careful about taking their own tablets. Moreover, close exposure to the other's cold might well override whatever protection was afforded to the twin taking vitamin C. For the forty-four pairs of twins living apart the average number of days of illness was 6.32 for the high-intake twins and 12.08 for the low-intake twins, corresponding to 48 percent protection by the extra 1000 mg of vitamin C per day.

In the other twin study, by Miller et al. (1977, 1978) forty-four pairs of identical twins were given 500, 750, and 1000 mg of vitamin C per day, depending on age, or a starch placebo. There was little difference in the amounts of illness of the vitamin-C twins and the placebo twins. All of these pairs of twins lived at home, and the same effects of mixing their tablets and exchanging their infections may have occurred.

Many other physicians have reported their observations that vitamin C seems to have value in helping to control the common cold, as well as other diseases. From a study of 2600 factory workers in Leipzig, Scheunert (1949) reported that an intake of either 100 mg or 300 mg of vitamin C per day decreased the incidence of respiratory diseases and other diseases by about 75 percent. Bartley, Krebs, and O'Brien (1953) found that the mean length of colds in subjects deprived of ascorbic acid was twice as great as for subjects not deprived. Fletcher and Fletcher (1951) stated that supplements of 50 mg to 100 mg of ascorbic acid per day increased the resistance of children to infection. Some value of small amounts of ascorbic acid was reported also by Barnes (1961), Macon (1956), and Banks (1965, 1968). Marckwell (1947) stated that there was a 50 percent chance of stopping a cold if enough ascorbic acid was taken: 0.75 g at once, followed by 0.5 g every three or four hours, continuing on later days if needed.

In the July-August 1967 issue of the magazine *Fact* there appeared an article entitled "Why Organized Medicine Sneezes at the Common Cold" by Dr. Douglas Gildersleeve, apparently a pseudonym for a physician who feared the consequences of writing heresy in a popular magazine. The author reported that he could suppress the symptoms of the common cold by making use of twenty or twenty-five times as much ascorbic acid as the 200 mg per day used by investigators whose reports he had read. In studies carried out on more than four hundred colds in twenty-five individuals, mostly his own patients, he had found the treatment with ascorbic acid in large amounts to be effective in 95 percent of the patients. The most frequent cold symptom, excessive nasal discharge, disappeared entirely on use of ascorbic acid, and other symptoms—sneezing, coughing, sore throat, hoarseness, and headache—were barely noticeable, if they were present at all. He reported that not one of the subjects ever experienced any secondary bacterial complications.

In this article Gildersleeve reported that in 1964 he wrote a paper in which he described his observations. He submitted the paper to eleven different professional journals, every one of which rejected it. One editor said to him that it would be harmful to the journal to publish a useful treatment for the common cold. He stated that medical journals depend for their existence on the support of their advertisers, and that more than twenty-five percent of the advertisements in the journals relate to patented drugs for the alleviation of cold symptoms or for the treatment of complications of colds.

Another editor said that he had rejected the paper because it was not correct. When Gildersleeve questioned him about this statement, he said, "Twenty-five years ago I was a member of a team of researchers that investigated vitamin C. We determined then that the drug was of no use in treating the common cold." He was not impressed when Gildersleeve told him that the amount of ascorbic acid that had been used in the early work was only one-twentieth of the minimum amount necessary to achieve significant results.

Explaining "Why Organized Medicine Sneezes at the Common Cold," Gildersleeve concluded: ". . . having worked as a researcher in the field, it is my contention that an effective treatment for the common cold, a cure, is available, that [it] is being ignored because of the monetary losses that would be inflicted on pharmaceutical manufacturers, professional journals, and doctors themselves."

Some other studies have addressed the therapeutic value of vitamin C in treating, as distinguished from preventing, the common cold. They confirm the experience reported by the pseudonymous Dr. Gildersleeve. In 1938 Ruskin reported his observations on more than one thousand patients to whom he had given an injection, sometimes followed by a second one, of

450 mg of calcium ascorbate as soon as possible after the onset of a cold. He found that 42 percent of the patients were completely relieved and another 48 percent were markedly improved. He concluded that "calcium ascorbate would appear to be practically an abortive in the treatment of the common cold." Several other somewhat similar reports are mentioned by Irwin Stone in his book *The Healing Factor: Vitamin C against Disease* (1972). Stone himself recommended taking 1.5 to 2 g of ascorbic acid by mouth at the first sign of a cold, with the dose repeated at twenty-minute to half-hour intervals until the symptoms have disappeared, which occurs usually by the third dose.

The physician Edmé Régnier of Salem, Massachusetts, reported in 1968 that he had discovered the value of the administration of large doses of ascorbic acid in the prevention and treatment of the common cold. For many years, beginning at the age of seven, he had suffered from repeated bouts of inflammation of the middle ear. He had tried a number of ways of controlling the infections, and after twenty years he tried the bioflavonoids (from citrus fruits) and ascorbic acid. He felt that this treatment had been of some benefit but not very great. He decided to try increasing the amount. After several trials he found that the serious and disagreeable manifestations of the common cold and the accompanying inflammation of the middle ear could be averted by the use of large amounts of ascorbic acid and that ascorbic acid alone was just as effective as the same amount of ascorbic acid plus bioflavonoids. He then initiated a study of twenty-one subjects with use of ascorbic acid alone, ascorbic acid plus bioflavonoids, bioflavonoids alone, or a placebo. This study extended over a period of five years. At first the subjects were kept ignorant of the preparations that they received, but later on (during the last year) it became impossible to continue the blind study, because a patient whose cold was developing recognized that he was not receiving the vitamin C that might have prevented it.

The method of treatment recommended by Régnier is the administration of 600 mg of ascorbic acid at the first signs of a cold (scratchiness of the throat, nasal secretion, sneezing, a chill), followed by an additional 600 mg every three hours or 200 mg of ascorbic acid every hour. At bedtime the amount ingested is increased to 750 mg. This intake, amounting to about 4 g of ascorbic acid per day, is to be continued for three or four days, reduced to 400 mg every three hours for several days, and then to 200 mg every three hours. Régnier reported that of thirty-four colds treated with ascorbic acid plus bioflavonoids, thirty-one were averted, and of fifty colds treated with ascorbic acid alone, as described above, forty-five were averted. He had no success in treating colds with bioflavonoids alone, or with a placebo.

He made the important observation that a cold that has been apparently aborted by the use of a large intake of ascorbic acid may return, even after a period of a week or more, if the ingestion of ascorbic acid is suddenly discontinued.

Even nearly 3 g per day for three days (2.66 g the first and second days; 1.33 g the third day) may not be effective if the treatment is delayed until after the cold has begun, as reported by Cowan and Diehl (1950). A similar lack of effectiveness of 3 g per day, starting after the cold had developed, was also reported by a group of seventy-eight British physicians (Abbott et al., 1968).

In a study carried out by the British Common Cold Research Unit in Great Britain (Tyrrell et al., 1977) with 1524 volunteers employed in industrial plants in several parts of England, each subject was given a vial containing ten effervescent tablets. Some of the vials contained 1000 mg of vitamin C per tablet, and others contained a placebo. The instructions were to take the tablets for 2.5 days, beginning when the first symptoms of a cold developed. The fraction developing a first cold was nearly the same, 31.1 percent for the vitamin-C group and 33.2 percent for the placebo group. No difference would be expected, since the two groups were on the same regimen until the first cold developed.

There was no difference in the duration of the colds. The lack of effect of taking 10 g of vitamin C during the first 2.5 days indicates that high doses of vitamin C should be taken until the cold is controlled. This finding corroborates Régnier's opinion on the likely return of aborted colds. If the cold is not completely suppressed, the rebound effect from the stopping of vitamin C intake may help in permitting it to run its full course.

One significant observation was made in the study by the Common Cold Research Unit. Of the 101 male vitamin-C subjects who experienced a first cold during the four months of the trial, 23 developed a second cold later on, whereas of the 98 similar male placebo subjects, nearly twice as many, 43, developed the second cold. This twofold difference has high statistical significance. The 10 g of vitamin C taken for the first cold may have had a strengthening effect on the immune system lasting a month or two. The difference in incidence of the second cold was not observed for the women in the study, possibly because vitamin-C depletion is not so serious for British women as for the men.

In a second Toronto study (Anderson el al., 1974), in which there were 2349 volunteers divided into eight groups, one group of 275 took 4 g of vitamin C on the first day of a cold and the second took 8 g on the first day, with no regular intake for either group. There was no clear benefit for the first group, but the authors point out that the 8-g therapeutic dose was associated with less illness than the 4-g therapeutic dose. The protective effect, measured by the decrease in number of days when individual symptoms were recorded, was about 5 percent for the single 4-g dose and 20 percent for the single 8-g dose.

The best study of the therapeutic effect of vitamin C was carried out by Asfora (1977), who gave 30 g of vitamin C or a placebo to 133 subjects (medical students, physicians, or clinic patients in Pernambuco) who had reported a developing cold. The vitamin C was given as effervescent 1000-mg tablets, with instructions that six should be taken each day (two at a time, three times a day) for five days; the placebo consisted of similar effervescent tablets. Some patients began on the first day of the cold, others on the second, and others on the third, as shown in the table below.

The number of subjects for whom the treatment may be said to have failed completely, in that they developed secondary bacterial infections

**Results of a controlled trial of the therapeutic value of 30 g of vitamin C (6 g per day for 5 days) beginning on the first, second, or third day of a cold.**

| Group | I | II | II | IV |
|---|---|---|---|---|
| Number of subjects | 45 | 30 | 17 | 41 |
| Male/female | 25/20 | 17/43 | 11/6 | 25/16 |
| Day of beginning vitamin C | 1 | 2 | 3 | placebo |
| % with bacterial complications | 13 | 20 | 41 | 39 |
| Average days of illness | 3.6 | 5.4 | 9.0 | >5* |
| With complications | 15.2 | 16.0 | 14.6 | >5* |
| Without complications | 1.82 | 2.71 | 5.10 | >5* |

*Not recorded

and were ill for an average of 15 days, was 13 percent for the first-day vitamin-C subjects, 20 percent for the second-day subjects, and 41 percent for the third-day subjects (also 39 percent for the placebo group). For the remaining subjects in each group, whose colds were without complications, the average number of days of illness was 1.82, 2.71, and 5.10 for the first-, second-, and third-day subjects. We see that 6 g of vitamin C per day, starting on the first or second day of the cold, stopped it for most of the subjects in this investigation.

We have now reviewed about thirty reported studies of the value of vitamin C taken in daily doses in preventing a cold from starting to develop or in reducing the severity of a cold. Some of the investigators have reported that both the incidence and the severity of the colds are decreased by the vitamin C. Thus Ritzel in his study of schoolboys who received 1 g of vitamin C per day reported a decrease in incidence (number of colds per subject) by 45 percent and also a decrease by 30 percent in the severity of individual colds (the number of days of illness per cold). Others have reported only a small decrease in incidence. Anderson has pointed out that with a small number of symptoms observable early in a cold, it is hard to decide whether the subject has a cold or not.

In the table on page 127 I have listed the results of sixteen trials, comprising all of the trials known to me that meet certain specifications. One is that ascorbic acid be given regularly over a period of time to subjects who were not ill at the start of the trial, with the subjects selected at random from a larger population. The study by Masek et al. (1972) is not included because the vitamin-C subjects were the workers in one mine and the placebo subjects were those in another, where the conditions affecting the health of the workers might have been either better or worse. In all but one of the studies a placebo, a tablet or capsule closely resembling the vitamin-C tablet or capsule, was given to the control subjects. The one exception was the carefully conducted and thorough study by Glazebrook and Thomson (1942), in which ascorbic acid was added to the food (cocoa or milk) of one or more of the seven divisions of boys that were served in seven different places in the dining hall.

The decrease in amount of illness per subject found in these sixteen controlled trials varies from 1 percent to 68 percent, and there is no clear indication that an intake of 1000 or 2000 mg per day gives greater

**Summary of results of controlled studies of amount of illness per subject in vitamin C subjects relative to placebo subjects**

| Study | % decrease in illness per person |
|---|---|
| * Glazebrook & Thomson (1942) | 50 |
| * Cowan, Diehl, Baker (1942) | 31 |
| * Dahlberg, Engel, Rydin (1944) | 14 |
| * Franz, Sands, Heyl (1956) | 36 |
| * Anderson et al. (1975) | 25 |
| Ritzel (1961) | 63 |
| Anderson, Reid, Beaton (1972) | 32 |
| Charleston, Clegg (1972) | 58 |
| Elliott (1973) | 44 |
| Anderson, Suryani, Beaton (1974) | 9 |
| Coulehan et al. (1974) | 30 |
| Sabiston & Radomski (1974) | 68 |
| Karlowski et al. (1975) | 21 |
| Clegg & Macdonald (1975) | 8 |
| Pitt & Costrini (1979) | 0 |
| Carr et al. (1981a, 1981b) | 48 |
| Average | 34 |

* 70 to 200 mg per day, average 31%; others, larger intakes, average 40%

protection than 70 to 200 mg per day. The studies giving the smallest and largest protective effects had soldiers as subjects. In the Pitt and Costrini study the marine recruits were in barracks in South Carolina. There was no protective effect against colds, but there was a significant protective effect against pneumonia. The Sabiston and Radomski study was carried out under more severe conditions, with soldiers living in tents in northern Canada, and the number of colds per subject was three times as great as for the South Carolina study. A possible explanation is that the amount of vitamin C in the rations of the marine recruits in South Carolina was much greater than that in the rations of the Canadian soldiers, providing greater protection for the marine recruits. It may be pertinent that in the 1975 study of Canadian subjects by Anderson, Beaton, Corey, and Spero there was a 25 percent protection, even though the intake of supplementary vitamin C was only one 500-mg tablet per week, equal to 70 mg per day. The average intake of vitamin C in the food in Canada is known to be less than that in the United States.

A principal reason for the failure of most of the controlled trials to show a large prophylactic or therapeutic effect is that the amounts of vitamin C taken are too small. It is as if the physicians and nutritionists reasoned, fallaciously, that since a tiny dose of vitamin C will cure scurvy, why should it take an astronomical dose to cure the common cold. Even so, the average of the sixteen values of the decrease in the amount of illness per person is 34 percent. For the five studies in which only 70 mg to 200 mg of ascorbic acid per day was given the average is 31 percent, and for the eleven in which 1 g per day or more was given it is 40 percent. We may conclude that even a small added intake of vitamin C, 100 mg or 200 mg per day, has considerable value, and that a larger intake probably has somewhat more value.*

The studies I have reviewed here fall short of the standards I have in mind not only because too little vitamin C was administered but also because the vitamin was not taken over a long enough period of time and biochemical individuality—different needs for different persons—was not considered. The factor of biochemical individuality is clearly shown in the illustration entitled "Vitamin C and schizophrenia" in Chapter 10. The fraction of a standard amount, 1.76 g, of vitamin C taken by mouth that is excreted in the urine during the next six hours varies from about 2 percent to about 40 percent. People representing these extremes might well respond differently to vitamin C taken to control the common cold.

Dr. Robert F. Cathcart, about whose work I shall have more to say in the next chapter, has had extensive experience in administering vitamin C to patients with colds. His observations on many thousands of patients have led him to conclude that the doses of vitamin C needed to control a viral disease depend on the nature of the disease and on the nature of the patient. In his 1981 report he suggests that you cannot cure a "100-gram cold" by taking a few grams of vitamin C.

The proper intake of vitamin C needed to control a viral infection, Cathcart found, is an intake just below the amount that causes a loose, watery bowel movement—increase in the intake of vitamin C to a sufficiently large amount does have a laxative effect, at first. This bowel-tolerance intake is said by him to be between 4 and 15 g per twenty-four hours for people in "ordinary good health," and to have much larger values

*In addition to the studies cited in this chapter, a number of others are discussed in my 1976 book, *Vitamin C, the Common Cold, and the Flu.* Some of these are the following: Masek, Neradilova, and Hejda, 1972; Wilson and Loh, 1973; Wilson, Loh, and Foster, 1976; Miller et al., 1977, 1978.

for the same persons, up to more than 200 g per twenty-four hours, when they are suffering from a viral disease. A similar observation with cancer patients was also made by Dr. Ewan Cameron.

We can now see how difficult it would be to carry out a proper trial of vitamin C and the common cold. The dose should be determined for each subject by the bowel-tolerance limit. It might be possible to formulate a suitable placebo with a bowel-tolerance limit, but it is clear that it would not be easy to carry out a controlled trial with the high intakes that are needed for 100 percent effectiveness.

I have received hundreds of letters from people who say that they have for years had freedom from colds after they began taking 500 mg, 1 g, 3 g, 6 g, or more vitamin C per day. We know that the 6 to 10 percent of people who never have colds must have enough vitamin C in their food. It is not unreasonable to believe that another 6 to 10 percent are close enough to this resistance that a supplement of 500 mg per day would protect them; another group might require 1000 mg per day, and others still more.

I believe that every person can protect himself or herself from the common cold. Catching a cold and letting it run its course is a sign that you are not taking enough vitamin C.

I am convinced by the evidence now available that vitamin C is to be preferred to the analgesics, antihistamines, and other dangerous drugs that are recommended for the treatment of the common cold by the purveyors of cold medicines. Every day, even every hour, radio and television commercials extol various cold remedies. I hope that, as the results of further studies become available, extensive educational efforts about vitamin C and the common cold will be instituted on radio and television, including warnings against the use of a dangerous drugs, like those about the hazards of smoking that are now sponsored by the United States Public Health Service, the American Cancer Society, the Heart Association, and other agencies.

# 14

## *Influenza and Other Infectious Diseases*

Though people often diagnose themselves as having "the flu," influenza is not the same disease as the common cold. Some of the signs and symptoms, such as increased nasal secretion, are similar, but influenza is a highly contagious, potentially life-threatening disease. Like the common cold, it is caused by a virus. The influenza viruses belong, however, to a different family from the cold viruses, and the two diseases manifest themselves in some significantly different ways.

The incubation time for influenza (time from exposure to onset of symptoms) is short, about two days. The onset usually is sudden. It is marked by chills, fever, headache, lassitude and general malaise, loss of appetite, muscular aches and pains, and sometimes nausea, occasionally with vomiting. Respiratory symptoms, such as sneezing and nasal discharge, may be present but are usually less pronounced than with the common cold. Coughing, without production of sputum, may occur, and hoarseness sometimes develops. The fever usually lasts for two to four days. In mild cases the temperature reaches 101°F to 103°F (38.3°C to 39.4°C) and in severe cases as much as 105°F (40.6°C).

Treatment consists of rest in bed, continuing for twenty-four to forty-eight hours after the temperature has become normal. Antibiotics may be used to control bacterial infections. The diet should be light, with a large intake (3000 to 3500 milliliters [ml] per day, about 7 pints) of water and fruit juices. Except during a pandemic, when an especially virulent strain infects most of the population in a country or several countries, almost all of the patients recover completely.

Influenza is an old disease. Hippocrates in his book *Epidemics* described a disease raging at Perinthos in Crete about 400 B.C. in such a way as to permit its identification as influenza. An influenza epidemic was reported in 1557-1558, and a pandemic spread throughout Europe in 1580-1581. Other epidemics or pandemics broke out in 1658, 1676, 1732-1733, 1837, 1889-1890, 1918-1919, 1933, and 1957, and a mild one in 1977-1978.

The most serious influenza pandemic was that of 1918-1919. It swept over the whole world in three successive waves, May to July 1918, September to December 1918, and March to May 1919. It is thought to have arisen in Spain, and it was popularly called the Spanish flu (Collier, 1974). It broke out almost simultaneously in all the European nations and probably was rapidly spread because of the movements of troops and because of wartime conditions. The first wave did not reach some parts of the world, including South America, Australia, and many islands in the Atlantic and Pacific Oceans. The second wave, which caused most of the deaths, covered the whole world except the islands of St. Helena and Mauritius. Between 80 and 90 percent of the people in most countries contracted the disease, and about twenty million died. The disease was clearly not the same as ordinary influenza, because in 1918-1919 most of the deaths occurred among young people, whereas in the preceding and following years most of the deaths from influenza were among the old.

From 1892 to 1918 it was thought that influenza was caused by a bacterium, called Pfeiffer's bacillus, that had been isolated from sputum or blood of influenza patients. Then in 1918 the French investigator Debré observed a similarity in the immune response of patients with influenza to those with measles, a viral disease, and concluded that influenza was probably also caused by a virus. Proof of this suggestion was immediately reported by Selter (1918) in Germany, Nicolé and Lebailly (1918) in Tunis, and Dujarric de la Rivière (1918) in France. The proof was obtained by forcing infected sputum and blood through a filter with pores so fine that no bacteria could pass through them. It was found that the filtered liquid put in the nasal passage of monkeys and of human volunteers caused them to develop the disease, which was accordingly ascribed to a "filterable" virus, the particles of which are much smaller than bacteria.

Isolation of strains of influenza virus, permitting thorough studies of their properties to be made, was achieved in 1933 by the British investigators Wilson Smith, Christopher Andrewes, and Patrick Laidlaw. An account of their procedure was published by Andrewes in 1965. During the influenza epidemic of 1933 Andrewes and Smith, both of the British National Institute for Medical Research, were working on influenza when Andrewes became ill with the disease. Smith had him gargle with salt water and used the solution in an attempt to infect rabbits, guinea pigs, mice, hedgehogs, hamsters, and monkeys, but without success. Laidlaw, in the same institute, had been able to infect ferrets with dog distemper; he found that Andrewes's garglings introduced into the noses of ferrets caused them to become ill with the flu. Later a way was found to infect mice with influenza.

In fact, there had for a long time been evidence that some strains of influenza virus infect certain animals, as well as human beings. Observers had noted that in the 1732 epidemic horses seemed to be suffering from the same disease as people. The virus that caused the 1918-1919 pandemic has been shown to be antigenically identical with porcine influenza virus (swine-flu virus). The virus was not studied during the pandemic itself; the methods for doing so were not developed until fifteen years later. In 1935, however, Andrewes showed that persons twenty years old or older had a high concentration of antibodies against swine-flu virus in their blood, whereas children younger than twelve had none. The clear conclusion is that swine-flu virus was infecting children at some time between 1915 and 1923, presumably 1918-1919.

Thorough studies have led to the classification of influenza viruses into several types, each with many strains. The types are A (with subtypes AO, Al, and A2), B, and C. All nonhuman-flu viruses are of type A. A person who has recovered from an infection with one type of the virus is immune to it for some time but not to the others.

Some protection against influenza is provided by the injection of a vaccine. The vaccine is prepared by growing the virus on embryonated (fertile) eggs, removing the allantoic fluid, which contains the crop of virus particles, and inactivating them by treatment with formaldehyde. The inactivated virus is no longer infective; that is, it is no longer able to stimulate the cells of a human being or other host to produce additional virus particles. It is, however, able to act as an antigen, causing the host to produce molecules of its specific antibody. This antibody can combine with active virus particles and neutralize them, thus protecting the immunized person against the disease.

Vaccines are usually made with strains of viruses that are prevalent in the country at the time. Immunity from the vaccination lasts for about one year, after which booster doses extending the protection for another year may be given. The protection provided by vaccination is estimated to be 70 to 80 percent. Its failure may usually be ascribed to infection by a strain of virus differing from the strains used in making the vaccine; new strains seem to be continually arising. The partial protection provided by vaccination is considered to be especially important for old people and people with chronic diseases.

There are some possible side effects of the vaccination. Persons with a history of sensitivity to eggs should not be given the vaccine. Some persons suffer from local or systemic reactions to the vaccine, but immediate reactions followed by death are very rare. Because of the possible side effects, physicians usually advise their patients to be vaccinated only when there is a special reason. The imminence of an epidemic may constitute such a reason, especially for persons who, because of age or illness, are deficient in their natural protective mechanisms and for persons who are occupationally exposed, such as those in hospitals and clinics.

The importance of influenza is made clear by a 1973 report by Schmeck, based on unpublished data from the National Center for Health Statistics. In the ranking of diseases according to their impact on health in 1971, influenza and pneumonia (which often is a sequel in influenza) came first in days of disability in bed in 1971 (206,241,000), with upper respiratory infections second (164,840,000) and heart disease third (93,137,000). In deaths, influenza and pneumonia rank fourth (56,000), behind heart disease (741,000), cancer (333,000), and cerebrovascular disease (208,000).

The best protection against the flu is one's natural defense mechanisms. These defense mechanisms seem to have protected about one-sixth of the people during the 1918-1919 pandemic, presumably for the most part those people whose defense mechanisms were operating most effectively. There is much evidence, discussed in connection with the common cold, that a good intake of vitamin C improves the functioning of the natural defense mechanisms to such an extent that a much larger fraction of the population would resist the infection. The proper use of vitamin C, together with vaccination when its use is indicated, should be effective in preventing an influenza pandemic or serious epidemic.

In 1976 there was fear that another swine-flu epidemic like the one in 1918-1919 would occur. The United States federal government appropriated $165 million to subsidize the preparation of vaccines, and many million people were vaccinated. The serious epidemic did not occur.

A sufficient number of the vaccinated persons suffered serious side effects from the vaccine to compel termination of the program. The worst of these side effects was the Guillain-Barré syndrome, a neuritis characterized by muscular weakness and sensory disturbances of the extremities.

The measures to be taken for the prevention and treatment of influenza through use of vitamin C are essentially the same as for the common cold. For most people the regular intake of 1 gram (g) or more per hour should be begun. Also, a high intake of vitamin C should not be used as an excuse for continuing to work until exhaustion sets in. A person who may be contracting a cold or influenza should go to bed, rest for a few days, and take plenty of fluids along with vitamin C, to have a much greater chance of avoiding serious illness. If you have a fever for more than a couple of days, or a very high fever, be sure to call your physician.

A good intake of vitamin C should prevent a secondary bacterial infection from beginning. If it does begin, your physician can control it by a suitable regimen with antibiotics. Some physicians might inject large amounts of sodium ascorbate.

Persons at special risk, such as those with heart, lung, kidney, and certain metabolic diseases, including diabetes, may be advised to be vaccinated against influenza, as may also doctors, nurses, and others exposed to the virus to more than the usual extent. They should also take vitamin C; it will protect against the side effects of the vaccination, as well as against the disease.

If an attack of influenza begins and is not stopped by vitamin C, you should continue to take the vitamin in large amounts. It should make the attack a light one, of short duration.

Vitamin C has value in preventing and treating not only the common cold and influenza but also other viral diseases and various bacterial infections. Its main mechanism of action is through strengthening the immune system, as was discussed in Chapter 12. It may also have a direct antiviral effect, in some way inactivating the virus. There are very few drugs that are effective against viral infections, so that the value of the indicated antiviral action of vitamin C is especially great. Most bacterial infections can be treated successfully with the appropriate antibiotics or other drugs, but vitamin C also has value as an adjunct to this treatment.

In 1935 Dr. Claus W. Jungeblut, working in the College of Physicians and Surgeons of Columbia University, was the first person to report that vitamin C, in concentrations that can be reached in the human body by a high intake, inactivates poliomyelitis virus and destroys its power of causing paralysis. He and other investigators showed that the vitamin inactivates herpes virus, vaccinia virus, hepatitis virus, and others (references to the early work are given by Stone, 1972). Jungeblut, who died in 1976, lived long enough to see greatly increased interest and activity in the field in which he pioneered.

The antiviral effect of vitamin C has also been studied by Murata and coworkers. Using viruses that infect bacteria as their model, they showed that these viruses are neutralized by a free-radical mechanism.

Dr. Fred R. Klenner, a physician in Reidsville, North Carolina, was stimulated by Jungeblut's report to use vitamin C in the treatment of patients with poliomyelitis, hepatitis, viral pneumonia, and other diseases (Klenner, 1948 to 1974). His suggested dose of sodium ascorbate by intravenous infusion for viral hepatitis is 400 to 600 mg per kilogram body weight; that is, 28 to 42 g for a 150-pound person, repeated every eight to twelve hours, and he has administered up to twice this amount for various viral diseases (Klenner, 1971, 1974).

In addition to the antiviral action of vitamin C, many investigators have reported that ascorbate inactivates bacteria. One of the earliest studies was that of Boissevain and Spillane (1937), who showed that an ascorbate concentration of 1 milligram (mg) per deciliter, which is easily reached in the blood, prevents the growth of cultures of the tuberculosis bacterium. Effectiveness of ascorbate in inactivating many other bacteria and their toxins has also been reported, including the toxins of diphtheria, tetanus, staphylococcus, and dysentery and the bacteria that cause typhoid fever, tetanus, and staphylococcus infections (references are given by Stone, 1972). The mechanism of the inactivation seems to be similar to that for viruses: attack by free radicals formed by ascorbate and molecular oxygen, catalyzed by copper ions (Ericsson and Lundbeck, 1955; Miller, 1969).

Klenner (1971), McCormick (1952), and others have reported a considerable degree of success in treating various bacterial infections in humans with large doses of vitamin C. This success may be attributed to some extent to the direct inactivation of the bacteria, for which evidence is presented in Chapter 13, but I think that for the most part it results from the action of the vitamin in increasing the power of the natural protective mechanisms of the body (Cameron and Pauling, 1973, 1974).

Hepatitis is inflammation of the liver caused by infections or toxic agents. It usually causes jaundice, a yellowness of the skin and the whites of the eyes resulting from an. excess of bile pigments in the blood. Toxic substances such as carbon tetrachloride and various drugs, as well as heavy metals, may cause toxic hepatitis. Vitamin C is of some value in preventing toxic hepatitis because it has rather general detoxifying capability by hydroxylating or glycosylating toxic organic compounds and by combining with heavy metals.

Infectious hepatitis may be caused by viruses or bacteria, usually by viruses introduced by fecally contaminated food or water. The usual treatment is bed rest for three weeks or more. Serum hepatitis (hepatitis B, inoculation hepatitis) is caused by a different virus, hepatitis B virus, and is usually transmitted to the patient by blood transfusions or use of unsterile hypodermic needles or dentists' drills. The incubation time is one to five months. Serum hepatitis occurs mostly in older people. It is more serious than infectious hepatitis, with mortality as high as 20 percent in some studies.

Dr. Fukumi Morishige in Japan became interested in vitamin C while he was a medical student: his thesis was on the value of the vitamin in accelerating the healing of wounds. When he became a thoracic surgeon and the head of a hospital in Fukuoka, Japan, he gave moderately large doses of vitamin C to some surgical patients who had received blood transfusions. He noticed that these patients did not develop serum hepatitis, whereas similar patients who did not receive the supplementary vitamin had a 7 percent incidence of the infection. In 1978 he and Murata reported their observations on 1537 surgical patients who had received blood transfusions in Torikai Hospital in Fukuoka between 1967 and 1976. Of the 170 patients who received little or no vitamin C, 11 developed hepatitis, an incidence of 7 percent, whereas of the 1367 patients who received from 2 to 6 g of vitamin C per day only 3 cases (all non-B) occurred, an incidence of only 0.2 percent. These numbers indicate that 93 patients were saved from the suffering and danger of hepatitis by the vitamin C (Morishige and Murata, 1978a).

A high intake of vitamin C protects the liver in several ways. It detoxifies poisonous substances that might cause toxic hepatitis. By this effect, it also helps to prevent damage to the liver from cigarette smoking and overindulgence in alcoholic drinks. By making the immune system more effective, it helps to prevent and control viral and bacterial infections of the liver.

The physician who has had the greatest amount of experience with vitamin C and viral diseases is Dr. Robert Fulton Cathcart III, of Los Altos, California.

Cathcart was for several years an orthopedic surgeon. In his practice he implanted in many patients a hip-joint prosthesis, a metal ball attached to a spike that fits inside the upper end of the femur and replaces the round part of this upper leg bone. This prosthesis had been developed by Austin Moore, an English investigator. Cathcart was troubled by the failure of the implant in many of the patients because of erosion of the hip socket into which the ball fits. He decided to find out why the prosthesis was not more successful. He examined many human hip bones and noticed that the ball at the top of the femur is not spherical but spheroidal, and he designed a new prosthesis conforming more closely to the shape of the femur. Many thousands of the Cathcart prostheses have now been implanted.

In 1971, shortly after my book *Vitamin C and the Common Cold* was published, Cathcart wrote me to tell how he had read the book and by following its recommendations had succeeded in controlling the serious respiratory infections and infections of the inner ear that had plagued him since childhood. He reported that a single dose of 8 g of vitamin C taken at the first sign of a cold usually stopped it, although often additional doses were needed.

He was so much impressed by the effectiveness of vitamin C that he gave up his practice as an orthopedic surgeon and became a general practitioner, specializing in the treatment of infectious diseases (Pauling, 1978). By 1981 he was able to report on his observations on 9000 patients treated with large doses of vitamin C (Cathcart, 1981).

Cathcart makes it his practice to establish for each of his patients their bowel-tolerance intake of vitamin C—the amount of vitamin C taken by mouth that is a little less than the amount that has a troublesome laxative effect. He found that vitamin C is most effective as an adjunct to appropriate conventional therapy, when needed, if it is ingested at the bowel-tolerance intake. This intake is different for different people and different for the same person at different times. Cathcart observed that the bowel-tolerance intake is usually very large for seriously ill patients and becomes smaller as the patient's health improves. He was astonished that for some severely ill patients the bowel-tolerance limit was more than 200 g per day. Within a few days, as the disease was controlled, the limit would fall toward the normal values, 4 to 15 g per day.

Having thus established a standard for administering vitamin C to his patients in a manner responsive to their biochemical individuality, Cathcart has accumulated a wealth of experience with this orthomolecular treatment of many different kinds of infection. He indicates that vitamin C has little effect on acute symptoms until doses of 80 to 90 percent of bowel tolerance are reached. He also has stated that suppression of symptoms in some instances may not be total but usually is very significant, and often the amelioration is complete and rapid.

It is known that many stressful conditions cause destruction of vitamin C and consequently low concentrations of the vitamin in the blood and other tissues, unless it is replaced by a high intake of the vitamin. Among these conditions are infectious diseases, cancer, heart disease, surgery, injury, cigarette smoking, and mental and emotional stress. The low level of vitamin C is called hypoascorbemia by Irwin Stone and induced scurvy or anascorbemia by Cathcart. Unless rectified, it leads to exacerbation of the trouble affecting the person. There is the possibility that the mechanism of the observed increased morbidity and mortality of men and women following the death of a spouse is the destruction of vitamin C by the stressful situation. This may be explained by extra demand for ascorbic acid in the adrenal glands for manufacture of the stress hormone, adrenalin, as shown in Chapter 8.

The possible consequences of induced anascorbemia have been described by Cathcart (1981) in the following words:

> The following problems should be expected with increased
> incidence with severe depletion of ascorbate; disorders of the
> immune system such as secondary infections, rheumatoid
> arthritis and other collagen diseases, allergic reactions to
> drugs, foods and other substances, chronic infections such
> as herpes, or sequelae of acute infections, and scarlet fever;

disorders of the blood coagulation mechanisms such as hemorrhage, heart attacks, strokes, hemorrhoids, and other vascular thromboses; failure to cope properly with stresses due to suppression of the adrenal functions such as phlebitis, other inflammatory disorders, asthma, and other allergies; problems of disordered collagen formation such as impaired ability to heal, excessive scarring, bed sores, varicose veins, hernias, stretch marks, wrinkles, perhaps even wear of cartilage or degeneration of spinal discs; impaired function of the nervous system such as malaise, decreased pain tolerance, tendency to muscle spasms, even psychiatric disorders and senility; and cancer from the suppressed immune system and carcinogens not detoxified; etc. Note that I am not saying that ascorbate depletion is the only cause of these disorders, but I am pointing out that disorders of these systems would certainly predispose to these diseases and that these systems are known to be dependent upon ascorbate for their proper function.

Not only is there the theoretical probability that these types of complications associated with infections or stresses could result from ascorbate depletion, but there was a conspicuous decrease in the expected occurrence of complications in the thousands of patients treated with oral tolerance doses or intravenous doses of ascorbate. This impression of marked decrease in these problems is shared by physicians experienced with the use of ascorbate such as Klenner (1949, 1971) and Kalokerinos (1974).

Infectious mononucleosis (glandular fever) is an acute infection that affects mainly young people and is sometimes epidemic in schools and colleges. It is characterized by swelling lymph nodes throughout the body and the appearance of abnormal lymphocytes in the blood. The patients, after an incubation period of five to fifteen days, have vague symptoms of headache, fatigue, fever, chills, and general malaise. Secondary throat infections and liver damage by clogging with lymphocytes sometimes occur, as well as problems with the spleen, nervous system, heart, and other organs. The disease sometimes runs its course in one to three weeks but often is troublesome for several months.

Cathcart has reported success in treating mononucleosis with large oral doses of vitamin C (see table on page 142). Here are his comments:

> Acute mononucleosis is a good example because there is such an obvious difference between the course of the disease, with and without ascorbate. Also, it is possible to obtain laboratory diagnosis to verify that it is mononucleosis being treated. Many cases do not require maintenance doses for more than 2 to 3 weeks. The duration of need can be sensed by the patient. I had ski patrol patients back skiing on the slopes in a week. They were instructed to carry their boda bags full of ascorbic acid solution as they skied. The ascorbate kept the disease symptoms almost completely suppressed even if the basic infection had not completely resolved. The lymph nodes and spleen returned to normal rapidly and the profound malaise was relieved in a few days. It is emphasized that tolerance doses must be maintained until the patient senses he is completely well, or the symptoms will recur.

During recent years a new disease has been recognized, acquired immune deficiency syndrome, usually called AIDS. It seems to be a viral disease, mainly transmitted by fecal matter during sexual contact but sometimes by blood transfusions. The patients are mainly promiscuous homosexual men, but there are some others, including a few children and infants. The patients develop secondary infections and a form of cancer, Kaposi's sarcoma, and the disease often results in death.

The success of vitamin C in controlling other viral diseases suggests that it be tried with AIDS. Dr. Ewan Cameron, Dr. Robert F. Cathcart, and I separately during the last three years made this proposal to appropriate medical groups, but with no response.

One study has been published. Cathcart (1984) examined ninety AIDS patients who had sought medical care from other physicians and who also took high doses of ascorbate on their own initiative, and he also treated twelve AIDS patients with high doses (50 to 200 g per day) of oral and intravenous ascorbate. From his limited observations he has concluded that vitamin C suppresses the symptoms of the disease and can reduce the incidence of secondary infections. It is evident that additional work along this line is needed.

Chemotaxis of phagocytes is an important part of the immune mechanism (Chapter 12). Chemokinesis is increased movement of the cells, either directed or random, in response to a chemical stimulus, and chemotaxis is increased movement in the right direction, toward the place where they are needed, such as the focus of an infection. Neutrophils are the leucocytes that are most chemotactically responsive—they arrive first at an inflammatory focus, followed by other phagocytic white blood cells.

There are many different causes of abnormal chemotaxis of phagocytes (Gallin, 1981). Many responsible genetic abnormalities are so serious that staphylococcus and other infections and skin problems appear in the first days of life, and most of these infants do not live very long. In several diseases, including rheumatoid arthritis and cancer, substances are released by the diseased tissues into the blood that interfere with the mobility of phagocytes.

Many investigators have reported that an increased intake of vitamin C improves the chemotactive response of phagocytes. One of many examples is Anderson (1981), who reported that 1 g of vitamin C per day gave improved neutrophil mobility in children with chronic granulomatous disease. Similar improvement has been reported in patients with asthma and tuberculosis. Patrone and Dallegri (1979) concluded that "Vitamin C represents the specific therapy for primary defects of phagocytic function in persons with recurrent infections."

The question of phagocytic function invites a digression here from infections to genetic disease. Patients with the recessive genetic disease called Chediak-Higashi disease suffer frequent and severe pyogenic (pus-forming) infections that result from abnormal chemotactic responsiveness of neutrophils and other phagocytic cells. These cells are able to move by means of the contraction of actin-myosin fibrils (similar to those in muscle) located in the front edge of the cell. Good locomotion of the cell is permitted by its structure, its stabilization by rods, called microtubules, that extend from the central region to the periphery. The genetic abnormality in Chediak-Higashi disease involves an abnormality in the protein tubulin that by aggregation forms the microtubules.

Ten years ago it was discovered that vitamin C enhances neutrophil chemotaxis (Goetzl et al., 1974). Several investigators have reported that increased intake of vitamin C by Chediak-Higashi patients protects them against infections, although it does not correct the abnormality in the

| Usual bowel-tolerance doses (Cathcart, 1981) | | |
|---|---|---|
| Condition | Grams per 24 hours | Number of doses per 24 hours |
| Normal | 4-15 | 4 |
| Mild cold | 30-60 | 6-10 |
| Severe cold | 60-100 | 8-15 |
| Influenza | 100-150 | 8-20 |
| ECHO, coxsackievirus | 100-150 | 8-20 |
| Mononucleosis | 150-200+ | 12-25 |
| Viral pneumonia | 100-200+ | 12-25 |
| Hay fever, asthma | 15-50 | 4-8 |
| Environmental and food allergy | 0.5-50 | 4-8 |
| Burn, injury, surgery | 25-150 | 6-20 |
| Anxiety, exercise, and other mild stresses | 15-25 | 4-6 |
| Cancer | 15-100 | 4-15 |
| Ankylosing spondylitis | 15-100 | 4-15 |
| Reiter's syndrome | 15-60 | 4-10 |
| Acute anterior uveitis | 30-100 | 4-15 |
| Rheumatoid arthritis | 15-100 | 4-15 |
| Bacterial infections | 30-200+ | 10-25 |
| Infectious hepatitis | 30-100 | 6-15 |
| Candida infections | 15-200+ | 6-25 |

tubulin molecules (Boxer et al., 1976, 1979; Gallin et al., 1979). This clear example of the value of vitamin C in controlling infectious diseases in these patients emphasizes its importance for the immune system.

Kartagener's disease is a recessive genetic disorder with low incidence (one in thirty thousand to forty thousand births) and an astonishing collection of manifestations. It is characterized by chronic bronchitis and infections of the sinuses and middle ears and a tendency to have chronic headache. Male patients are sterile and have immobile spermatozoa; many patients show *situs inversus,* with the heart on the right side and some or all of the other internal organs in the right-left reflected positions.

These facts raise the question of how the large-scale chirality of the human body is determined. Why do most people have the heart on the left side? What has gone wrong with the patients with Kartagener's disease who have *situs inversus?*

In the discussion of right-handed and left-handed amino acids in Chapter 9 it was pointed out that the proteins in the human body are all built of L-amino acids. One of the principal ways of folding the polypeptide chains (linear sequences of amino-acid residues) in proteins is the alpha helix. The alpha helix is required by the handedness of the L-amino-acid residues to be a right-handed helix, like an ordinary screw. The diameter of an amino acid is only about one hundred-millionth of that of a human being, but a segment of alpha helix may be one hundred times as long, thus carrying the message of handedness to structures as large as one-millionth of the diameter of the body.

Another way of transferring chirality to larger structures was discovered in 1953, when I pointed out that a globular protein molecule, built of perhaps ten thousand atoms, could have two mutually complementary sticky patches on its surface such as to cause it to combine with similar molecules to produce a large helix in the form of a tube (Pauling, 1953). Such a structure, in units such as the microtubules, can carry handedness throughout a cell.

The spermatozoon normally swims by using its tail as a propeller, with a corkscrew motion. The corkscrew (helix) might be either right-handed or left-handed. Its handedness in a normal spermatozoon is determined by little protuberances, called dynein arms, which stick out from the tail to either the right or the left. These dynein arms are missing from the spermatozoa of patients with Kartagener's disease; the tails then do not know which way to twist, the spermatozoa do not swim, and the patients are sterile (Afzelius, 1976).

In the same way the cilia in the bronchi are unable to wave back and forth to keep the bronchi clear, and the patients are accordingly especially susceptible to bronchitis and associated infections. The tendency to have chronic headaches may result from a defect of the cilia of the epithelial membrane lining the ventricles of the brain and the canal of the spinal cord.

The nature of the structures that determine the chirality of the organs, placing the heart on the left side, is not known, but it is likely that they resemble the dynein arms of the sperm tails. Their abnormality for Kartagener patients might leave the positioning of the heart and other organs to chance, so that half of them would show *situs inversus*.

These patients have abnormal neutrophil chemotaxis that is related to a microtubule abnormality. There is the possibility that their resistance to bacterial infection might benefit from an increased intake of vitamin C, as do the patients with Chediak-Higashi disease, but this has not yet been demonstrated.

I have been astonished, as have other people, that in the last quarter of the twentieth century a single substance would be recognized to be helpful no matter what disease a person is suffering from. The reason that vitamin C is such a substance is that by its involvement in many biochemical reactions in the human body it makes the body's natural defenses more powerful, and it is these natural defenses that provide most of our resistance to disease. Our bodies can fight disease effectively only when we have in our organs and body fluids enough vitamin C to enable our natural protective mechanisms to operate effectively. The amount required is, of course, much larger than the amount that has been recommended by the authorities in medicine and nutrition in the past.

# 15

## *Wounds and Their Healing*

A wound is an injury to the body caused by physical means, with disruption of the normal continuity of body structure. Accidents and surgical operations cause wounds. Broken bones are wounds. Wounds cause about 150 million visits to physicians per year in the United States. About 75 million people per year suffer injuries, and about 20 million surgical operations are carried out. These numbers show that any factor that can increase the rate of healing of wounds and decrease the length of stay in hospitals can be very valuable.

It was observed long ago that when a sailor developed scurvy, old scars from wounds that had been incurred twenty years earlier would break open. Since the healing of wounds requires the generation and laying down of collagen at the site, it would seem wise to call upon vitamin C in its role in the synthesis of collagen (Chapter 9). Murad and his coworkers, who demonstrated the eightfold increase in collagen production in tissue cultures supplied with vitamin C, concluded their paper with this observation: "The clinical implications of this study are appreciable. The importance of ascorbate in wound healing has been recognized for years. Ascorbate is concentrated in wounded tissues and rapidly utilized during wound healing. Tensile strength of wounds and incidence of wound dehiscence are related to ascorbate levels. Because humans are dependent on dietary sources for ascorbate, deficiency is common in the elderly as well as sick and debilitated persons, who most commonly undergo surgical treatment. Such patients may need supplemental ascorbate for optimal wound healing."

This is a fine statement, but I shall criticize the last sentence, which reflects the astonishing and often irrational conservatism of the medical establishment in its attitude toward vitamins. Why say "may need supplemental ascorbate," and why only "sick persons" (elderly, sick, debilitated persons)? The evidence shows clearly that every person needs supplementary ascorbate for optimum wound healing.

An experimental wound in a subject who for seven months had been on a diet containing no vitamin C failed to heal and then healed normally when the subject was given 1 gram (g) per day of the vitamin for ten days (Lund and Crandon, 1941). Several investigators have reported that surgical wounds do not heal in patients whose blood plasma concentration of ascorbate is less than 2 milligrams (mg) per liter, corresponding to an intake of less than 20 mg per day (references are given in the reviews by Schwartz, 1970). One patient with bilateral hernia and plasma concentration only 0.9 mg per liter was given 100 mg of ascorbic acid per day after the herniorrhaphy on one side; after the second operation he was given 1100 mg per day. The skin and fascia wounds on the first side healed poorly, whereas those on the second side healed well, with breaking strength three to six times that for the first side (Bartlett, Jones, and Ryan, 1942).

Bourne in 1946 showed that the scar tissue in guinea pigs was much stronger with a high intake of vitamin C (see illustration below), and Collins et al. in 1967 reported that gingival wounds healed in eight days for guinea pigs with a daily intake of 20 mg of vitamin C, twelve days for

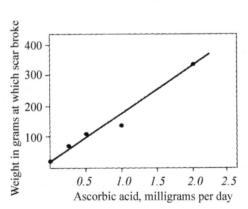

*Vitamin C and scar tissue. A 1946 study showed that scar tissue in guinea pigs was much stronger with a high intake of vitamin C. The points on the graph show the strength of scar tissue in guinea pigs that had been given no vitamin C, 0.25 mg, 0.5 mg, 1 mg, and 2 mg per day. The scars had been formed during a seven-day period after the cuts, one-quarter inch long, had been made. The scar tissue is four times as strong for an intake of 2 mg per day as for 0.25 mg per day (Bourne, 1946). Similar results for humans have been reported by Wolfer, Farmer, Carrol, and Manshardt (1947).*

those with a daily intake of 2 mg, and seventeen days for those receiving no supplementary vitamin. Ringsdorf and Cheraskin (1982) reported a 40 percent decrease in the time of healing standard gingival wounds in human volunteers who received a supplement of 1 g of vitamin C per day. These authors conclude from their review of the published evidence and from their own work that daily doses of 500 to 3000 mg of vitamin C significantly accelerate healing for persons recovering from surgery, decubital ulcers, and leg ulcers caused by hemolytic anemia.

I estimate that the length of stay in the hospital could be decreased by an average of two days by the proper use of supplementary vitamin C, not only through its strengthening of the immune system but also through its acceleration of the process of healing of surgical wounds, broken bones, burns, and other injuries. If we take $500 per day as the average cost of hospitalization, the saving in the cost of health care for the forty million patients with short-term stays in hospitals achieved by the administration of between 1 and 20 g of vitamin C per day would be $20 billion per year, and in addition millions of patients would be spared unnecessary suffering.

It is deplorable that this way of decreasing suffering and saving money is being ignored by organized medicine, and by many individual physicians and surgeons.

It is not only by failing to act that many physicians and surgeons do harm to their patients. Often the patient who arrives in the hospital is prevented from receiving the supplementary vitamin C and other vitamins and minerals that he or she has been taking, just when they are needed the most.

The value of vitamin C in promoting wound healing was recognized in the 1930s, when studies were made with guinea pigs, and it was recognized that the requirement of vitamin C for the synthesis of collagen might be the major mechanism of this action. I remember that in 1941 Dr. Thomas Addis, professor of medicine in Stanford Medical School, prescribed supplementary vitamins and minerals for all his patients. Thirty years later I asked the physicians and surgeons in medical schools and hospitals that I was visiting to tell me what their practice was about prescribing vitamin C for their patients. One surgeon told me that he had all of his patients take 500 mg of vitamin C per day, but usually I received no response, and

I formed the opinion that vitamin C was prescribed less in 1971 than in 1941. I think that during the last few years more physicians and surgeons have begun the routine prescribing of vitamin C, but I have not been able to obtain statistical information about this matter. From the reports made to me by patients, however, it is clear that many physicians and surgeons now recognize the value of supplementary vitamin C.

If you are injured or have to have a surgical operation, be sure to insist on being given the optimum amount of vitamin C.

There have been many observations that vitamin C concentrates at the site of an injury and is destroyed. If supplementary amounts of the vitamin are not given to the patient, the concentrations in the plasma, serum, whole blood, and white cells drop to low levels. Crandon et al. (1961) in their study of 287 surgical patients found that the vitamin C concentration in the leucocytes and platelets (buffy coat) and in the plasma decreased after surgery by about 20 percent. Similar results have been reported by other investigators (Coon, 1962; Irvin and Chattopadhyay, 1978; McGinn and Hamilton, 1976). Mukherjee, Som, and Chatterjee (1982) found a large decrease in ascorbate concentration in the plasma and blood, over 50 percent, after trauma or surgery for 40 patients and some increase in the concentration of the oxidation product dehydroascorbic acid. Sayed, Roy, and Acharya (1975) studied 1434 patients and found a decrease in leucocyte concentration following surgery of 19 percent for the patients whose surgical wounds were not infected and by 30 percent for those whose wounds were infected.

It was observed long ago that peptic ulcers are associated with a deficiency of vitamin C (Ingalls and Warren, 1937; Portnoy and Wilkinson, 1938). The gastric juice in the stomach is acidic and corrosive. It contains enzymes such as pepsin to attack the proteins in the food and in this way to continue the process of digestion that was started in the mouth by chewing and by the action of the enzymes in the saliva. Since the walls of the stomach contain proteins, there is the possibility that the gastric juice might attack them. Sometimes the protective structures break down in some spot and the gastric juice begins its attack, causing an ulcer in the stomach (a gastric ulcer) or in the adjacent intestine (a duodenal ulcer). The formation of these ulcers can be initiated by aspirin, cortisone, cincophen, and other drugs, which sometimes cause gastric hemorrhage.†

Many later reports of vitamin C and ulcers have been published, showing that an increased intake of the vitamin has both prophylactic and therapeutic value. A discussion of the evidence with references to the literature has been presented by Irwin Stone (1972).

A pressure sore (bed sore, decubitus ulcer) is an ulcer overlying a bony prominence that has been under pressure from a bed, wheelchair, or other object. These ulcers plague paraplegics and debilitated persons. They are hard to handle, and surgical treatment is often needed.

In 1972 Burr and Rajan reported their observations on ninety-one paraplegics and forty-one control subjects (patients without pressure sores), with the controls and the patients with pressure sores each divided into four subgroups (male and female, smokers and nonsmokers). In each of the eight subgroups the concentration of vitamin C in the leucocytes was highest for the controls and lowest for the patients with pressure sores. Also in each of the six categories the concentration was much lower for the smokers than for the nonsmokers.

A double-blind controlled trial with twenty surgical patients with pressure sores was reported in 1974 by Taylor et al. Ten of the subjects, selected at random, were given 1 g of vitamin C each day, and the other ten were given a placebo. After one month there was an average reduction in pressure-sore area by 84 percent for the vitamin-C patients, with six completely healed, and by 43 percent for the placebo patients, with three completely healed. The investigators point out that their results have high statistical significance in showing the acceleration of healing of pressure sores by 1 g per day of vitamin C. A larger intake should be even more effective.

More than thirty years ago it was reported that vitamin C and other vitamins in large doses have much value in the treatment of burns (Brown, Farmer, and Franks, 1948; Klasson, 1951; Yandell, 1951). It is, of course, reasonable that vitamin C should help in this healing process because of its being required for the synthesis of collagen, which is a principal component of scar tissue and of skin. The investigators usually administered about 2 g of vitamin C per day, orally or by intravenous infusion, and in addition applied dressings of a 5 percent or 10 percent aqueous solution of the vitamin. Other vitamins were administered in daily amounts: 20,000 International Units (IU) of vitamin A, 20 to 50 mg of $B_1$, 20 mg of $B_2$, 150 to 250 mg of niacin, 2000 IU of vitamin D, and 1 mg of vitamin K.

Excellent results in the treatment of burns with vitamin E, both orally and topically, have also been reported (Shute and Taub, 1969). Vitamin E also has value in converting keloids (hard irregular excrescences on the skin, often the result of burns) into skin of normal texture.

Supplementary vitamin C has value in preventing and healing gastric ulcers and in the healing of wounds and burns. Intakes as small as 1 g per day have been found to have a significant effect. The optimum intake, of several grams per day, can be expected to be even more effective.

Much suffering and loss of life can be prevented by the proper use of vitamin C. I remember that fifty years ago I asked one of my graduate students about the condition of his father, who had undergone abdominal surgery some time before. He said that his father was declining in health (and in fact died not long afterward), because the surgical incision would not heal. There is little doubt that he was deficient in vitamin C. I regret that I did not know enough about vitamin C at that time to enable me to suggest that he be given vitamin C and other vitamins. Now, fifty years later, there is no excuse for a surgical patient not to be given good amounts of supplementary vitamin C.

# 16

## *Muscular Activity*

The function of the muscles in the human body is to do work, powered by the energy released by the oxidation of foods, especially the carbohydrates and fats. In doing work a muscle contracts, decreasing its length and increasing its width in such a way as to keep its volume constant. Good health requires good muscular activity. It should be no surprise to the reader who has come this far to learn that vitamin C has a part in maintaining the integrity and function of muscle tissue.

Muscle tissue contains 20 to 30 percent protein. The contractile material is the protein actomyosin, which is itself composed of two fibrous proteins, actin and myosin. The molecular mechanism of muscular contraction is now known, largely through the work of the British biologist H. E. Huxley. A muscle consists of myosin molecules that are aggregated into filaments with the head ends of the molecules pointing in two opposite directions. The actin molecules are attached to a plate, from which they extend on both sides. In an extended muscle the ends of the actin filaments just reach the ends of the myosin filaments. The end of a myosin molecule is attracted to the complementary regions on the surfaces of the actin molecules by specific interatomic forces, and as a result the myosin filaments, in the course of contraction of the muscle, creep along down the channels between the actin filaments, with successive myosin molecules shifting from one actin molecule to the next.

In its contraction the muscle has done work. Energy must be supplied to break the bonds between the heads of the myosin molecules and the complementary regions of the actin molecules. This energy is supplied by the oxidation of foods, especially fats. The oxidation takes place inside the mitochondria, which are small structures inside the muscle cells and participating in their metabolism. The energy of the oxidation is used to produce the high-energy molecules adenosine triphosphate (ATP) from adenosine diphosphate (ADP) and phosphate ion. The high-energy ATP molecules then diffuse into the contracted muscle and use their energy to change the structure of the actin and myosin complementary regions in such a way that they no longer attract one another, permitting the muscle to relax into its extended state. These regions then revert to their active structures and the muscle is ready to contract again, when instructed by a nervous impulse.

One of the substances involved in muscular activity is carnitine. It is one of many orthomolecular substances in the human body—substances normally present and required for life. Its molecules are small, containing only twenty-six atoms, its formula being $(CH_3)_3N^+CH_2CH(OH)CH_2COO^-$. It was discovered in 1905 by two Russian scientists, Gulewitsch and Krimberg, who were studying muscle. They found that the substance is present to the extent of about 1 percent in the juice from red meat, with a smaller amount in that from white meat, and named it from *carnis,* the Latin word for "flesh" or "meat." It was then discovered that carnitine is required to move molecules of fat into the mitochondria, where they are oxidized to provide the energy of muscular activity. A molecule of carnitine in the cytoplasm outside the mitochondrion combines with a molecule of fat and a molecule of coenzyme A to make a complex that can penetrate the mitochondrion wall. Inside the mitochondrion, the complex liberates the carnitine, which can move outside to repeat its action of serving as a shuttle to carry more molecules of the fuel into the mitochondrion.

The rate at which the fat is made available as fuel for the muscle is determined by the amount of carnitine in the muscle. This makes carnitine an important substance.

We obtain some carnitine from various foods, especially red meat. This may explain why red meat has the reputation of increasing muscular strength and why beef extract, made from the soluble constituents of beef meat, was for a century a popular drink (beef tea).

We are also able to synthesize carnitine from lysine, one of the amino acids that are present in the polypeptide chains of the many proteins in our bodies and that we obtain in good amount by digesting the proteins in our food. Studies on animals have shown that most of the carnitine has been synthesized by the animal from lysine, with only about one-fifth coming from the food (Cederblad and Linstedt, 1976; Leibovitz, 1984). Similar studies have not been carried out for human beings, but there is the possibility that many people would achieve greater muscular strength by an increase in their carnitine levels.

A gene mutation resulting in loss of the ability to convert lysine into carnitine has been reported by Engel and Angelini (1973). The patients are extremely fatigued and have extraordinary muscular weakness. For some patients the disease is controlled by a high intake, several grams a day, of L-carnitine (for references see Leibovitz, 1984).

In his 1984 book about carnitine Brian Leibovitz discusses the results of his own studies and those of other investigators of the value of supplementary carnitine in improving strength, health, and athletic performance and in leading to decreased obesity. His recommended dietary intake of L-carnitine is 500 milligrams (mg) per day. He also points out that there is some evidence that the mirror-image form, D-carnitine, which does not occur in nature, has been observed to have some toxic reactions. Only the L form is effective in increasing muscular power. Accordingly only half of a dose of the D, L mixture would be effective, and the other half might be harmful. I have found in the December 1984 issue of *Prevention* magazine three advertisements for D, L-carnitine and none for L-carnitine, but Leibovitz lists six companies that sell the pure L isomer.

The optimum intake of vitamin C and of other vitamins and minerals might increase the amount of L-carnitine synthesized from lysine to obviate the need for any supplementary carnitine. The conversion of lysine to carnitine takes place through five successive biochemical reactions, each catalyzed by a specific enzyme. The second and fifth of these reactions involve hydroxylation, for which vitamin C is needed. Accordingly the amount of carnitine that is made in the human body depends on the intake of vitamin C. This explains the fact that sailors who were developing scurvy showed lassitude and muscular weakness as the first signs of their disease, and why Ewan Cameron's debilitated cancer patients in Vale of Leven Hospital said "But Doctor, I now feel so strong" a few days after they began their intake of 10 grams of vitamin C per day.

The other nutrients involved in the conversion of lysine to carnitine are the amino acid methionine, vitamin $B_6$, and iron.

There are muscle fibers everywhere in the body. Leucocytes swim through the contraction of their actin-myosin fibrils. The heart beats through muscular contraction. The role of vitamin C in benefitting the heart is the subject of the next chapter.

Much backache, low-back pain, is caused by muscular weakness and by deterioration of the collagenous substances in the joints. Nearly every person suffers occasionally from back pain, sometimes caused by too heavy a load on the back muscles, and about 50 percent of people more than sixty years old have chronic back trouble. Surgery is needed in case of a ruptured intervertebral disk or certain other conditions.

The preceding discussion of vitamin C in relation to both collagen and muscle suggests that a high intake of this vitamin might often provide significant control of back problems. In 1964 Dr. James Greenwood, Jr., clinical professor of neurosurgery in Baylor University College of Medicine, reported his observations on the effect of an increased intake of ascorbic acid in preserving the integrity of intervertebral disks and preventing back trouble. He recommended the use of 500 mg per day with an increase to 1000 mg per day if there was any discomfort or if work or strenuous exercise was anticipated. He said that evidence from most patients indicated that muscular soreness experienced with exercise had been greatly reduced by these doses of ascorbic acid, but it increased again when the vitamin was not taken. He concluded, from observation of more than five hundred cases, that "it can be stated with reasonable assurance that a significant percentage of patients with early disk lesions were able to avoid surgery by the use of large doses of vitamin C. Many of these patients after a few months or years stopped their vitamin C and symptoms occurred. When they were placed back on the vitamin the symptoms disappeared. Some, of course, eventually came to surgery" (Greenwood, 1964). Greenwood has informed me when he visited me at my home in California that he has continued to find vitamin C helpful in controlling problems with the lower back. Larger intakes than the 500 or 1000 mg per day that he first recommended have even greater value.

# 17

# *The Heart*

Heart disease (rheumatic fever and rheumatic heart disease, hypertensive heart disease, ischemic heart disease, acute myocardial infarction, and other forms) is the principal cause of death in the United States, responsible for about 48 percent of all deaths, with related diseases (stroke, hypertension, atherosclerosis, and other diseases of arteries, arterioles, and capillaries) responsible for another 10 percent. In 1986 about 1,400,000 people in the United States will die of these diseases. I believe that the death rate from these diseases at every age could be decreased greatly, probably cut in half, by the proper use of vitamin C and other nutrients.

There is no doubt that heart disease is related to the diet. In the 1976 congressional hearings on the relation between diet and disease the nation's top health officer, Dr. Theodore Cooper (Assistant Secretary for Health in the Department of Health, Education and Welfare) stated that "While scientists do not yet agree on the specific causal relationships, evidence is mounting and there appears to be general agreement that the kinds and amount of food and beverages we consume and the style of living common in our generally affluent, sedentary society may be the major factors associated with the cause of cancer, cardiovascular disease, and other chronic illnesses."

About thirty years ago it was recognized that there is a correlation between the incidence of heart disease and the amount of cholesterol in the blood. Cholesterol is a lipid, soluble in fats and oils, with chemical formula $C_{27}H_{46}O$. It is manufactured in all cells of animals, especially the liver, but is not found in plants. Human beings synthesize about 3000 to 4000 milligrams (mg) per day and receive a somewhat smaller amount in their food, mainly from eggs and animal fat. Cholesterol is found in all the tissues of the human body, especially the brain and spinal cord. People with a high percentage of cholesterol in the blood have an increased incidence of cardiovascular disease.

High blood cholesterol was found to cause fatty deposits in blood vessels throughout the body, narrowing these vessels and reducing the flow of blood through them. The decreased blood flow can lead to heart disease and diseases of the circulatory system. It was recommended by the medical authorities that people decrease their intake of eggs and animal fat. For twenty years there was no change in the mortality from cardiovascular diseases in the United States. Since 1970 there has been some decrease, but it is not known whether it is the result of a change in diet or some other cause, perhaps the larger increase in the intake of supplementary vitamin C and other vitamins since 1970.

Later studies have shown that there are several correlations between cardiovascular disease and constituents of the blood. Most of the cholesterol in the blood is not free; instead, it is attached to the molecules of certain serum proteins that have an affinity for fatlike substances, forming lipoprotein molecules. Some of these molecules have a low density: they are called beta-lipoprotein, or low-density lipoprotein, and those with higher density are called alpha-lipoprotein, or high-density lipoprotein. The two kinds of lipoproteins can be separated by spinning a sample of blood in an ultracentrifuge, and their amounts can be measured. For many years most of the emphasis has been on the cholesterol in the low-density lipoprotein or on the total cholesterol, which is more easily measured, and the high-density lipoprotein was usually ignored. It has now been found that the incidence of cardiovascular disease tends to increase with increase in the amounts of total blood cholesterol, low-density lipoprotein (LDL) cholesterol, and triglycerides, and to decrease with the amount of high-density lipoprotein (HDL) cholesterol. These correlations can be understood from the functions of LDL and HDL. LDL carries cholesterol through the bloodstream, where it may attach itself to cells and form atherosclerotic plaques, whereas HDL picks it up and carries it to the gall bladder, where it is converted into bile acids that are then eliminated into the intestines through the bile duct.

The amounts of cholesterol in the blood and tissues are determined by the rate at which it is synthesized in the liver (from acetate and other precursors), the rate at which it is obtained from food, the rate at which it is converted into bile acids and excreted into the intestines, and the rate at which the bile acids are reabsorbed in the lower bowel and then reconverted into cholesterol. A steady state is set up between the rate of destruction (conversion to bile acids) and the other three rates. All of these rates are affected by the genotype of the person, the nature of the diet, and other factors.

We see that it should be possible to change the steady-state level in the blood by varying any one of these four rates. An interesting and important study of this sort, with use of a drug, cholestyramine resin, was completed by the National Heart Institute in 1984. Cholestyramine resin is an artificial macromolecular substance (consisting of very large molecules) that is insoluble in water and when taken by mouth is retained in the feces and then eliminated. It has the property of combining with bile acids and thus preventing their reabsorption into the blood and reconversion into cholesterol. In this way its ingestion leads to some decrease in the amount of cholesterol in the body.

The study, which took ten years, cost $150 million. I think that it was worthwhile for the National Heart Institute to spend this amount, because the study gave a definite result, the amount of benefit that we might expect from stopping the reabsorption of the bile acids in the lower bowel. In comparison with the cost of medical treatment of patients with heart disease, more than $100 billion per year, the cost of the investigation was trivial.

Each of the 1900 cholestyramine patients, chosen by lot from the 3800 men in the study, was supposed to take a spoonful (4 grams [g]) of the resin granules six times per day. The 1900 controls in the double-blind study were supposed to take the same amount, 24 g per day, of another resin that does not combine with the bile acids. Compliance in each group was about two-thirds, an average of 16 g of resin each day. I am not astonished by the low compliance; it is a nuisance to have to take a spoonful of granules six times a day, for years, especially when there are occasional side effects of constipation, diarrhea, and nausea.

In its principal finding, this study showed that the cholestyramine subjects had an average lowering of total blood cholesterol by 8.5 percent more than the controls, and their death rate from heart disease was 25 percent less. The investigation of the effect of cholestyramine resin provides what seems to be a reliable value of the effect of reducing blood cholesterol. In this study it was found that the percentage decrease in the death rate from heart disease was three times the percentage decrease in the cholesterol level.

In December 1984 a panel of experts convened by the National Institutes of Health (NIH) issued a report that included the recommendation that adults thirty years old or older with total cholesterol levels 240 mg per deciliter or more, younger adults with levels above 220 mg per deciliter, and children with levels above 185 mg per deciliter take steps to reduce the level, through changing the diet or by cholesterol-lowering drugs. The drugs may have serious side effects, and changing the diet has limited value.

The 1984 panel of the National Institutes of Health recommended decreasing the amount of eggs and animal fat in the diet to a cholesterol intake of 250 to 300 mg per day. Also, in the 1977 report "Dietary Goals for the United States" prepared by the staff of the Select Committee on Nutrition and Human Needs, U.S. Senate (Senator George McGovern, chairman), one of the six dietary goals is "Reduce cholesterol consumption to about 300 mg per day." But it has been known since 1970 from the multimillion-dollar Framingham study of diet in relation to heart disease that restricting the intake of cholesterol does not reduce the cholesterol level in the blood. In this study the men and women had average cholesterol intakes of 702 and 492 mg per day, respectively. (One egg provides about 200 mg.) The average serum concentrations for men and women with higher than average intakes were found to be 237 and 245 mg per deciliter, respectively, and those for men and women with lower than average intakes were nearly the same, 237 and 241 mg per deciliter. Thus there was no effect of decreased intake of cholesterol on the concentration in the blood. The explanation of this rather surprising result is that human beings, of course, synthesize cholesterol in their own cells, in the amount of around 3000 or 4000 mg per day, and there is a feedback mechanism that decreases the rate of synthesis of the substance when the intake is increased. It is regrettable that Senator George McGovern's committee and the NIH panel should be giving unreliable information and advice to the American people such as to tend to deprive them of a reasonable amount of such good foods as eggs, meat, and butter.

The fat-in-food cholesterol-in-the-bloodstream idea† is dying hard, as noted in Chapter 6. During the last decade it has become increasingly evident that the great hope of thirty years ago that heart disease could be controlled by limiting the intake of saturated fat (as in meat and butter) and cholesterol (in meat and eggs) and increasing that of unsaturated fat, especially polyunsaturated fat (margarine, certain vegetable oils) had failed. A thoughtful study of the evidence was published in *The New England Journal of Medicine* in 1977 by Dr. George V. Mann of Vanderbilt University School of Medicine. In his opening paragraph he writes that "Foundations, scientists, and the media, both lay and scientific, have promoted low fat, low cholesterol, polyunsaturated diets, and yet the epidemic continues unabated, cholesteremia in the population is unchanged, and clinicians are unconvinced of efficacy. . . . And yet the oil and spread industry advertises its products with claims and promises that make these foods seem like drugs. The vibrant certainty of scientists claiming to be authorities on these matters is disturbing." He mentions that in the 1950s the diet-heart enthusiasts exerted pressure on physicians, who "were overwhelmed by this assault, arising from both their waiting rooms and their professional journals. A low fat, low cholesterol diet became as automatic in their treatment advice as a polite goodbye."

In his 1976 article "Is It True What They Say About Cholesterol?", Dr. Mark D. Altschule discussed the hypothesis that the ingestion of foods, such as eggs, that contain cholesterol increases the risk of heart disease. He said that "Today an awesome collection of powerful agencies, public and private, put forward statements that assert or imply its truth." He then discussed eight clinical trials, carried out in the United States, England, and Scandinavia and published between 1965 and 1972. Most of these studies failed to show that a change in the amount of cholesterol in the diet had any significant effect on the incidence of heart disease.

These results and other similar results have caused Mann and others to reach the conclusion that the emphasis on the intake of fats and cholesterol during the last thirty years has been misguided and fruitless. The way is now clearing for the recognition of the decisive work of John Yudkin and of those who have followed up on his demonstration (Chapter 6) that it is the increase in the consumption of the sugar sucrose that has brought on the pandemic of heart and circulatory disease in the prosperous industrial countries of the world.

Along with the reduction of sucrose in the diet there is another measure everyone can take to reduce the risk of heart disease from elevated cholesterol levels in the blood: that is the intake of supplemental vitamin

C. An increased intake of vitamin C decreases total cholesterol, LDL cholesterol, and triglycerides, and increases HDL cholesterol; in all these ways it helps protect against heart disease.

Total cholesterol is regulated by vitamin C in several ways. Ginter (1973) in Czechoslovakia showed that a high intake of the vitamin increases the rate of removal of cholesterol from the blood by its conversion into bile acids, which are excreted with the bile into the intestines (many additional references are given by Turley, West, and Horton, 1976). This conversion involves hydroxylation reactions, for which ascorbate is in general required. A good dose of vitamin C taken before breakfast can act as a laxative and speed up the elimination of the waste material in the bowel, thus decreasing the reabsorption of the bile acids and their reconversion to cholesterol. A high-fiber diet probably also has value because of a similar effect.

The discovery that a high HDL level helps prevent cardiovascular disease was made long ago (Barr, Russ, and Eder, 1951) and has been verified in many recent studies, such as the Tromsö Heart Study in Norway (Miller et al., 1977) and a study in Hawaii (Rhoads, Gulbrandsen, and Kagan, 1976). In several recent studies it has been verified that an increased intake of vitamin C increases the HDL level (Bates, Mandal, and Cole, 1977; Hartz et al., 1984; Glover, Koh, and Trout, 1984).

In an early study by I. A. Myasnikova in 1947 she reported that serum cholesterol concentrations in humans with high cholesterol could be lowered by the increased intake of vitamin C. Ginter found in one study with patients with average initial plasma cholesterol level of 263 mg per deciliter that intake of 1 g of vitamin C per day resulted in three months in an average decrease in this level by 10 percent and a decrease in triglycerides by 40 percent (Ginter, 1977). In a study of patients with an average initial cholesterol level of 312 mg per deciliter who were given 3 g of vitamin C for three weeks the decrease in the cholesterol level was 18 percent and that in triglycerides was 12 percent (Fidanza, Audisio, and Mastroiacovo, 1982).

Little change, however, is observed for men and women with low or normal cholesterol values, 132 to 176 mg per deciliter, by taking 1 or 3 g of the vitamin per day for four to twelve weeks (Johnson and Obenshain, 1981; Khan and Seedarnee, 1981; Elliott, 1982). The explanation of this difference has been discussed by Ginter through a study of 280 men and women divided into fourteen groups on the basis of the initial cholesterol level (Ginter, 1982). When 300 to 1000 mg of vitamin C was given to the subjects, their average cholesterol levels changed by amounts ranging from +5 percent to -19 percent, as shown in the illustration on page 162. The heavy line in the figure corresponds to the linear regression line given by Ginter. His conclusion, which agrees with the results of other investigators, is that vitamin C has little effect on the cholesterol level in the normal range, below about 200 mg per deciliter, but has a large effect in decreasing high levels by 10 to 20 percent.

If we accept the 1984 statement by the National Institutes of Health Panel that for each 1 percent decrease in the cholesterol level there would result a 2 percent decrease in cardiovascular mortality or the cholestyramine result of 8.5 percent decrease in cholesterol associated with a 25 percent decrease in cardiovascular mortality, we may conclude that an increased intake of vitamin C might lead to a 20 to 60 percent decrease in the mortality rate for the people at risk.

There is evidence from epidemiological studies of the health of populations to support this conclusion. These studies have shown quite clearly that a diet including fresh fruits and vegetables is beneficial to the health. The effort has been made to analyze the diets in relation to their effect on health in order to determine what nutrients in the ingested foods are most important in decreasing the death rates. Of all of the twenty-five factors considered in the San Mateo County study conducted by Chope and Breslow, the intake of vitamin C was found to be the most important in decreasing the death rate (Chope and Breslow, 1955). The people in the study who had been receiving 50 mg or more per day had an age-corrected death rate only 40 percent of that of the people who had been receiving less than 50 mg per day. Most of the deaths, as with the population as a whole, were from cardiovascular disease.

An epidemiological study by Knox of a very large population in England gave similar results (1973). He found, as had been known before, that a high intake of calcium is associated with protection against ischemic heart disease and cerebrovascular disease and also that a still greater protective effect—greater than that for any other factor—is associated with an increased intake of vitamin C. In an attempt to obtain evidence about the mortality rate among users of vitamin supplements a prospective six-year study was made of 479 elderly California respondents to a 1972 questionnaire carried in *Prevention* magazine (Enstrom and Pauling, 1982). The subjects had an average daily intake of about 1 g of vitamin C, as well as larger than usual intakes of vitamin E and vitamin A, and they followed other good health practices. Relative to the expected 1977 rate for U.S. whites, their standardized mortality rate for cardiovascular diseases (which caused 58 percent of all deaths), was 75 percent for males, 46 percent for females, 62 percent for both sexes. The values for all causes of death were 78, 54, and 68 percent of the expected national rate for that year. These observations indicate that these health-conscious elderly Californians have a life-style, including taking supplementary vitamins, that is correlated with a 38 percent decrease in cardiovascular mortality and a 24 percent decrease in mortality from other causes.

These epidemiological studies and other similar ones strongly support the conclusion that a significant amount of protection against cardiovascular

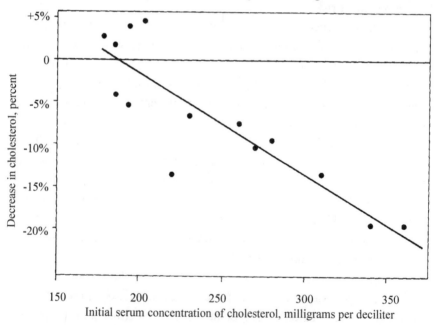

*Vitamin C and cholesterol. The fourteen dots show the average percentage change in total cholesterol concentration in the blood serum for fourteen groups of twenty subjects each with different average initial values. (Redrawn from Figure 9 of Ginter, 1982.)*

disease can be achieved by increasing the intake of vitamin C above the 60 mg Recommended Daily Allowance of the U.S. Food and Nutrition Board.

Much evidence has been reported recently about the value of eating fish, either lean fish or fat fish, in decreasing the incidence of coronary heart disease. In one study (Kromhout et al., 1985) it was found that subjects who ate no fish had an age-standardized death rate from coronary heart disease 2.5 times as great as that for subjects who ate 1 ounce (28.3 grams) or more per day. Part of the effect can be attributed to the fish oils (Phillipson et al., 1985; Lee et al., 1985).

Hundreds of millions of dollars have been spent by the National Institutes of Health, the American Heart Association, and other agencies in support of studies of cardiovascular disease in relation to LDL and HDL cholesterol, triglycerides, saturated fats, and unsaturated fats. Very little attention has been paid to vitamin C and other vitamins. I think that these agencies have been betting on the wrong horse.

It is fortunate that vitamin C is not a drug—it is an orthomolecular substance, normally present in the human body and required for life, and it has extremely low toxicity. You do not need to have a physician's prescription or the approval of the medical establishment to use it in the best way to improve your health and to prevent heart disease. Your knowledge may even be greater and your judgment better than theirs.

# 18

## *Cardiovascular Disease*

For the control of the atherosclerotic pathology that underlies the cardiovascular diseases in their several manifestations there is another vitamin that has demonstrated its efficacy, administered alone and with vitamin C. This is vitamin E (tocopherol), one of the fat-soluble vitamins. It was discovered in 1922 by Herbert M. Evans, professor of biochemistry in the University of California, and his coworker Katherine Scott Bishop. They showed that it is necessary for full health in rats, but the question of whether or not it is needed for humans was not settled until recently. Only in 1968 did the U.S. Food and Nutrition Board finally decide that it is essential to human nutrition and set the recommended daily allowance for an adult at 30 international units (IU).

By 1980, however, the Recommended Daily Allowance (RDA) had been reduced by the board to 10 IU. The board has described the basis of its decision in the following words:

> Inasmuch as there is no clinical or biochemical evidence that vitamin E status is inadequate in normal individuals ingesting balanced diets in the United States, the vitamin E activity in average diets is considered satisfactory. . . . The values [of the RDA] in the table should be considered as average adequate intakes in the United States, but the adequacy of these intakes will vary if the PUFA (polyunsaturated fatty acid) content of the diet deviates significantly from that which is customary. . . . Evidence that normal persons benefit from supplements above the recommended allowance is largely subjective.

The Food and Nutrition Board has accordingly rejected all of the evidence that will be presented here—or perhaps it considers that people who may die of cardiovascular disease or have other problems that are helped by vitamin E are not "normal persons." Since more than half of all people in the United States die of cardiovascular disease, this attitude seems to me to be irrational. As late as 1980 the board had not learned about the difference between the minimum intake and the optimum intake of an essential nutrient.

During the last sixty years a keen controversy has persisted over the possible value of vitamin E in far larger amounts than 10 IU per day for controlling or curing many serious diseases, including coronary heart disease and peripheral vascular disease. The controversy centers around the Canadian physician Dr. R. James Shute and his two sons, Dr. Evan V. Shute and Dr. Wilfrid E. Shute, who had begun using vitamin E in the treatment of disease in 1933. Their claims of success were contradicted by many other physicians, especially in the years around 1948, and for thirty-seven years since then the stand taken by nearly all medical authorities has been that vitamin E in amounts greater than the RDA of 10 IU has no value in improving health or in preventing or controlling disease. It is my opinion that the authorities are wrong about vitamin E, as they were about vitamin C.

When vitamin E was isolated from wheat germ oil in 1936, it was found to be a mixture of several similar substances, which are called alpha-tocopherol, beta-tocopherol, gamma-tocopherol, delta-tocopherol, and so on. Each of these can occur as the D form or the L form. They all have biological activity and antioxidant power but in different amounts. Vitamin E capsules often contain pure D, L-alpha-tocopheryl acetate, for which 1 milligram (mg) equals 1 IU. They may, however, contain a mixture of tocopherols or their esters, in relative amounts such as to give the biological effect corresponding to the number of IU stated on the label. The various biological and antioxidant effects do not change in quite the same way from one tocopherol to another, so that the number of IU is only a rough measure of the activity of vitamin E. Wilfrid Shute recommended that alpha-tocopherol (or alpha-tocopheryl acetate) be used in controlling heart disease, but the other tocopherols taken in the same dosage (measured in IU) probably have essentially the same value.† The relative vitamin-E activities of the several tocopherols have been determined by animal studies, especially the effectiveness in permitting normal reproduction in the rat.

Pure vitamin E is an oil, practically insoluble in water but soluble in oils and fats. It is found in many foods (butter, vegetable oils, margarine, eggs, fruits, and vegetables). In 1956 it was discovered that patients in a state hospital who for several years had lived on a diet containing only 3 IU of vitamin E showed an increased fragility of their red blood cells, caused by oxidation of the unsaturated fatty acids in the cell membrane. Vitamin E acts as an antioxidant and prevents or reverses the oxidation, being itself oxidized in the process. Vitamin C, which is also an antioxidant, can restore the vitamin E to its original state.

A diet high in unsaturated fatty acids, especially the polyunsaturated ones, can destroy the body's supply of vitamin E and cause muscular lesions, brain lesions, and degeneration of blood vessels. Care must be taken not to include a large amount of polyunsaturated oil in the diet without a corresponding increase in the intake of vitamin E.

In 1950 the Council on Pharmacy and Chemistry of the American Medical Association published a report on vitamin E, including the following statements:

> More than three years ago stories appeared concerning
> a remarkable new treatment for patients with circulatory
> disease. The treatment was said to have been discovered by
> some investigators in London, Canada. It was alleged that
> large doses of vitamin E, or alpha tocopherol, could effect
> remarkable recoveries in patients with a wide variety of
> cardiovascular disorders who had not been benefitted by
> more orthodox therapy. . . . The first announcement of the
> possible effectiveness of alpha tocopheryl acetate in coronary
> heart disease appeared as a letter, signed by A. Vogelsang
> and E. V. Shute, in *Nature* (1946, 157:772). Subsequently a
> series of articles appeared in the *Medical Record (Surgery,
> Gynecology, and Obstetrics,* 1948, 86:1) that varicose
> ulcers, thrombophlebitis, early gangrene of the extremities,
> thromboangiitis obliterans, and cerebral thrombosis respond
> to vitamin E therapy. The disease most recently reported
> by Vogelsang of the Shute Institute to respond to vitamin E
> therapy is diabetes *(Medical Record,* 1948, 161:363; *Journal*

*of Clinical Endocrinology,* 1944, 8:883). . . . The lay press
already has devoted considerable space to the claimed virtues
of vitamin E. ... It is regrettable that the hopes of sufferers
from heart disease and other cardiovascular conditions, as
well as those of countless diabetic persons, should be falsely
raised by unbridled enthusiasm.

This attitude of unhealthy skepticism has persisted for thirty-five years.
In 1977 the leading U.S. authority on old-fashioned nutrition, Dr. Jean
Mayer, president of Tufts University, stated that "Because of the variety of
the deficiency signs in various animals, enormous doses of vitamin E have
been tried in a great many human diseases, from habitual abortion to heart
disease and muscular dystrophy. The experiments were not a success. So
doctors went back to the position that we need vitamin E, but only in
moderate amounts," (Mayer, 1977.) Mayer also describes the use of large
amounts of vitamin C to control the common cold as a "fad," started by
me, and suggests that no one should ever take more than the RDA, quoting
several of the fallacious arguments discussed in Chapter 13.

Harmful side effects from very large doses of vitamin E have not been
reported.† In this respect it differs from the various drugs, such as aspirin
(to mention one of the less dangerous), that are widely used in treating
the diseases for which the Shutes claim that vitamin E is valuable. The
fact that vitamin E is safe and the fact that the Shutes claim that it has
value in treating coronary heart disease and several other diseases should
have caused the skeptical medical authorities to carry out a thorough
investigation by means of a number of large double-blind trials, in which
patients in one group, selected at random, receive the vitamin, and those in
another group receive a placebo. But in fact these thorough investigations
have not been carried out, thirty-nine years after the original claims were
made.

It has been argued that it was the duty of the Shutes to carry out these
double-blind studies themselves, but the basic principles of medical ethics
have made it impossible for them to do so. They themselves were convinced
of the great value of vitamin E in 1946. A physician has the moral duty
to give to each patient the treatment that he or she believes to have the
greatest chance of healing the patient. Hence it was the duty of the Shutes

to continue to use vitamin E for all their patients with the diseases that they had found vitamin E to control. To have kept this beneficial treatment from half of their patients would have been immoral.

It would not be immoral, however, for a skeptic, a physician who believes that vitamin E has no value, to carry out a double-blind study of this sort. It is not the Shutes but rather the other members of the medical profession who have failed in their duty, by not having made extensive studies of vitamin E, when there was strongly suggestive evidence that this nontoxic, safe, natural substance has some value, probably even great value, in controlling diseases that each year cause about 200 million patient-days of bed disability and 1 million deaths in the United States.

In addition to many papers published in medical journals since 1946, the Shutes have described their methods and results in two books, *Vitamin E for Ailing and Healthy Hearts,* by Wilfrid E. Shute and Harold J. Taub (1969) and *The Heart and Vitamin E,* by Evan Shute and his staff (1956, 1969). The diseases discussed in separate chapters of these books include coronary and ischemic heart disease and the accompanying angina, rheumatic fever, acute and chronic rheumatic heart disease, high blood pressure, congenital heart disease, peripheral vascular disease, arteriosclerosis, Buerger's disease, varicose veins, thrombophlebitis, arterial thrombi, indolent ulcer, diabetes, kidney disease, and burns. They believe that vitamin E in doses of between 50 IU and 2500 IU per day has value in treating all of these diseases. The vitamin E is given by mouth. An ointment (3 percent vitamin E in petroleum jelly) is also used for burns and ulcers and some forms of pain.

Wilfrid Shute states that in the twenty-two years before 1969 he had treated thirty thousand cardiovascular patients. The records of hundreds of them have been published. For the most part, the only "control cases" have been provided by the record of the patient himself before he began vitamin E. For example, one patient, an elderly physician with diabetes, had severe ulceration and impairment of the circulation in one leg, so serious as to indicate that amputation was necessary. The leg was amputated. Ulceration and impairment of the circulation developed in the other leg. He then learned of the Shutes. Vitamin E was administered. After some months the other leg was healed, and amputation was avoided.

Another patient, age fifty-eight in 1951, had a coronary occlusion with posterior infarction. After two weeks in the hospital he was sent home but was not able to work. After six months he was seen by Wilfrid Shute, who placed him on 800 IU of vitamin E per day. Within ten weeks he was free of symptoms and had returned to work. Seventeen years later he had an attack of auricular fibrillation, which was soon controlled with oxygen. He was in good condition in 1968, at age seventy-six.

There are scores of such case histories in the books. They do not constitute proof, but there is no doubt that Wilfrid Shute and Evan Shute were convinced that vitamin E is the most important substance in the world. I confess to having the same feeling about vitamin C.

Some years ago I was prompted by an article in *Consumer Reports* to check the published studies of vitamin E and heart disease. *Consumer Reports* is a publication that purports "to provide consumers with information and counsel on consumer goods and services, to give information on all matters relating to the expenditure of the family income, and to initiate and to cooperate with individual and group efforts seeking to create and maintain decent living standards." It has millions of readers. For many products its advice may be good, but for the vitamins it is completely unreliable. It makes no tests of vitamins but relies upon some anonymous authority whose judgment seems to me to be untrustworthy.

In its January 1973 issue, *Consumer Reports* had an article entitled "Vitamin E: What's Behind All Those Claims for It?" The writer of the article gave a long list of diseases for which therapeutic claims for vitamin E have been made (those mentioned by Wilfrid and Evan Shute, as listed above, and also acne, aging, and others) and concluded with the statement, "We have been unable to unearth valid scientific evidence that vitamin E helps any of the long list of ailments catalogued on page 62." He then wrote that the only therapeutic use of vitamin E established by a well-controlled clinical trial is the treatment of hemolytic anemia in certain premature babies and that some doctors prescribe it as a precautionary measure in a few relatively rare diseases involving fat absorption.

The article concluded, "Otherwise, the use of vitamin E as a dietary supplement or as a medication for common ailments is at best a waste of money. But far more serious, it could lead to postponing proper medical treatment in favor of worthless self-medication. And the cost of that may be incalculable."

The conclusions are said to be based on published reports of various trials of vitamin E by physicians, to which reference is made in the article. I made a careful examination of every one of these published reports, and I found that they do not justify the conclusion reached by *Consumer Reports*. My conclusion is that their medical authority, the writer of the article, lacked the ability to evaluate the evidence properly.

*Consumer Reports* had listed several studies of vitamin E and coronary heart disease that had been carried out around 1949. All were said to have given negative results, refuting the claims made by the Shutes. I decided that the studies were all unreliable because they used too small an amount of the vitamin or used it for too short a time or for some other reason. For example, the study that is described as "perhaps the most sophisticated" was carried out by Donegan, Messer, Orgain, and Ruffin, of Duke University School of Medicine (Donegan et al., 1949). It involved twenty-one patients with cardiovascular disease, who were followed for five to twenty months. During alternate months each patient received vitamin E (150 to 600 IU per day) or a placebo. The patients were seen once a month. There was little difference in their condition after a month of vitamin E than after a month of placebo.

It is known, however, that two or three months of vitamin E intake is needed for it to become effective. It is stored in the fat, and depletion of the body store occurs only slowly. Hence, the patients would not have changed very much in their store of vitamin E during the alternate months. This study, like the others, does not provide any refutation of the claims made by the Shutes.

Dr. Alton Ochsner, the great heart surgeon who died in 1981, published several papers on his success in treating blood clots (thromboembolism and thrombophlebitis) with vitamin E (Ochsner, DeBakey, and DeCamp, 1950; Ochsner, 1964). Ochsner stated: "In all [surgery] patients in whom venous thrombosis [a blood clot in a vein] might develop, for a number of years we have routinely prescribed alpha tocopherol (vitamin E) 100 international units, three times a day, until the patient is fully ambulatory. . . . Alpha tocopherol is a potent inhibitor of thrombin [blood clotting factor] that does not produce a hemorrhagic tendency [as anticoagulant drugs tend to do] and therefore is a safe prophylactic against venous thrombosis."

Another piece of testimony was overlooked by *Consumer Reports*. This is the work of Dr. Knut Haeger of the Department of Surgery of Malmö Hospital, Sweden, who described his observations of 227 patients with peripheral occlusive arterial disease (1968). Of these patients 104 (average age 60.0 years) received 300 to 600 IU of vitamin E per day, with no other treatment, and 123 (average age 59.4) received either vasodilators, antiprothrombin, or multivitamins.

There were no significant differences among the groups of patients given the last three different treatments. After two to seven years of observation, several differences were observed between the vitamin E patients and the other patients. Nine of the vitamin E patients died during the study, and 19 of the other group (8.7 percent versus 15.4 percent). One of the 95 surviving vitamin E patients had to have a leg amputated, and 11 of the 104 surviving patients of the other group (1.05 percent versus 10.58 percent; statistically significant at the 99-percent level of confidence). The patients with peripheral or occlusive arterial disease after walking some distance suffered from sharp pains in the calves of the legs, because of an insufficient supply of oxygen to the muscles. Of the vitamin E patients, 75 percent increased their walking distance by 50 percent, as compared with 20 percent of the other patients; 38 percent of the vitamin E patients more than doubled their walking distance, as compared with only 4 percent of the other patients. The subjective feeling of improvement was much greater for the vitamin E patients than for the others.

A number of other studies have given similar results. Boyd and Marks (1963) reported on 1476 patients with general atherosclerosis who had been treated with vitamin E for ten years. They found that the ten-year survival rate for these patients was higher than that found in any similar studies of patients who had not received vitamin E.

My conclusion from the evidence summarized above and other reports in the medical literature, developed by able physicians other than the Shutes, is that there is no doubt that vitamin E has great value in controlling peripheral vascular disease, which often occurs together with heart disease and with diabetes, and also in preventing and treating blood clots (thromboembolism and thrombophlebitis). In addition, I believe that there are sound arguments that support the claims made by the Shutes about the value of vitamin E for preventing and controlling coronary heart disease and other diseases.

Haeger pointed out that the sharp pains in the calves of the legs that are experienced by patients with peripheral occlusive arterial disease after they have walked some distance are analogous to the sharp heart pains (angina) of patients with coronary heart disease. In each instance the pain results from a deficiency of oxygen—the working muscle has used up the oxygen faster than it can be brought to the muscle of the leg or heart through the clogged arteries. There is no doubt that the muscle pain is relieved by vitamin E (as are also the muscle cramps that some people experience). It is, accordingly, reasonable that the angina of the patient with heart disease would also be relieved by vitamin E, as described by Wilfrid Shute and Evan Shute in their books.

It was recognized more than fifty years ago that a low intake of vitamin E leads to muscular dystrophy, a disorder of the skeletal muscles characterized by weakness similar to that caused by a deficiency of vitamin C (the studies of vitamin E and muscular dystrophy have been discussed by Pappenheimer, 1948). The difficulty in walking experienced by patients with peripheral occlusive arterial disease may result in part from a low vitamin-E concentration in the muscles and in part from a decreased rate of delivery of oxygen to them. The damage to the muscles when vitamin E is in short supply may be the result of oxidation of the unsaturated lipids, which are protected by the fat-soluble antioxidant vitamin E when it is present in sufficient concentrations.

Several kinds of hereditary muscular dystrophies are known. For the most part their nature is not thoroughly understood, and there is no specific therapy recommended for them. Myasthenia gravis is treated by inhibitors of cholinesterase, corticosteroids, and surgical removal of the thymus gland. The medical authorities do not mention the possible value of vitamins in controlling muscular dystrophies. The evidence about the involvement of vitamin E and vitamin C as well as $B_6$ and other vitamins in the functioning of muscles suggests that the optimum intakes of these nutrients should be of value to the patients. So far as I know, no careful study of an increased vitamin intake for patients with hereditary muscular dystrophy has been reported.

Vitamin E, the fat-soluble antioxidant vitamin, and vitamin C, the water-soluble antioxidant vitamin, collaborate in protecting the blood vessels and other tissues against damage by oxidation. They slow down the process of deterioration of the body with the passage of time and help to prevent cardiovascular disease. They have value as an adjunct to appropriate conventional therapy in the treatment of cardiovascular disease and other diseases.

In this book I have restricted my discussion almost exclusively to vitamins and other orthomolecular substances, with only occasional mention of drugs. I make an exception in this chapter to discuss a nonorthomolecular procedure—EDTA (ethylene diaminetetra-acetic acid) chelation prophylaxis—for atherosclerosis and the consequent diseases of the heart and peripheral circulatory system.† One reason is that this prophylactic treatment seems to me to have a quite rational scientific basis, and the evidence of its value seems to me to be strong. The other reason is that most people would neither learn the truth about it nor receive good advice from their physicians. Most physicians have heard about EDTA treatment, but advise against it on the basis of some false ideas, as discussed below.

EDTA is used widely in analytical chemistry and chemical industrial processes, such as dyeing and the manufacture of soaps and detergents, where even very small concentrations of heavy metal ions in the water interfere with the reactions. It acts by combining strongly with these ions and thus sequestering them. This process is called chelation.

EDTA is used in medicine, with approval by the Food and Drug Administration, for treatment of persons poisoned with cadmium, chromium, cobalt, copper, lead, manganese, nickel, radium, selenium, tungsten, uranium, vanadium, or zinc. It is usually administered by slow intravenous infusion of a solution containing 3 grams (g) of the calcium disodium salt. The poisonous metal ions combine more strongly with EDTA than does the calcium ion and replace it in the complex and are then eliminated in the urine.

EDTA also has value in helping to control cardiovascular disease, including atherosclerosis, occlusive arterial disease, and heart disease resulting from a decreased supply of oxygen to the heart muscles. For this purpose a solution of 3 g of sodium EDTA in 500 milliliters (ml) of

Ringers solution, normal saline solution, or dextrose solution, often with some added sodium ascorbate, is administered by intravenous infusion over a period of three hours. The usual course of prophylactic treatment consists of twenty such infusions, usually two per week for ten weeks. There is evidence that such a treatment helps to eliminate atheromatous plaques.

In the development of atherosclerosis the first step consists of laying down a mass of loosely aggregated connective tissue (collagen fibrils and mucopolysaccharides, often with some fibroblast cells) on the inner wall of the artery. The process may be initiated by a small lesion in the wall. Cholesterol and other lipids then begin to accumulate in the plaque, with a small amount of calcium. Later, as the plaque grows, it incorporates more calcium and becomes harder. By diminishing the size of the lumen of the artery it leads to decrease in the flow of blood to the tissues, to increase in blood pressure, and to damage to the heart and other organs because of the restricted supply of oxygen.

The main way in which EDTA operates to improve the cardiovascular system may be by removing calcium ions from the plaques. The cholesterol could then more easily be removed by the high-density lipoprotein. Other ways in which EDTA chelation might be beneficial have been discussed by Dr. Bruce W. Halstead in his 1979 book *The Scientific Basis of EDTA Chelation Therapy.*

Halstead discusses the toxicity of EDTA at length. When the amount and the rate of administration are controlled in the recommended manner, the substance shows few side effects. Decrease in calcium concentration is corrected by administration of calcium compounds.

Halstead says that during the thirty years before 1979 more than 150,000 patients in the United States received more than two million treatments by EDTA chelation therapy, mainly for cardiovascular disease, and that when it is properly administered it can be used with safety. Both he and Walker (1980) recommend that it be administered only by a physician thoroughly trained in EDTA chelation therapy.

Chelation therapy is far safer and much cheaper than having a by-pass operation. There seems to be a reasonable chance that this treatment would obviate the need for the operation.

When I testified in 1984 at the hearing of an orthomolecular physician, the assistant attorney general of the State of California, who was the prosecutor, asked me if I knew that EDTA chelation therapy for controlling cardiovascular problems had not been approved by the Food and Drug Administration. My answer was "Yes, I know that. I also know that the same EDTA therapy is approved by the FDA for heavy-metal detoxification, and that the reason it does not have FDA approval for cardiovascular problems is that no one has tried to get it. Many years ago Abbott Laboratories, which owned the U.S. patent rights, dropped its application for FDA approval for treating arteriosclerotic disease, for financial reasons—the patent would expire too soon. No one else could afford to apply."

Despite the facts that this therapy for cardiovascular disease lacks FDA approval because pharmaceutical companies are not interested in obtaining it and that there is no legal bar to its use by physicians for this purpose, there has been a good bit of harassment by the government of physicians who use this therapy (Halstead, 1979; Walker, 1980). This harassment has the support of some medical societies, and, like the similar harassment of orthomolecular physicians, it seems to be based largely on ignorance and bias.

# 19

## *Cancer*

Cancer, including neoplasms of the lymphatic and hematopoietic (blood-cell-forming) systems, is the cause of 22 percent of all deaths in the United States. Each year about 600,000 people develop cancer, and most of them, more than 420,000, die of the disease. The amount of suffering associated with cancer is much greater than that for most other diseases. It is for this reason that the federal government has emphasized research on cancer and has allocated several hundred million dollars per year for cancer research, reaching $1 billion this year.

Despite the great amount of money and effort expended in the study of cancer, progress during the last twenty-five years has been slow. A significant increase in survival time after diagnosis was achieved about thirty years ago, largely through improvements in the techniques of surgery and anesthesia. During the last twenty-five years some improvement in treatment of certain kinds of cancer has been achieved, mainly through the use of high-energy radiation and chemotherapy, but for most kinds of cancer there has been essentially no decrease in either incidence or length of time of survival after diagnosis, and it has become evident that some new ideas are needed, if greater control over this scourge is to be achieved.

One new idea is that large doses of vitamin C may be used both to prevent cancer and to treat it. The most important work along this line has been carried out by Dr. Ewan Cameron, formerly chief surgeon in Vale of Leven Hospital, Loch Lomondside, Scotland, and now medical director of the Linus Pauling Institute of Science and Medicine.† I have had the good fortune of having been associated with Dr. Cameron in his clinical research in this area during the last fourteen years. Accounts of our work are given in the book *Cancer and Vitamin C* (1979)† and the published papers cited in the references section and are summarized later in this chapter. Another surgeon who has made important contributions in this field is Dr. Fukumi Morishige, of Fukuoka, Japan.

Irwin Stone in his 1972 book *The Healing Factor: Vitamin C against Disease* discussed the early reports that doses of vitamin C of 1 to 4 grams (g) per day, sometimes given together with an increased intake of vitamin A, seemed to have value in controlling cancer in some patients. This work was done largely by German physicians in the period between 1940 and 1956. Despite the indication that these doses of vitamin C were of value in the treatment of cancer, the early studies did not lead to a thorough examination of the possible virtues of vitamin C in that connection. Some favorable results were also reported in studies with animals, but the early work in this field too was not followed up.

In 1951 it was reported that patients with cancer have usually a very small concentration of vitamin C in the blood plasma and in the leucocytes of the blood, often only about half the value for other people. This observation has been verified many times during the last thirty years. In 1979 Cameron, Pauling, and Brian Leibovitz listed thirteen studies, all showing large decreases in both plasma and leucocyte concentrations. The level of ascorbic acid in the leucocytes of cancer patients is usually so low that the leucocytes are not able to carry out their important function of phagocytosis, of engulfing and digesting bacteria and other foreign cells, including malignant cells, in the body. A reasonable explanation of the low level of vitamin C in the blood of cancer patients is that their bodies are using up the vitamin in an effort to control the disease. The low level suggests that they should be given a large amount of the vitamin in order to keep their bodily defenses as effective as possible.

Only one of the early reports on vitamin C and cancer dealt with the use of large doses of vitamin C over as long a period as eighteen months. In 1954 Dr. Edward Greer, of Robinson, Illinois, published a report about a remarkable patient who apparently controlled his cancer (chronic myeloid leukemia) over a period of two years by the oral intake of very large amounts of vitamin C. This patient, an elderly executive of an oil company, had a number of concurrent illnesses. He developed chronic heart disease in September 1951 and was described in May 1952 as having alcoholic cirrhosis of the liver and polycythemia (an increased number of circulating red blood cells). In August 1952 the diagnosis of chronic myeloid leukemia was established and verified by an independent hematologist. In September 1952, after extraction of some of his teeth, he was advised to take some vitamin C to promote healing of his gums. He immediately began to take very large amounts, from 24.5 g to 42 g per day (seven 500-milligram [mg] tablets taken seven to twelve times a day). He said that he set this regime for himself because he felt so much better when he took these very large doses. The patient repeatedly remarked about his feeling of well-being, and he continued in active employment. On two occasions Greer insisted that the vitamin C be stopped. Both times when the patient did so his spleen and liver became enlarged, soft, and tender, his temperature rose to 101 degrees, and he complained of general malaise and fatigue, typical leukemic symptoms. His signs and symptoms rapidly improved when he resumed the intake of vitamin C. He died of acute cardiac decompensation in March 1954, at age seventy-three. His spleen was then firm, and the leukemia, polycythemia, cirrhosis, and myocarditis had shown no progression during the eighteen months since he began his intake of large doses of vitamin C. Greer concluded that "the intake of the huge dose of ascorbic acid appeared to be essential for the welfare of the patient."

In 1968 Cheraskin and his associates described a synergistic effect of supplemental ascorbate on the radiation response in patients with squamous-cell carcinomas of the uterine cervix. Twenty-seven patients were given 750 mg of ascorbic acid per day, beginning one week before the radiation treatment and continuing until three weeks after its termination; in addition they received a vitamin-mineral supplement and general nutritional advice (decrease in intake of sucrose). The controls were twenty-seven similar patients who did not receive the vitamins or nutritional advice. Radiation therapy was equally vigorous for the two groups. The response to the radiation was significantly higher for the nutritionally treated patients (average score 97.5) than for the controls (average score 63.3). Thus there is some evidence that cancer patients undergoing radiotherapy have an increased requirement for ascorbic acid and that satisfying this increased requirement protects against some of the harmful effects of irradiation as well as potentiating the therapeutic response.

The late Dr. William McCormick of Toronto appears to have been the first to recognize that the generalized connective-tissue changes that attend scurvy are identical with the local connective-tissue changes observed in the the immediate vicinity of invading neoplastic cells (McCormick, 1959). He surmised that the nutrient (vitamin C) known to be capable of preventing such generalized changes in scurvy might have similar effects in cancer. The evidence that cancer patients are almost invariably depleted of ascorbate lent support to his view.

There are some other interesting associations between scurvy and cancer. The historical literature contains many allusions to the increased frequency of "cancers and tumors" in scurvy victims. A typical autopsy report of James Lind (Lind, 1753) contains phrases such as "all parts were so mixed up and blended together to form one mass or lump that individual organs could not be identified," surely an eighteenth-century morbid anatomist's graphic description of neoplastic infiltration. Conversely, in advanced human cancer, the premortal features of anemia, cachexia, extreme lassitude, hemorrhages, ulceration, susceptibility to infections, and abnormally low tissue, plasma, and leucocyte ascorbate levels, with terminal adrenal failure, are virtually identical with the premortal features of advanced human scurvy.

Epidemiological evidence indicates that cancer incidence in large population groups is inversely related to average daily ascorbate intake. Of the several different published investigations, all giving essentially the same result, I mention the work of the Norwegian investigator Bjelke who in 1973 and 1974 published accounts of the exhaustive studies that he had made of gastrointestinal cancers by means of a dietary survey by mail and a case-controlled study. His work, which involved more than thirty thousand people in the United States and Norway, included a determination of the consumption of various foods, as well as smoking habits and other factors. He found a negative correlation between the consumption of fruits, berries, vegetables, and vitamin C and the incidence of gastric cancer, whereas starchy foods, coffee, and salted fish were positively correlated. The two most important factors were, he concluded, the total intake of vegetables and the intake of vitamin C. The greater the intake of vegetables and of vitamin C, the smaller is the incidence of cancer.

In 1973 I went to the National Cancer Institute to show a dozen top specialists there the case histories of the first forty patients with advanced cancer in Vale of Leven Hospital, Loch Lomondside, Scotland, who had been treated with 10 g of vitamin C per day by Dr. Ewan Cameron; my objective was to ask these specialists to carry out a controlled trial of vitamin C. They were not impressed by the evidence or the possibility that some control over cancer could be achieved by using large doses of this vitamin as an adjunct to appropriate conventional therapy. My wife, who had accompanied me, said afterwards that she had never before seen a group of medical researchers with less interest in new ideas. They told me that the National Cancer Institute would not do anything with vitamin C until studies had been made with animals.

Those specialists did suggest, however, that I apply to the National Cancer Institute for a grant to provide support for our Institute in California to carry out such a study. I at once applied to the institute for a grant to support studies of vitamin C in relation to cancer in mice and guinea pigs. It was approved as scientifically sound by the institute's consultants, but it was turned down. My next seven applications met the same fate. Finally the National Cancer Institute made a grant to us that provided partial support for a careful study of vitamin C in relation to spontaneous breast cancer in mice that we conducted in our institute in Palo Alto from 1981 to 1984. This study is by far the most carefully carried out and reliable animal study of vitamin C and cancer that has ever been made (Pauling et al., 1985).

The mice used in this investigation, strain RIII, begin to develop palpable breast tumors at about age forty weeks. Formation of the tumors involves a virus that is transmitted from mother to daughter in the maternal milk. The rate at which the first tumor develops after the end of the lag period is constant—that is, after that age the tumorless mice have the same chance each week of demonstrating the first tumor.

In our study we had seven groups of mice, fifty in each group, eating carefully prepared food containing percentages of 0.076, 1.86, 2.9, 4.2, 8.0, 8.1, or 8.3 of added ascorbic acid. They began these diets at age 9 weeks and continued it to age 114 weeks. Mice burdened with tumors were killed to prevent suffering. We found that the lag period increased steadily with increasing intake of vitamin C, from age 38 weeks for 0.076 percent C to age 52 weeks for 8.3 percent C. Also, the rate of appearance of the first tumor among each group of mice decreased steadily in percentage, from 2.7 per week for 0.076 percent C to 0.7 per week for 8.3 percent C. The biostatistical evaluation of the results shows that the confidence level of the conclusion that increased amounts of vitamin C in their food leads to decreased incidence of spontaneous breast cancer in this strain of mice is extremely high. The chance that the observations are the results of a statistical fluctuation is only about one in a million.

The overall result is that the age at which the tumor appears increases greatly with increased intake of vitamin C. This age for half the mice to develop a tumor (the median age) increases from 66 weeks for the smallest amount of the vitamin to 120 weeks for the largest amount. Development of the cancer is delayed in the RIII mouse strain from middle age to extreme old age.

Similar results with skin cancer in mice caused by irradiation with long-wavelength ultraviolet light (similar to sunlight) were obtained in an earlier study in our institute (supported by contributions by many people, not by the National Cancer Institute) (Pauling, Willoughby, et al., 1982). Other animal studies made by various investigators, usually with much smaller groups, have given less reliable results.

It has been recognized for many years that patients with cancer have a decreased level of vitamin C in the blood and also that these patients, especially children with cancer, have a high tendency to develop infections. Infection is a major cause of morbidity and of mortality in children with cancer, partially because the anticancer therapy damages the immune mechanism.

The low level of vitamin C in the blood should, of course, be rectified for all cancer patients by a high intake of the vitamin. This high intake should function to provide some protection against infectious diseases and should be a valuable adjunct to conventional therapy in the treatment of the infectious diseases as well as of the cancer itself. These facts about vitamin C, infection, and cancer seem never to have been learned or to have been forgotten by many physicians. An example is a recent article on infections in children with cancer by Hughes (1984). This article mentions eleven factors as indicators of increased susceptibility of infectious disease in a child with malignancy. One of these factors is malnutrition. There is some discussion of the effect of the anticancer therapy and the type and extent of the malignancy on the natural defense mechanisms of the body, but there is no discussion of vitamin C and other nutrients in strengthening the defense mechanisms and essentially no discussion or recommendations about nutrition. There is no mention in the article of the fact that cancer patients have a decreased level of ascorbate in the blood, which should be rectified.

Ascorbate in the human body has rather wide powers to destroy toxic substances. It collaborates with enzymes in the liver to react with these substances, often by hydroxylating them, converting them into other substances that are not toxic, for elimination then in the urine. We do not yet have information about the extent to which the optimum intake of vitamin C can provide protection against the carcinogenic substances in our foods, drinks, and environment that get into our bodies, but some examples show that this effect may be large.

Nitrites and nitrates in foods such as bacon and other preserved meats react in the stomach with amino compounds in the stomach contents to form nitrosamines, which are carcinogenic and which cause cancer of the stomach. A good intake of vitamin C destroys the nitrites and nitrates and prevents stomach cancer. A vigorous effort is being made now to reduce the amounts of nitrites and nitrates in foods, as a way of controlling cancer. Increased intake of vitamin C can also help to achieve this end.

It has also been reported that the cancers that often appear in the bladders of cigar smokers and other users of tobacco regress if the patient ingests a sufficient amount of ascorbic acid, 1 g per day or more. Schlegel, Pipkin, Nishimura, and Schultz (1970) found the ascorbic-acid level of the urine to be about half as great for smokers as for nonsmokers and to be low for patients with bladder tumors. They also found with mice that implantation in the bladder of a pellet containing 3-hydroxyanthranilic acid (a derivative of the amino acid tryptophan) caused bladder tumors to develop if the mice were receiving a normal diet but not if they had extra ascorbic acid in their drinking water. The authors suggest that the ascorbic acid prevents the oxidation of 3-hydroxyanthranilic acid to a carcinogenic oxidation product. They state, "There seems to be reason to consider the beneficial effects of an adequate ascorbic acid level in the urine (corresponding to a rate of intake of 1.5 g per day) as a possible preventive measure in regard to bladder tumor formation and recurrence" (Schlegel, 1975; Schlegel et al., 1967, 1969). They also call attention to investigations indicating that ascorbic acid may have a beneficial effect on the aging process of atherosclerosis, the hardening and thickening of the walls of the arteries (Willis and Fishman, 1955; Sokoloff and others, 1966).

It was reported by Dr. Robert Bruce, director of the Toronto branch of the Ludwig Cancer Research Institute, in 1977 that there are mutagenic and presumably carcinogenic substances in the intestinal contents of human beings. Later he and his associates reported that a good intake of vitamin C greatly reduces the amount of these substances (Bruce, 1979). In this way, and also by reducing the residence time of the waste material in the body, as we discussed in Chapter 10, a proper intake of vitamin C helps to protect the lower bowel against cancer.

Colonic polyposis is a genetic disease characterized by the formation of large numbers of polyps in the colon and rectum. These polyps are benign tumors, but their presence has long been recognized as a premalignant condition. According to Willis (1973), "Victims of familial polyposis are almost certain to die of carcinoma of the colon or rectum at an early age." There is, however, now hope for them. Studies by DeCosse et al. (1975), Lai et al. (1977), and Watne et al. (1977) with sixteen persons with familial polyposis gave the result that the regular intake of 3 grams of vitamin C per day caused the polyps to disappear in half of the patients. There is a real possibility that a larger intake, of 10 or 20 g per day, would control the disease in others.

Before we met each other and began our collaboration, Ewan Cameron had carried out operations on hundreds of patients with cancer in his surgery in Scotland. Like many other people, he thought that this disease, which causes so much suffering, needed a fresh approach. He gathered a large amount of information about cancer and formulated a new theory on its causation, which he published in a book, *Hyaluronidase and Cancer,* in 1966. In this book he suggested that a significant amount of control over cancer might be achieved by strengthening the natural defense mechanisms of the human body. In particular, he mentioned that malignant tumors are known to produce an enzyme, hyaluronidase, that attacks the intercellular cement of surrounding tissues, weakening this cement to such an extent as to permit invasion of the tissues by the neoplasm. He suggested that some way might be found to strengthen the intercellular cement and in this way to build up the natural defense mechanisms of the body to such an extent as to resist attack by the malignant cells. For several years he tried giving various hormones and other substances to patients with advanced cancer in the hope of achieving this result, but he did not succeed in finding any substance or mixture of substances that was effective.

I read his book and was much impressed by his argument. I had been working on vitamin C in relation to the common cold and other diseases, and in 1971 I had the idea that the known property of ascorbic acid of increasing the rate of synthesis of collagen would permit large doses of vitamin C to strengthen the intercellular cement by the increased synthesis of collagen fibrils, which are an important part of this intercellular cement. I mentioned this idea in an address that I gave at the dedication of the Ben May Laboratory for Cancer Research in Pritzker Medical School, University of Chicago. By then, Cameron had independently reached the tentative conclusion that ascorbate might be involved in the synthesis of the naturally occurring hyaluronidase inhibitor and had already begun cautiously to prescribe ascorbate to dying cancer patients under his care. In November 1971 he read an account of my address in the *New York Times*. We immediately corresponded, and this marked the beginning of a long and productive association.

Whereas Cameron had been disappointed in his trials of various hormones, he immediately thought that the treatment with vitamin C was of considerable benefit to the patients, and during the next ten years he gave the vitamin in large doses to several hundred patients with advanced cancer, almost all of them being patients for whom the conventional methods of treatment had been tried and found to be of no further benefit. He and his coworkers published several papers on their observations. In one paper they reported that the vitamin C seemed to control pain quite effectively, so that patients who had been receiving large doses of morphine or diamorphine could stop taking the narcotic drug (Cameron and Baird, 1973). He also published a detailed report on the first fifty patients with advanced cancer to be treated with large doses of vitamin C (Cameron and Campbell, 1974), and a paper on one patient who seemed to recover completely from cancer when treated with vitamin C, in whom, however, the cancer returned when the intake of vitamin C was stopped, and who again recovered completely when the treatment with vitamin C was resumed. This patient continues to take vitamin C, 12.5 g per day, and after twelve years seems to be in excellent health (Cameron, Campbell, and Jack, 1975).

The first observation made by Cameron was that most of the ascorbate-treated patients entered upon a period of increased well-being and general clinical improvement. The benefits enjoyed by a majority of these patients included, in addition to increased well-being, relief from pain, a decrease in malignant ascites (cells shed from the tumors, potentially initiators of new tumors and so the agents of metastasis) and malignant pleural effusions, relief from hematuria, some reversal of malignant hepatomegaly and malignant jaundice, and decrease in the red-cell sedimentation rate and in the serum seromucoid level, all accepted indicators of lessening malignant activity. It was thus possible to conclude that both the increase in well-being and the apparent increase in survival time resulted from a significant attack by the ascorbate, either directly or by way of the natural protective mechanisms of the body, on the malignancy itself.†

By 1973 it seemed to Cameron and me that a controlled trial should be carried out, in which half of the patients, selected by tossing a coin or by some more sophisticated randomizing process, received 10 g of vitamin C each day and the others received a placebo. By that time, however, Cameron had become so convinced of the value of vitamin C to patients with advanced cancer that he was unwilling for ethical reasons to withhold it from any patient to whom he had the power to give it; accordingly he could not carry out such a trial with his patients. I then went to the National Cancer Institute to suggest that it carry out such a trial, as mentioned earlier in this chapter.

Even though we could not carry out a double-blind randomized clinical trial, we could carry out a controlled trial. The Vale of Leven Hospital is a large one, with 440 beds, and it registers about 500 new cancer patients each year. Although Cameron was the senior consultant surgeon in administrative charge of the 100 surgical beds, he was in direct medical charge of only some of these cancer patients. At first none of the other physicians or surgeons gave large doses of vitamin C to their patients, and even in later years many of the Vale of Leven cancer patients have not received this treatment. Thus there have been other cancer patients closely similar to the ascorbate-treated patients, receiving the same treatment, except for the ascorbate, from the same medical and surgical staff, in the same hospital. These patients could serve as the controls.

In 1976 we reported the survival times of one hundred terminal cancer patients given supplemental ascorbate and those of a control group of one thousand patients of similar initial status who had been treated by the same clinicians in the same hospital and who had been managed identically except for the supplemental ascorbate. The one thousand controls thus provided ten control patients for each ascorbate-treated patient, matched as to sex, age, primary tumor type, and clinical status of "untreatability." We employed an outside doctor, who had no knowledge of the survival times of the ascorbate-treated patients, to examine the case histories of each of the control patients and to record for each of them the survival time—the time in days between the date of abandonment of all conventional forms of treatment and the date of death.

The results were surprising, even to us (see illustration on facing page) (Cameron and Pauling, 1976). By 10 August 1976 all of the one thousand control patients had died, whereas eighteen of the one hundred ascorbate-treated patients were still living. On that date the average time of survival after the date of "untreatability" was 4.2 times as great for the ascorbate-treated patients as for their matched controls. The one hundred ascorbate-treated patients have lived on the average more than three hundred days longer than their matched controls, and in addition it is our strong clinical impression that they have lived happier lives during this terminal period. Moreover, a few of them continue to survive, still taking their daily doses of sodium ascorbate, and some of them might well be considered to have been "cured" of their malignant disease, in that they are free of overt manifestations of cancer and are leading normal lives.

We considered this to be a remarkable achievement, bearing in mind that if the mortality of cancer could be decreased by 5 percent the lives of twenty thousand American cancer patients would be saved each year.

Because of the importance of the problem of cancer, we made a second examination of the case histories of the Vale of Leven patients in 1978, again with one hundred ascorbate-treated patients and one thousand matched controls (Cameron and Pauling, 1978a, 1978b). Ten of the original one hundred ascorbate-treated patients, mainly with rare forms of cancer for whom it had been difficult to find sets of exactly matched controls, were replaced by new ones, and the one thousand matched controls were independently selected, without regard as to whether or not they had been selected before (about half of them were in the earlier set). Some of the results of this study are given in the illustrations on pages 188-89. The one hundred ascorbate-treated patients and their matched controls (same type of primary tumor, same sex, and same age to within five years) were divided into nine groups, based on the type of primary tumor; for example, 17 ascorbate-treated patients and 170 controls with cancer of the colon. (The ninth group, not shown in the figures on pages 188-89, included patients with types of cancer other than those shown in the illustrations not cited.) Survival times were measured from the date when the patient was

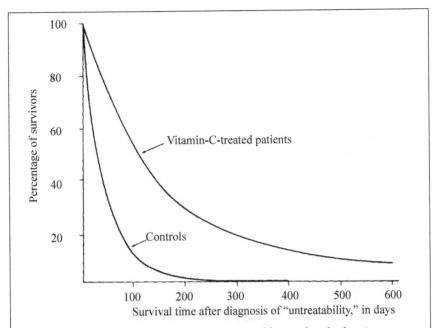

*Vale of Leven study. Upon being judged untreatable, one hundred patients under the care of Ewan Cameron at the Vale of Leven Hospital in Scotland were treated with vitamin C, usually 10 g per day. Their survival times are here compared to a control group of one thousand patients matched by age, sex, and site of cancer to the experimental group. At all the times plotted, the vitamin-C-treated patients were surviving in a much larger percentage than the controls, with no controls surviving past day 500.*

determined to be "untreatable"; that is, when the conventional therapies were deemed to be no longer effective—at this date or a few days later ascorbate treatment was begun. In 1978 the mean survival times for the nine groups were between 114 and 435 days greater for the vitamin-C groups than for the corresponding control groups, an average of 255 days for all groups, and were continuing to increase because 8 percent of the vitamin-C patients were still alive, and none of the controls were.

A similar study was carried out in the Fukuoka Torikai Hospital in Japan during the five years beginning 1 January 1973 (Morishige and Murata, 1979), with results, shown in the illustration on page 190, similar to those obtained in Vale of Leven Hospital.

More recently, two controlled trials have been carried out in the Mayo Clinic. This Mayo work has been publicized as refuting the Vale of Leven and Fukuoka Torikai studies. The record shows, however, that the Mayo

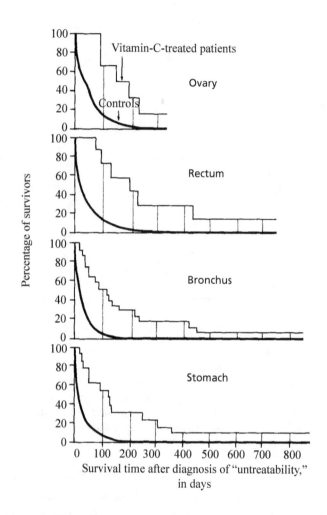

*Vale of Leven survival times. For cancers with eight different primary sites in the Vale of Leven study (summarized in the figure on page 187) the survival times of the vitamin-C-treated patients are compared to those of their matched controls. Survival is measured from the day the patient was judged untreatable. In conventional cancer statistics, survival for five years (1826 days) is recorded as "cure."*

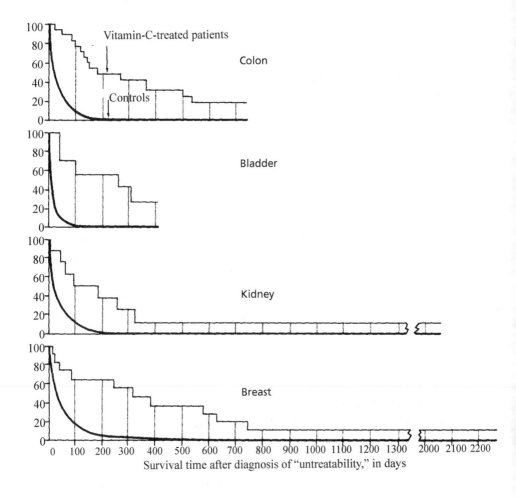

Survival time after diagnosis of "untreatability," in days

Clinic doctors did not follow the protocols of those studies.† That work has, therefore, only small relevance to the question of how great the value of vitamin C is for cancer patients.

The first Mayo Clinic study (Creagan et al., 1979) showed only a small protective effect of vitamin C. Cameron and I attributed this reported result to the fact that most of the Mayo Clinic patients had already received heavy doses of cytotoxic drugs, which damage the immune system and interfere with the action of vitamin C, and the fact that the controls were also taking vitamin C in much larger amounts than were the controls in Scotland or Japan. Only 4 percent of the Vale of Leven patients had received prior chemotherapy.

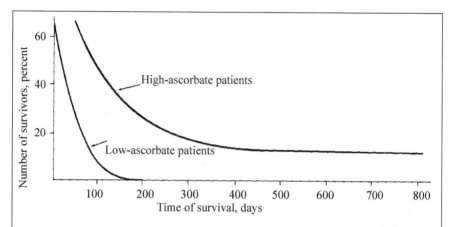

*Fukuoka Torikai Hospital study. Matched experimental and control subjects received large amounts of vitamin C (5 grams or more per day, averaging 29 grams per day) and small amounts (4 g per day or less) respectively, upon being judged untreatable. Patients in the control group had all died by day 200, when 25 percent of the high-intake group were still alive. The six still alive on 10 August 1978, indicated by the long extension past 400 days, had survived an average of 866 days after being judged untreatable. (Adapted from Morishige and Murata, 1978b.)*

In our studies the vitamin-C patients took large amounts of the vitamin, without stopping, for the rest of their lives or until the present time, some for as much as fourteen years. In the second Mayo Clinic Study (Moertel et al., 1985), the vitamin-C patients received the vitamin for only a short time (median 2.5 months). None of the vitamin-C patients died while taking the vitamin (amount somewhat less than 10 g per day). They were, however, studied for another two years, during which their survival record was no better than that of the controls, or even somewhat worse. The Moertel paper and a spokesman for the National Cancer Institute, who commented on it (Wittes, 1985) both suppressed the fact that the vitamin-C patients were not receiving vitamin C when they died and had not received any for a long time (median 10.5 months). They announced vigorously that this study showed finally and definitely that vitamin C has no value against advanced cancer and recommended that no more studies of vitamin C be made.

Their results provided no basis whatever for this conclusion, because in fact their patients died only after being deprived of the vitamin C. To the extent that their study showed anything, it is that cancer patients should not stop taking their large doses of vitamin C. Yet the study was heralded upon publication as one that reflected adversely on the Cameron-Pauling work.

When this Mayo Clinic paper appeared, 17 January 1985, Cameron and I were angry that Moertel and his Mayo Clinic associates, the spokesman for the National Cancer Institute, and also the editor of *The New England Journal of Medicine* had managed to prevent us from obtaining any information about their results until a few hours before their publication. Six weeks earlier Moertel refused to tell me anything about the work, except that their paper was going to be published. In a letter to me he promised that he would arrange for me to have a copy of the paper several days before publication, but he broke that promise.

The misrepresentation by Moertel and his associates and by the National Cancer Institute spokesman has done great harm. Cancer patients have informed us that they are stopping their vitamin C because of the "negative results" reported by the Mayo Clinic.

It is not often that unethical behavior of scientists is reported. Fraud committed by young physicians doing medical research has been turned up several times in the last few years. Improper representation of the results of clinical studies, as in the second Mayo Clinic report, is especially to be condemned because of its effect in increasing the amount of human suffering.

The Mayo Clinic paper stimulated a vigorous response from the public addressed to Cameron and me. The first two letters reached me five days after the publication of the paper. The following excerpts are quoted with permission of the writers.

One letter was written to Moertel, the principal Mayo Clinic investigator, by a man in Utah, who sent a copy to me. It was written the day after publication, and the entire letter reads as follows:

Dear Dr. Moertel:

In March 1983 my right lung was removed due to cancer. The X-ray showed no spread and no follow-up treatment was given.

On May 8, 1984 a cat-scan showed metastasis to the brain, two small tumors on front of brain, right side and left side, 3 cm. Also one large tumor at the back, 6 cm.

The prognosis was terminal with about a year to live. The treatment was radiation at LDS Hospital, Salt Lake City which would shrink and control the tumors for a while, but not eradicate them.

I immediately went on a nutritional program which included Vitamin C. I went to my bowel tolerance level of 36 grams a day.

On July 9th another cat-scan was done at LDS Hospital and the tumors were completely gone. I just finished a follow-up cat-scan and chest X-ray which showed no sign of cancer.

I feel strongly that the Vitamin C (and other nutrients) together with the radiation removed the tumors. I am still on 36 grams daily and plan to be indefinitely and feel the Vitamin C has played an important part of my miraculous cure.

In the book "Cancer and Vitamin C" by Ewan Cameron and Linus Pauling, they *do not* suggest the use of vitamin C alone to cure cancer but only to augment traditional treatments.

My records are open for verification. I realize you do not like case histories, but X-rays and doctors reports plus real results are pretty good proof.

I do not know how much Vitamin C you gave in your blind studies, but each person's requirements are different. Therefore, any amount short of bowel tolerance levels, which could not be done in a blind study such as yours, is useless.

It is my hope that if you are truly interested in the cancer patient you will reconsider your position.

The second letter was written to me by an eighty-one-year-old man in San Francisco. Here are some excerpts from his letter:

This letter is essentially about the use of your basic theories concerning cancer and vitamin C. As I wrote before, I had surgery for colorectal cancer on 4 September, 1980. It had metastasized to the liver where a tumor about 35 mm in diameter was found. It was not operable under the circumstances. I started reading on the subject and taking injections of 5-FU at the same time. I knew you had written on vitamin C and the common cold but was unaware of your work with Dr. Cameron on cancer in Scotland.

In the literature, I quickly found that metastasized cancer to the liver was tantamount to a death sentence, survival rates ranging from a few weeks to 18 months. In most studies, untreated metastases had a survival period averaging 6.1 months. I also quickly became convinced that the fluorinated pyrimidine 5-FU was nothing more than a placebo. I decided to quit taking it. The oncologist I was seeing did not object and ordered a liver scan. This showed that the tumor had grown from 35 mm to 52 millimeters in diameter while I was taking the injections.

By nature, I am a sanguine man and since fifteen, I have known that life would be the death of me yet. Gathering all my material together and using your thinking on the subject as a guide, I worked out a regime based on vitamin C, vitamin E and other dietary supplements.

The second liver scan, after I ingested 10-12 grams of vitamin C daily for three months, showed no change in the size or texture of the liver lesion. It was there, all right, but it had not grown. I continued my self-treatment, looked for a medical doctor who could help me. I found myself faced with an ocean of ignorance on the part of the medical fraternity as to the immensely complex process by which the human body absorbs and uses the materials upon which it exists. And profound indifference as to what I was doing. I know 12 doctors personally, most of them I consider friends. Five of them tell me that they had one course in nutrition for a single semester in medical school. The other seven had no course at all. None asked me anything about what I was doing.

I continued the liver scans, one each three months. The lesion remained the same until the ultrasound scan of 15 October, 1984. To my surprise, this scan showed a decrease amounting to 32% in the cubic content of the tumor. Because of the nature of the finding, the series was run twice. Once by the technician and then by the doctor in charge of the laboratory to make sure of an accurate finding. The tumor had also begun to be infiltrated with calcium.

During all of this time, I have been reasonably healthy with no sign of cancer, working at one thing or another and sailing our boat on the Bay. I have a chest x-ray each year because the normal path of the decrease is from the liver to the lungs. My lungs are clear.

In your writing, you suggest that the intake of ascorbic acid be moved up until one becomes uncomfortable and then to back down a bit. In your letter to me, you proposed 25 grams of C daily. I have been taking 36 grams daily for more than two years now. In divided portions, I have no difficulty with this.

I have planned on writing you for more than a year, but pure sloth has caused me to put it off. The present spur to my intent is the article read at breakfast two days ago about the Mayo Clinic procedure. I think that this is a shabby business indeed. Mayo is the last place I would want to see used for a study of vitamin C under any conditions. They are flawed because of the manner in which they did their first so-called study. What is needed should be obvious to a blind man. That is, nothing short of a series of massive tests, using thousands of patients with scores of different kinds of cancer. And these grouped in various stages of this degenerative disease. It would have to be a national effort as no clinic, hospital or teaching university could possibly carry it out on the necessary scale.

I am sure that you are absolutely right in saying that vitamin C, while not a cure for cancer, is a vital and potent adjunct in the management and control of the disease. And it is a fact that any form of chemotherapy will damage the body's own immune system. In my case, I must have achieved a dandy immune system or my cancer would long ago have reached one of the lymph glands.

That the tumor on my liver has become non-invasive is obvious. That it will stay that way is not obvious. Knowing

that it is there puts me in the position of living under the
sword of Damocles. I am reasonably certain that I shall die of
cancer . . . if I do not die of old age first. I was 81 years of age
on January 16, 1985.

These letters are representative of scores of letters that Cameron
and I have received. Such evidence may be dismissed as anecdotal
when compared to the statistical evidence from large-scale trials—with
inadequate intakes of vitamin C. The anecdotes nonetheless should
challenge conscientious investigators to run large-scale trials with intakes
of vitamin C as prescribed by Cameron.

In Chapter 26 I have more to say about the behavior of Moertel and his
colleagues in illustration of the difference between vitamins and drugs.

Based upon the results of our studies, Cameron and I have recommended
that a high intake of vitamin C be taken by every cancer patient, as an
adjunct to appropriate conventional therapy and beginning as early in the
course of the disease as possible.

How many people could be helped in this way? The quantitative
information that we have is based mainly on the observation of patients
with advanced cancer in Scotland who received 10 g of vitamin C per
day. As the result of observations on several hundred patients, Cameron
reached the following conclusions about the effects of administering this
amount of vitamin C to patients with advanced cancer:

- Category I. No response of tumors, but usually improvement in well-
  being—about 20%
- Category II. Rather small response—about 25%
- Category III. Retardation of growth of tumors—about 25%
- Category IV. No change in tumor (standstill)—about 20%
- Category V. Tumor regression—about 9%
- Category VI. Complete regression—about 1 %

Better results are obtained with intakes greater than 10 g per day.

In our book *Cancer and Vitamin C,* Cameron and I stated our conclusion
that "This simple and safe treatment, the ingestion of large amounts of
vitamin C, is of definite value in the treatment of patients with advanced

cancer. Although the evidence is as yet not so strong, we believe that vitamin C has even greater value for the treatment of cancer patients with the disease in earlier stages and also for the prevention of cancer."

The last sentences in that book are the following:

> With the possible exception of during intense
> chemotherapy, we strongly advocate the use of supplemental
> ascorbate in the management of all cancer patients from as
> early in the illness as possible. We believe that this simple
> measure would improve the overall results of cancer treatment
> quite dramatically, not only by making the patients more
> resistant to their illness but also by protecting them against
> some of the serious and occasionally fatal complications of
> the cancer treatment itself. We are quite convinced that in the
> not too distant future supplemental ascorbate will have an
> established place in all cancer-treatment regimes.

We have now had the opportunity to observe patients who have taken 10 g or more per day of vitamin C during intense chemotherapy. It seems clear that there is benefit from the vitamin C, which controls to a considerable extent the disagreeable side effects of the cytotoxic chemotherapeutic agents, such as nausea and loss of hair, and that benefit seems to add its value to that of the chemotherapeutic agent. We now recommend a high intake of vitamin C, in some cases up to the bowel-tolerance limit (Chapter 14), beginning as early as possible.

There are many advantages to using vitamin C as an adjunct to appropriate conventional therapy in the treatment of cancer patients. Vitamin C is inexpensive. It has no serious side effects, but instead improves the appetite, controls the feeling of misery that plagues cancer patients, improves the general health, and gives the patient a greater capacity to enjoy life. For every patient there is the chance that through its use, together with the appropriate conventional therapy and good intakes of other nutrients, the disease can be kept under control for many years.

# 20

## *The Brain*

Of all of the organs in the human body, the brain is the most sensitive to its molecular composition. The proper functioning of the brain is known to require the presence of many different kinds of molecules in the right concentrations. This is the physical, the molecular environment of the mind. The physiology of the brain tends always to maintain that environment constant. In persons suffering from scurvy the concentration of vitamin C in the brain is kept high even when there is almost complete depletion in the blood and other tissues. So sensitive is the brain that if a person is deprived of oxygen for a few minutes, the brain dies (as is shown by a flat electroencephalic curve), while the other organs survive.

In considering the health of the rest of the body, we have encountered the biochemical individuality that sets each person singularly apart from every other (Chapter 10). Can it be argued that they do not differ in the amounts of critical substances supplied to the brain? We must ask then what part the molecular environment of each mind plays in establishing the singularity of each individual's personality.

This simple question leads us to the possibility that the brain may suffer a localized cerebral avitaminosis or other localized cerebral deficiency disease. There is the possibility that some human beings have a sort of cerebral scurvy, without any of the other manifestations, or a sort of cerebral pellagra, or cerebral pernicious anemia. It was pointed out by Zuckerkandl and Pauling (1962) that every vitamin, every essential amino acid, and every other essential nutrilite represents a molecular disease, which our distant ancestors learned to control, when it began to afflict them, by selecting a therapeutic diet, and which has continued to be kept under control in this way. The localized deficiency diseases mentioned above may be compound molecular diseases, involving not only the original lesion, the loss of the ability to synthesize the vital substance, but also another lesion, one that causes a decreased rate of transfer across a membrane, such as the blood-brain barrier, to the affected organ, or an increased rate of destruction of the vital substance in the organ, or some other perturbing reaction. These deficiencies in the supply or synthesis of crucial molecules may manifest themselves in symptoms diagnosed as psychosis of one kind or another to be treated by attempts to modify the patient's behavior or personality.

In the ninth edition of the *Encyclopaedia Britannica* (1881) insanity is defined as a chronic disease of the brain inducing chronic disordered mental symptoms. The author of the article, J. Batty Tuke, M.D., lecturer on insanity, School of Medicine, Edinburgh, then stated that this definition

> possesses the great practical advantage of keeping before the
> student the primary fact that insanity is the result of disease of
> the brain, that it is not a mere immaterial disorder of the intellect.
> In the earliest epochs of medicine the corporeal character
> of insanity was generally admitted, and it was not until the
> superstitious ignorance of the Middle Ages had obliterated the
> scientific—though by no means always accurate—deductions of
> the early writers that any theory of its purely psychical character
> arose. At the present day it is unnecessary to combat such a
> theory, as it is universally accepted that the brain is the organ
> through which mental phenomena are manifested, and therefore
> it is impossible to conceive of the existence of an insane mind in
> a healthy brain.

By 1929, when the fourteenth edition of the *Encyclopaedia Britannica* was published, the situation had changed, largely because of the development of psychoanalysis by Sigmund Freud. The earlier definition of insanity was deleted and was replaced by discussions from two points of view: that of the materialistic school, who held that structural changes in the brain are involved, and that of the psychogenic school, who held that insanity is the result of abnormalities of the ego and that the structural changes in the brain observed in certain forms of insanity are caused by a perverted mentality.

Even now, half a century later, when we have extensive knowledge of the action of psychotropic drugs, brain tumors, brain injuries, slow viruses, protein starvation, and other factors affecting the function of the brain, there are still practitioners of psychoanalysis who ignore the brain and attempt only to treat the ego.

When the use of vitamin $B_3$ was introduced (by drinking milk, 1920 on, or eating bread made from flour fortified with the vitamin, 1940), it cured thousands of pellagra patients of their psychoses, as well as of the physical manifestations of their disease. For this purpose, only small doses are required; the Recommended Daily Allowance (RDA) of the National Research Council is 17 milligrams (mg) per day (for a 70-kilogram [kg], 154-pound, male).† In 1939 Cleckley, Sydenstricker, and Geeslin reported the successful treatment of nineteen patients, and in 1941 Sydenstricker and Cleckley reported similarly successful treatment of twenty-nine patients, with severe psychiatric symptoms by use of moderately large doses of nicotinic acid (0.3 to 1.5 grams [g] per day). None of these patients had physical symptoms of pellagra or any other avitaminosis. More recently many other investigators have reported on the use of nicotinic acid and nicotinamide for the treatment of mental disease. Outstanding among them are Dr. Abram Hoffer and Dr. Humphry Osmond, who since 1952 have advocated and used nicotinic acid in large doses, in addition to the conventional therapy, for the treatment of schizophrenia. Their work, which ignited my interest in vitamins, will be discussed more fully later in this chapter.

A deficiency of vitamin $B_{12}$, cobalamin, whatever its cause (pernicious anemia, a genetic lack of the factor in gastric juice that is needed to transport the vitamin into the blood; or infestation with the fish tapeworm *Diphyllobothrium*, whose high requirement for the vitamin results in deprivation for the host; or excessive bacterial flora with a high requirement for the vitamin) leads to mental illness, often more pronounced than the physical consequences. The mental illness associated with pernicious anemia often appears years before the anemia develops. All of these manifestations of severe $B_{12}$ deficiency are, of course, controlled by the administration of the vitamin in adequate amounts.

There is also epidemiological evidence that even only moderate deficiency of $B_{12}$ may lead to mental illness. Edwin, Holten, Norum, Schrumpf, and Skaug (1965) determined the amount of $B_{12}$ in the serum of every patient over thirty years old admitted to a mental hospital in Norway during a period of one year. Of the 396 patients, 5.8 percent (23) had a pathologically low concentration, less than 101 picograms per milliliter (ml), and the concentration in 9.6 percent (38) was subnormal (101 to 150 picograms per milliliter). The normal concentration is 150 to

1300 picograms per milliliter. The incidence of pathologically low and subnormal levels of $B_{12}$ in the serums of these patients, 15.4 percent, is about thirty times that in the general population, about 0.5 percent (estimated from the reported frequency of pernicious anemia in the area, 9.3 per 100,000 persons per year). Other investigators have also reported a higher incidence of low $B_{12}$ concentrations in the serums of mental patients than in the population as a whole and have suggested that $B_{12}$ deficiency, whatever its origin, may lead to mental illness.

These observations indicate that an increased intake of vitamin $B_{12}$, as well as of other vitamins, should be a part of the treatment of every mentally ill person. The vitamin can be effectively taken by mouth, except by those persons with pernicious anemia, for whom injections are needed.

An interesting investigation of the relation between intelligence, as indicated by the results of standard mental ability tests, and the concentration of ascorbic acid in the blood plasma has been reported by Kubala and Katz (1960). The subjects were 351 students in four schools (kindergarten to college) in three cities. They were initially divided into the higher-ascorbic-acid group (with more than 1.10 mg of ascorbic acid per 100 milliliters of blood plasma) and the lower-ascorbic-acid group (less than 1.10 mg per 100 milliliters) on the basis of analysis of blood samples. By matching pairs on a socioeconomics basis (family income, education of father and mother), seventy-two subjects in each group were selected. It was found that the average measured intelligence quotient (IQ) of the higher-ascorbic-acid group was greater than that of the lower-ascorbic-acid group in each of the four schools; for all seventy-two pairs of subjects the average IQ values were 113.22 and 108.71, respectively, with an average difference of 4.51. The probability that a difference this great would be found in a similar test on a uniform population is less than 5 percent; hence the observed difference in average IQ of the two groups is statistically significant.

The subjects in both groups were then given supplementary orange juice during a period of six months, and the tests were repeated. The average measured IQ for those in the initially higher-ascorbic-acid group had increased very little (by only 0.02), whereas that for the lower group had increased by 3.54 IQ units. This difference in increase is also statistically significant, with a probability that it is just a statistical fluctuation of less than 5 percent in a uniform population.

The study was continued through a second school year with thirty-two pairs (sixty-four subjects), with similar results. The relation between the average measured IQ and the average blood-plasma ascorbic-acid concentration for these sixty-four subjects tested four times during a period of months is shown in the illustration below. These results indicate that the IQ is raised by 3.6 units when the blood-plasma ascorbic-acid concentration is increased by 50 percent (from 1.03 to 1.55 mg per 100 milliliters). This increase would for many people result from increasing the intake of ascorbic acid for an adult by 50 mg per day (from 100 to 150 mg per day).

Kubala and Katz conclude that some of the variance in intelligence-test performance is determined by the "temporary nutritional state of the individual, at least with regards to citrus or other products providing ascorbic acid." They suggest that "alertness" or "sharpness" is diminished by a decreased intake of ascorbic acid.

There is no indication in the illustration cited that maximum mental ability has been reached at the value 1.55 mg of ascorbic acid per 100 milliliters of blood plasma. This concentration corresponds for a 70-kg adult to the daily ingestion of about 180 mg of ascorbic acid. I conclude that for maximum mental performance the daily allowance of ascorbic acid should be at least three times the 60 mg recommended by the U.S. Food and Nutrition Board and at least nine times the 20 mg recommended by the corresponding British authority. Still larger intakes might have an additional effect.

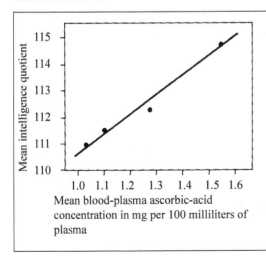

*Vitamin C and IQ. Relation between mean intelligence quotient and mean concentration of vitamin C in the blood plasma is shown for sixty-four school children. Four tests were made of each child over a period of eighteen months. The plasma vitamin-C concentration was changed by giving all the subjects extra orange juice during certain months. (Redrawn from Figure 1 of Kubala and Katz, 1960.)*

People differ from one another in their ability to fit into the world, to get along with other people, and to make their own living by contributing to the work needed to keep the world going. For many people inability is inborn, and shows up in childhood as mental retardation, slowness to learn, an impairment of the ability to think clearly. The problem of mental retardation is a very serious one. About fifteen million people in the United States are mentally deficient, including about two million classed as severely deficient. The cost of taking care of the more severely retarded ones I estimate at more than $50 billion per year. Mental retardation is a cause of suffering not only to the retarded person but also to his or her family.

Many causes of mental retardation are now known, and for a few it is known how to prevent or modify the genetic damage. An example is phenylketonuria (PKU), which results from the inability to make the enzyme that catalyzes the conversion of the amino acid phenylalanine into another amino acid, tyrosine. Both of these amino acids are present in the proteins in our food. A child with PKU has an excess of phenylalanine and a deficiency of tyrosine in the blood. This condition interferes with the proper development and functioning of the brain, leading to mental retardation. If the PKU infant shortly after birth is given a special diet low in phenylalanine and is kept on the diet for several years, the severe mental retardation does not occur.

Down's syndrome (trisomy 21, mongolism) is the result of a genetic abnormality in which the cells of the person contain three, rather than two, of one of the smaller chromosomes, number 21. Persons suffering from this disease thus tend to produce 50 percent more than usual of many different kinds of enzymes, programmed by the hundreds of genes on this chromosome. As a result, such persons show many abnormalities. They are small in stature; have an abnormally large size and unusual shape of the head; abnormalities in shapes of the hands and feet; a large, protruding tongue; and the slanted eyes under epicanthal folds that caused the disease originally to be called mongolism. About one-third suffer from congenital heart disease, and they have an increased incidence of acute leukemia; these problems often result in early death. Those who survive to adulthood show accelerated aging and usually die between forty and sixty.

People with Down's syndrome are placid and affectionate, and the infants rarely cry. They are severely retarded mentally, with IQ usually about 50. The incidence in births to young mothers is about one in two thousand, rising to about one in twenty-two for mothers more than forty years old. Persons with Down's syndrome constitute the largest group of institutionalized mental retardates.

An important medical and scientific problem is that of finding a way of treating these genetic abnormalities, starting in infancy, that would prevent much of the mental retardation and also the physical abnormalities, such as small stature and unusual appearance. I believe that we can now see that this goal can in part be reached by nutritional and other orthomolecular measures. Even a partial decrease in the severity of mental retardation can be very important. Increase in IQ from 50 to 70 (low normal) means the difference between a life of dependency on others and a life of independence and self sufficiency.

Dr. Ruth F. Harrell, of Old Dominion University, Norfolk, Virginia, and her collaborators Ruth Capp, Donald Davis, Julius Peerless, and Leonard Ravitz have reported the results of their double-blind study of the effect of administering a mixture of nineteen vitamins and minerals to sixteen mentally retarded children between five and fifteen years old (six boys and ten girls) (Harrell el al., 1981). Their initial IQ values, averages of measurements by three or more psychologists, varied from 17 to 70, with mean a value of 47.7. The subjects were assigned randomly to two groups. During the first four months of the double-blind study the six subjects in group 1 were given six vitamin-mineral tablets each day, and the ten subjects in group 2 were given six placebo tablets; then for four additional months every subject received the vitamin-mineral tablets.

Harrell had been inspired by having read the suggestions by Professor Roger J. Williams of the University of Texas, who in 1933 had discovered pantothenic acid, that an increased intake of important nutrients might help control some genetic diseases (Williams, 1956). She had then carried out a trial experiment with a severely retarded seven-year-old boy who was in diapers, could not speak, and had an estimated IQ of 25 to 30. A biochemist, Dr. Mary B. Allen, devised the formulation of vitamins and minerals given in the table on page 204. On this treatment the boy soon

---

**Daily doses of supplementary vitamins and minerals (six tablets).**

| | | |
|---|---:|---|
| Vitamin A palmitate | 15,300 | IU |
| Vitamin D (cholecalciferol) | 300 | IU |
| Thiamine mononitrate | 300 | mg |
| Riboflavin | 200 | mg |
| Niacinamide | 750 | mg |
| Calcium pantothenate | 490 | mg |
| Pyridoxine hydrochloride | 350 | mg |
| Cobalamin | 1 | mg |
| Folic acid | 0.4 | mg |
| Vitamin C (ascorbic acid) | 1500 | mg |
| Vitamin E (d-a-tocopheryl succinate) | 600 | IU |
| Magnesium (oxide) | 300 | mg |
| Calcium (carbonate) | 400 | mg |
| Zinc (oxide) | 30 | mg |
| Manganese (gluconate) | 3 | mg |
| Copper (gluconate) | 1.75 | mg |
| Iron (ferrous fumarate) | 7.5 | mg |
| Calcium phosphate ($CaHPO_4$) | 37.5 | mg |
| Iodide (KI) | 0.15 | mg |

The daily dose was 6 tablets. The tablets also contained microcrystalline cellulose, povidone, stearic acid, sodium silicoaluminate, hydroxypropylmethylcellulose, propylene glycol, silica gel, polyethylene glycol, titanium dioxide, oleic acid, and tribasic sodium phosphate as excipients. The placebo tablets contained lactose, microcrystalline cellulose, stearic acid, povidone, propylene glycol, hydroxypropyl-methylcellulose, titanium dioxide, and oleic acid.

---

began to talk and in a few weeks began to read and write and to act like a normal child. Two years later he was getting along well in school subjects and had an estimated IQ of 90. Allen had also administered another orthomolecular substance, thyroid, to her patients, and fourteen of the sixteen in the Harrell study also received thyroid, in amounts of 30 to 120 mg per day.

The main results are shown in the illustration on page 205. The group that received the supplement for eight months showed a steady increase in average IQ, from 46 to 61. The other group showed no change during the first four months, when the placebo was given, and then an increase from 49 to 59 during the next four months, when the vitamin-mineral supplement was given.

From these results we may conclude that there is a reasonable chance that a child with severe mental retardation could by vitamin-mineral

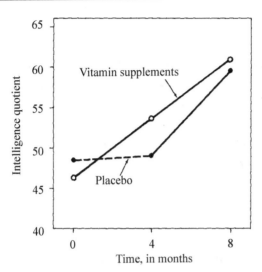

*Vitamin C and mental retardation. Retarded people who received vitamin-mineral supplements over an eight-month period showed an average increase in IQ of 15 points (from 46 to 61). A control group that received no supplements for the first four months showed no change in IQ. When the controls were given vitamin-mineral supplements for four months, they showed an average increase in IQ of 10 points (from 49 to 59) approaching the experimental groups. (Adapted from Harrell et al., 1981.)*

supplementation beginning early in life achieve an increase in IQ of 20 points or more. The largest individual increases reported by Harrell et al. were 24 points (42 to 66) in eight months and 21 points (50 to 71) in four months, enough gain to put those persons in a position to become self-sufficient. The improved nutritional status resulting from taking the vitamin-mineral supplement, with about thirty times the RDA for vitamin C and good amounts of other nutrients, would benefit anyone taking it, and it is my recommendation that this improved nutritional regimen be followed by every retarded child. The cost of 180 tablets, one month's supply, is less than $10, and is accordingly small compared with the other expenses involved in caring for a mentally retarded person.

Three of the subjects in the study by Harrell et al. suffered from Down's syndrome. Their initial IQ values were 42, 59. and 65, and the increases with intake of the vitamin-mineral supplement and thyroid (for the first two) were 24 and 11 (in eight months) and about 10 (in four months), respectively.

There is no accepted conventional treatment for Down's syndrome. The physician who has made the greatest effort to ameliorate that condition is Dr. Henry Turkel, of Detroit, Michigan. He has reported on his work in a paper communicated to the Select Committee on Nutrition and Human Needs for the United States Senate, Senator George McGovern, Chairman (Turkel, 1977), and in a book. *New Hope for the Mentally Retarded— Stymied by the FDA* (Turkel, 1972). In 1940 he had begun treating Down's syndrome patients with tablets that he had developed. The tablets contain mainly orthomolecular substances—ten vitamins, nine minerals, one amino acid (glutamic acid), choline, inositol, para-aminobenzoic acid, thyroid, unsaturated fatty acids, and digestive enzymes. These substances should improve the health of the patients. In addition his preparation contains several drugs, given in smaller dosages than those usually prescribed. One of the drugs is pentylenetetrazole, which stimulates the central nervous system. Another is aminophylline, a heart stimulant. I do not know enough about drugs to permit me to comment on their value for these patients, but there is the possibility that their action as stimulants is beneficial.

I know Dr. Turkel, and I can testify as to his sincerity and conviction.† The results that he reports are striking. Many of the children show a reduction of the developmental anomalies, especially of the bones. Their appearance changes in the direction of normality. Their mental ability and behavior improve to such an extent that they are able to hold jobs and support themselves. Rapid growth (increase in height) occurs during the period when the tablets are being taken, and the growth stops during the periods when they are not taken.

My conclusion is that there is little danger that this treatment or treatment with the supplementary nutrients would do harm, and there is evidence that the patients would receive significant benefit. There are about 300,000 people with Down's syndrome in the United States. I think that all—especially the younger ones—should try nutritional supplementation to see to what extent it benefits them.

Turkel treats Down's syndrome patients in Michigan, but he is not allowed by the Food and Drug Administration to ship his tablets across state lines. In 1959 he filed a new-drug application with the FDA (necessary because his tablets contain some drugs). The application was turned down, and his later efforts were also unsuccessful. The director of the National Institute of Neurological Diseases and Blindness, referring to Turkel's treatment of Down's syndrome patients, wrote that "On theoretical grounds, and based on known effects of these drugs, which consist of vitamins, minerals, and other medications, our advisors have stated that, although they are not harmful, they doubt that the drugs would be of specific value in treating mongolism" (Turkel, 1972, p. 123). The FDA in rejecting the new-drug application stated that "The known facts concerning mongolism preclude any reasonable hope that your products would be of benefit in this condition, which is caused by a defect in the basic cell structure. This finding, considered together with the long history of inability of medical science to find a treatment or cure for mongolism, suggests that this condition is beyond hope of successful treatment by the kind of preparations that you wish to recommend for this purpose" (Turkel, 1972, p. 119).

I think that this attitude of the National Institutes of Health (NIH) and FDA is the result of ignorance, bias, misunderstanding of the nature of vitamins and other orthomolecular substances, and lack of hope or vision— they seem to have the conviction that nothing new can be discovered.

Autism is a genetic disease that manifests itself in the first one or two years of life in about one child in three thousand (80 percent are boys). The autistic child remains alone, not developing social relationships with his parents or other people. He has language problems, refusing to speak or using language in an odd way. He adheres to rituals, resists change, and has an unusually strong attachment to objects. His IQ is usually low, and he may develop seizures. Those with higher IQ benefit somewhat from psychotherapy and special education.

There is no accepted conventional therapy for autism. Several investigators, however, have reported that vitamin supplementation has value. The most significant work has been done by Dr. Bernard Rimland, a psychologist who is director of the Institute for Child Behavior Research, San Diego, California (Rimland, 1973; Rimland, Callaway, and Dreyfus, 1977).† Through their parents, Rimland arranged for 190 autistic children to be studied for twenty-four weeks. The parents of each child were required to obtain the cooperation of the child's physician or another local doctor to provide on-site medical supervision and to complete monthly reports on the child's status under the vitamin treatment. Many parents found such strong resistance from the physicians that they were required to withdraw; this reduced the number of children in the reported study from an original 300 to 190.

After the tablets were gradually introduced over five weeks, the children took ten per day for twelve weeks. There was then a no-treatment period of two weeks, followed by doses of ten tablets per day for two weeks. The daily intake of nutrients provided by the ten tablets was 1000 mg of vitamin C, 1000 mg of niacinamide, 150 mg of pyridoxine, 5 mg of thiamine, 5 mg of riboflavin, 50 mg of pantothenic acid, 0.1 mg of folic acid, 0.01 mg of vitamin $B_{12}$, 30 mg of para-aminobenzoic acid, 0.015 mg of biotin, 60 mg of choline, 60 mg of inositol, and 10 mg of iron. The cost of the vitamins was about $10 per month.

The parents and physicians made regular reports, which were analyzed for the amount of improvement when the vitamins were taken and for deterioration during the no-treatment interval. The conclusion was that 86 of the 190 children (45 percent) showed great improvement, very good improvement, or significant improvement; 78 (41 percent) showed some smaller amount of improvement; 20 (11 percent) showed no change; and 6 (3 percent) deteriorated. Thus about three-quarters of the children were benefitted by the nutritional supplement, and only 3 percent were made worse.

There were indications that vitamin $B_6$ was especially important, and a double-blind study of fifteen children was then carried out (Rimland et al., 1977). During the study the children continued to take the same vitamins, minerals, and drugs as before the study began. Each child during one period received either vitamin $B_6$ (75 to 800 mg per day, different for different children) or a placebo, and then during a second period the placebo or the $B_6$. Ten of the fifteen children were judged to have benefitted from the $B_6$ (average score +24), one showed no change, and four deteriorated (average score -16). The investigators concluded that vitamin $B_6$ seems to be a safe agent with potential value in the management of autistic children. My opinion, based on these Rimland studies and others, is that orthomolecular treatment with vitamins and minerals should be tried for every autistic child as having the possibility of leading to significant improvement without danger of leading to harmful side effects that act as a deterrent to the trial of a drug.

Epilepsy is a recurrent disorder of the brain that involves brief attacks of altered consciousness, usually a convulsive seizure with loss of consciousness and with jerking of the extremities. Convulsive seizures can be caused by drugs and by lack of oxygen, but the cause of most epileptic seizures is not known. About 2 percent of the American people are affected. Conventional treatment is the use of anticonvulsant drugs (diphenylhydantoin, phenobarbital, several others). This treatment usually is effective, but the side effects of the drugs can be troublesome.

In her study of nutritional supplements and mental retardation Harrell noticed that three of the children who were seizure-prone had no seizures during the four to eight months during which they received the vitamin-mineral supplement. She studied seven more seizure-prone children by giving them the supplement for one month, during which they had no seizures. Her application to the National Institutes of Mental Health for a grant to support a more extensive study was turned down.

The nutritional treatment should be tried with children subject to seizures. It provides general healthful benefit, and for many it might control the problem of the seizure-prone children as well as the drugs do, without the disagreeable side effects.

Affective disorders are a form of mental illness involving a feeling or emotion or disturbance evidenced in inappropriate response and reaction to the objective circumstances at the time. Schizophrenic disorders are forms of affective disorders that tend to be chronic and that involve various psychotic symptoms, such as delusions, hallucinations, and deteriorated functioning over long periods of time. Nearly everyone has periods of sadness, depression, and grief following a death or disappointment, and periods of elation following success and achievement. It is only when the periods last too long, the mood is too extreme, and the person does not respond to reassurance and other efforts to help that he or she can be described as psychotic and suffering from an affective disorder. Schizophrenia and other affective disorders are the major mental illnesses. It is estimated that about 12 percent of men and 18 percent of women suffer from some form of clinically significant affective disorder during their lifetimes, and about 2 percent have one or more schizophrenic episodes.

Affective disorders—depressions, elations, schizophrenic episodes—have a variety of causes, such as drugs (steroidal contraceptives, other steroids, L-dopa, reserpine, cocaine, sedatives, amphetamines, and others) or disease (influenza, hepatitis, mononucleosis, encephalitis, tuberculosis, syphilis, multiple sclerosis, cancer, and others). Other causes include vitamin deficiencies ($B_1$, $B_3$, $B_6$, $B_{12}$) or allergic responses to foods, chemicals, and other environmental factors (Hoffer and Osmond, 1960; Hawkins and Pauling, 1973; Cheraskin and Ringsdorf, 1974; Philpott, 1974; Pfeiffer, 1975; Dickey, 1976; Lesser, 1977). The best way to control these psychoses is by finding and eliminating the causes. Improved nutrition is also often helpful.

Manic depression is usually treated with compounds of lithium. This element is present in the earth's crust in only a small amount, 0.01 percent, far smaller than sodium, 2.8 percent, or potassium. 2.6 percent. The lithium ion may influence the central nervous system by interfering with the motion of sodium ions and potassium ions. Lithium is not known to be required for life and probably should not be called an orthomolecular substance.

During the last two decades large numbers of young people have developed psychoses because of the use of mood-changing drugs—uppers, downers, cocaine and harder drugs, probably also marijuana. Many of them have recovered to the point where they could lead normal lives by the regular intake of vitamins and minerals in the optimum amounts.

The first double-blind study in the field of psychiatry was that carried out by Osmond and Hoffer in the Saskatchewan Hospital and University Hospital, Saskatoon, which I cited in Chapter 3. Osmond and Dr. John H. Smythies had formulated the hypothesis that schizophrenia might be caused by the production in the body of a substance with psychological properties similar to those of mescaline and lysergic acid diethylamide (LSD), perhaps by methylation reactions similar to that involved in the conversion of noradrenaline to adrenaline. It is known that a methylating agent, the amino acid methionine, when taken in large amount by a schizophrenic person exacerbates his or her illness. Osmond and Hoffer had the idea that a substance that picks up methyl groups might prevent these methylation reactions from producing the harmful substances. They knew that niacin, vitamin $B_3$ (nicotinic acid or nicotinamide), is such a demethylating agent, and they also knew that it is remarkably free of toxicity, so that large amounts can be taken. In early 1952 they administered niacin to half a dozen schizophrenic patients, with good results. One patient was a seventeen-year-old boy who was excited, overactive, silly, deluded, and sometimes hallucinating. He responded to some extent to electroconvulsive therapy and insulin-coma treatment, which, however, had to be stopped because he developed facial palsy. Toward the end of May he was lying naked in bed, incontinent and hallucinating. There was nothing else Osmond and Hoffer could do for him (the tranquilizers used today had not yet been discovered), so on May 28 they began giving him 5 g of niacin and 5 g of vitamin C per day. He was better the next day, almost normal ten days later, went home in July, and was still well ten years later.

Osmond and Hoffer then set up their double-blind experiment with thirty schizophrenic patients, some of whom, selected at random, were given a placebo, others nicotinic acid, and others nicotinamide, in the amount of 3 g per day for thirty-three days. During the next two years the placebo group was well during only 48 percent of the time, whereas the other two groups were well 92 percent of the time (Osmond and Hoffer, 1962). After 1952 they continued to give niacin to some of the hospitalized patients, some of whom continued to take it after their discharge. The record of the niacin patients was uniformly better than that of the others. For example, the number of the niacin patients still well after five years was 67 percent, about twice that of the others, 35 percent.

I have talked with many orthomolecular psychiatrists. The average amounts of niacin administered is about 8 g per day, with an equal amount of vitamin C and usually also good amounts of other nutrients. There seems to be agreement with Osmond's estimate that about 20 percent of patients hospitalized for the first time with acute schizophrenia and given orthomolecular treatment have another attack requiring hospitalization, whereas with only conventional treatment their number is about 60 percent. There is little doubt that this vitamin supplementation, as an adjunct to appropriate conventional treatment, has great value.

The orthomolecular treatment of schizophrenia has not yet been generally accepted, although it is used in a few psychiatric hospitals. In 1973 a committee of the American Psychiatric Association published a report, *Megavitamin and Orthomolecular Therapy in Psychiatry,* in which arguments were presented to support the conclusion that megavitamin and orthomolecular therapy has no value in the treatment of schizophrenia or other mental diseases. I pointed out that this report contained many incorrect statements and logical errors (Pauling, 1974b). This bias against vitamins and lack of respect for the facts are not found in the 1976 report of megavitamin therapy of the Joint University Megavitamin Therapy Review Committee to the minister of Social Services and Community Health of the Province of Alberta, Canada. The report presents a balanced account of the evidence and a number of recommendations about further investigations (McCoy, Yonge, and Karr, 1976). The 1979 report on nutrition and health of the Council on Scientific Affairs of the American Medical Association, on the other hand, ignores the question of the value of vitamin supplements except to say that the public is being misled by extravagant claims.

Much information about nutrition in relation to mental disease is given in the thirty-one articles by thirty-seven authors in the 1973 book *Orthomolecular Psychiatry: Treatment of Schizophrenia* (Hawkins and Pauling, 1973). One chapter describes the results of giving a mixture of three vitamins (C, $B_3$, and $B_6$) by mouth to acute schizophrenic patients and control subjects and then measuring the amounts excreted in the urine. Low excretion of a vitamin is thought to indicate a special need for that vitamin. Nearly all of the schizophrenic patients (94 percent) were low excretors of one or more of the vitamins, far more than the 62 percent of the controls. The authors concluded that deficiency in any one of these three vitamins could increase the probability of an attack of schizophrenia. Other authors emphasized that there are many kinds of schizophrenia, and that different patients may be benefitted by improving their nutritional status in many different ways, with optimum intakes of niacin, ascorbic acid, thiamine, pyridoxine, other vitamins, minerals, and other nutrients.

In 1970 I was walking along Main Street in the small town of Cambria, on the coast of California, when a passing car stopped and the driver got out and ran back to me. She said, "Dr. Pauling, I owe my life to you. I am twenty-six years old. Two years ago I was contemplating suicide. I had suffered miserably from schizophrenia for six years. Then I learned about vitamins when someone told me about your paper on orthomolecular psychiatry. The vitamins have saved my life."

There are now many orthomolecular psychiatrists. Many interesting papers are published in the *Journal of Orthomolecular Psychiatry.*† I believe that improved nutrition should be a part of the treatment of every person with mental problems, and I am glad that progress is being made in this direction.

# 21

## *The Allergies*

Many people suffer from asthma, hay fever, allergic rhinitis, allergic bronchitis, or some other hypersensitivity reaction, to such substances as house dust, pollen, other environmental factors, or certain foods or drugs. That they can be helped to some extent to control their problems by the proper intake of vitamin C and other nutrients was pointed out long ago by several investigators (Korbsch, 1938; Holmes and Alexander, 1942; Holmes, 1943; Leake, 1955; other references are given by Stone, 1972). The established role of vitamin C in strengthening the immune system suggests that it should have value in managing hypersensitivity reactions, which are essentially immune reactions. Many recent studies affirm this proposition and show that the vitamin has such value at daily doses of 500 milligrams (mg) or somewhat more. A careful study of the effect of still larger doses has yet to be made.

An important molecular actor in hypersensitivity reactions is histamine. This is a small molecule, containing only seventy atoms, its formula being $C_5H_9N_3$. It is closely related to histidine, one of the essential amino acids. Histamine is stored in granules of the cells in many tissues, especially of the skin, lungs, and stomach, and it is released from these granules when an antigen (such as the antigenic molecular groups of pollen grains that cause hay fever) combines with its specific antibody. Its release may also be triggered by the stimulus of certain drugs or by disruption of the tissues.

When histamine is released, it combines with specific proteins and starts the reactions that are characteristic of hypersensitivity. In the skin the capillaries are dilated, and their walls become permeable to fluid, producing a wheal (a flat burning or itching eminence, such as is caused by a mosquito bite) and redness. The arterioles are dilated, permitting a larger flow of blood to the affected region. Dilation of the blood vessels in the brain may cause headache. Contraction of smooth muscles in response to histamine may cause restriction of the bronchi and difficulty in breathing.

The heart may be affected, with stronger contractions and more rapid beat. Itching is caused by the effect of histamine on nerve endings.

Many drugs, called antihistamines, are known that are often effective in counteracting the histamine released in a hypersensitivity reaction. They have much value, but, as with most drugs, they must be used with caution because of the possible harmful side effects, such as drowsiness, dizziness, headache, nausea, lack of appetite, dryness of the mouth, and nervousness. They exert their antihistaminic function by competing with histamine for the specific sites on the protein molecules through which histamine exerts its effects.

The many reports, beginning nearly fifty years ago, about the value of vitamin C as an adjunct to other treatments in the control of hypersensitivity reactions caused researchers to study the interaction of this vitamin and histamine. In 1975 Chatterjee and his associates showed that when guinea pigs are put on a diet containing no vitamin C, the blood level of histamine started to rise on the third day and reached a high level by the fourteenth day, when they were beginning to show signs of scurvy (Chatterjee et al., 1975b). They suggested that one of the functions of vitamin C is to regulate the amount of histamine in the body by converting it into another substance, hydantoin-5-acetic acid, which then decomposes into normal metabolic products (Subramanian, 1978). The conversion involves a hydroxylation reaction, for which vitamin C is required. It is evidently the destruction of vitamin C in this process that results in its deficiency for other vital functions and brings on incipient scurvy.

Dr. C. Alan B. Clemetson has carried out an important study of the relation between vitamin C and histamine in the blood of four hundred men and women in New York. The concentration of vitamin C in the blood ranged from the dangerously low value of 0.00 to 0.19 mg per deciliter (for fourteen) to a high of 2.5 (for two), with a median of 0.8, which corresponds to the intake of about 100 mg of the vitamin per day. The histamine concentration varied over more than a threefold range, with a striking dependence on the level of vitamin C, as shown in the illustration on page 216. The slope of the curve shows that for values of ascorbate concentration from 1.0 to 2.5 mg per deciliter there is no change in the histamine concentration. Most people who ingest 250 mg of vitamin C per day or more have plasma concentrations in this range, and I consider this to be the normal range (Pauling, 1974c). The results with histamine support this conclusion, in that the homeostatic (feedback) mechanisms that operate to keep the histamine concentration constant, at its optimum value, are achieving this goal in this range.

For smaller values of the ascorbate level, however, the histamine level rises rapidly. Chatterjee et al. (1975b) have suggested that the vasodilating action of histamine may be responsible for some of the manifestations of scurvy. Remarking that scurvy may be partly due to histamine intoxication, Clemetson has observed that it may be more than a coincidence that inflammation, such as that produced by histamine, seems to resemble localized scurvy.

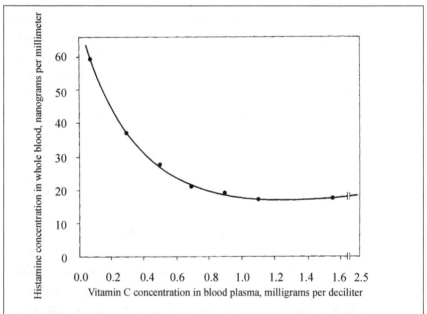

*Vitamin C and histamine in blood. In a study of four hundred people, Alan B. Clemetson demonstrated the effectiveness of vitamin C in lowering the histamine concentration in the blood. Histamine is shown by the scale at the left, vitamin C by the scale on the bottom. The points indicate the average concentration of histamine, corresponding to increasing concentration of ascorbate in the blood plasma, in milligrams per deciliter, for the ranges 0.00 to 0.19, 0.20 to 0.39, 0.40 to 0.59, and so on. The point plotted at the far right shows the average concentration of histamine for concentrations of ascorbate from 1.2 to 2.5 milligrams per deciliter. (Adapted from Clemetson, 1980.)*

Additional evidence has been provided by Nandi et al. (1976), who reported that in rats and guinea pigs stress induced by vaccine treatment, fasting, and exposure to heat or cold increased the production of histamine (measured in gastric mucosa and urinary excretion). Treatment with vitamin C decreased the urinary excretion significantly.

These observations provide strong support for the conclusion that an increased intake of vitamin C has value in helping to control hypersensitivity problems.

Clemetson (1980) also compared histamine and vitamin C levels in 223 pregnant women and a number of nonpregnant women. He found that the pregnant women had lower levels of vitamin C and higher levels of histamine than the others. One woman developed partial separation of the placenta (*abruptio placentae*) and vaginal bleeding in the thirty-fifth week of pregnancy. Her plasma ascorbate level was very low, 0.19 to 0.27 mg per deciliter, and her blood histamine level was high, 35 to 38 mg per milliliter. She was given 1000 mg of vitamin C per day, the bleeding stopped, and she was delivered of a healthy child at forty weeks. Two other *abruptio placentae* patients had plasma ascorbate levels of 0.38 and 0.25 and histamine levels of 44 and 55, respectively. Clemetson states that ascorbate and histamine levels should be obtained for pregnant women, and supplementation with vitamin C should be given when it is needed.

Anaphylactic shock is a sudden, acute reaction to an antigen, mainly through histamine release in a hypersensitized person. The person develops hives (urticaria) and has difficulty in breathing and may lose so much liquid from the blood by seeping through the walls of the blood vessels as to nearly stop the circulation of the blood. Among the antigens that cause anaphylaxis are foreign proteins, such as those in horse serum (giving rise to serum sickness); any one of many drugs (penicillin in penicillin-sensitive persons); and substances introduced by snake bites (rattlesnakes, cottonmouths, cottonheads, coral snakes), Gila monster bites, spider bites (especially by the black widow spider and violin spider, sometimes by other spiders, nearly all of which are venomous), and bee stings. A single bee sting may cause death. About four times as many deaths in the United States are caused by bee stings as by snake bites. Persons known to be at risk should carry a kit containing epinephrine and an antihistamine.

Human beings, monkeys, and guinea pigs, which do not synthesize vitamin C, are more susceptible to anaphylactic shock than other animals. It was discovered nearly fifty years ago that a high intake of vitamin C protects guinea pigs against anaphylaxis (Raffel and Madison, 1938; many other studies have been made). Fred R. Klenner has reported on the effective treatment of snake bite by the intravenous infusion of sodium ascorbate (1971). It would be wise for persons who might be exposed to agents that could cause anaphylaxis to ingest regular high doses of vitamin C.

Asthma (bronchial asthma) is a disease characterized by difficulty in breathing because of the spasmodic contraction of the bronchi, recurring at intervals and accompanied by a wheezing sound, a sense of constriction in the chest, a cough, and expectoration. An attack is often subsequent to exposure to an allergen, but sometimes it results from psychosocial stress (emotional upset) or other stresses, viral respiratory disease, or inhalation of cold air, gasoline fumes, fresh paint, or cigarette smoke, or from change in the barometric pressure. About half of the persons with this disease have it in a severe and troublesome form. It can usually be controlled by drugs, which, of course, have disagreeable and harmful side effects.

Reports of the value of vitamin C for the control of asthma began around 1940. There is now good evidence that vitamin C has such value as an adjunct to conventional therapy. Some of the older studies gave negative results, perhaps because of the use of too small an amount of the vitamin for too short a time. Most of the recent studies have shown that the vitamin has a significant effect. For example, a reduced airflow caused by inhalation of histamine aerosol (Zuskin, Lewis, and Bouhuys, 1973), flax dust (Valic and Zuskin, 1973), or textile dust (Zuskin, Valic, and Bouhuys, 1976) was partially controlled for several hours by 500 mg of vitamin C. Ogilvy, Du Bois, and their collaborators at Yale University then carried out several studies with methacholine, a drug that induces constriction of the bronchi and decreased airflow in both healthy persons and asthmatics. Six healthy young men given methacholine either by aerosol inhalation or by mouth showed bronchoconstriction that decreased the airflow by about 40 percent, whereas the amount of decrease was only 9 percent when they ingested 100 mg of vitamin C one hour before the administration of the drug (Ogilvy et al., 1978, 1981). Similar results were obtained with asthmatic patients (Mohsenin, Du Bois, and Douglas, 1982).

In a recent double-blind study of forty-one asthmatic Nigerian patients (Anah, Jarike, and Baig, 1980) twenty-two were given 1 gram (g) of vitamin C per day, and nineteen were given a placebo, for fourteen weeks during the rainy season, when the asthma is exacerbated by respiratory infections. The vitamin-C subjects had less than one-quarter as many asthmatic attacks during this period as the placebo subjects, and the attacks were less serious. All of the thirteen vitamin-C patients who had no attacks during the fourteen weeks had at least one attack during the eight weeks after the vitamin was stopped.

Anderson et al. (1980) reported on their study of ten white asthmatic children in Pretoria, South Africa. These children, who initially had bronchial asthma and showed exercise-induced bronchoconstriction, were given 1 g of vitamin C per day and were assessed clinically and immunologically for six months. They showed increased neutrophil chemotaxis, improved lung function, and greater transformation of lymphocytes under antigenic stimulation, and they all were free of severe asthmatic attacks during the six months.

These investigations support the conclusion that an increased intake of vitamin C has value for asthmatic patients.

Hay fever (pollinosis) is an acute inflammation of the mucous membrane of the nostrils that is usually caused by windborne tree, grass, or weed pollens. Itching, sneezing, production of a watery nasal secretion, and flow of tears occur during the pollen season. Antihistamines and other drugs are used to control the problem. The sufferers often try to avoid the guilty pollen and sometimes move to a different part of the country—where they may have the bad luck to find another kind of pollen that is as bad as the original culprit.

One of the early reports about the value of vitamin C in controlling hay fever was that of Holmes and Alexander (1942), who reported that 200 mg per day was often effective. The matter was made confusing, however, by other investigators, who reported that they observed no benefit. This situation has not changed very much. For example Kordansky, Rosenthal, and Norman (1979) studied the effect of vitamin C on ragweed-induced bronchospasm in six ragweed-sensitive asthmatic adults and reported that 500 mg had no protective effect. This amount is probably too small, and a long period of administration may be needed. In 1949 Brown and Ruskin studied sixty hay fever patients and reported that about 50 percent of those taking 1 g of vitamin C per day and about 75 percent of those taking 2.25 g per day showed improvement. For forty-seven years I have observed one subject who suffered greatly for decades from hay fever caused by ragweed and olive pollen and has for the last twelve years found much relief by taking 3 g of vitamin C per day.

I suggest that persons suffering from hay fever should take about this amount regularly and should increase their intake to the bowel-tolerance level (Chapter 14) during the pollen season.

Sometimes the immune reaction turns upon its own body; antibodies form against antigens in the cells of the patient. Among these auto-immune diseases are systemic lupus erythematosis, myasthenia gravis, glomerulonephritis, and pemphigus. Little information is available about the possible value of high doses of vitamin C in helping to control these diseases.

# 22

## Arthritis and Rheumatism

Arthritis is inflammation of a joint. More than one hundred different kinds of arthritis have been characterized, with many different causes. Gout, for example, is caused by the formation of crystals of sodium hydrogen urate in the joint. Infectious agents such as gonococcal bacteria or the viruses of mumps or hepatitis may also cause inflammation of the joints, as can other diseases, drugs, allergens, and cancer.

Rheumatoid arthritis and osteoarthritis are readily distinguished. In rheumatoid arthritis the swollen joints in the fingers are soft and tender; in osteoarthritis they are hard and usually not tender. The joints near the end of the fingers are usually involved in osteoarthritis, but not those closer to the wrist, whereas in rheumatoid arthritis it is the wrist and parts of the hand other than the ends of the fingers that are affected.

Rheumatism (fibromyositis) comprises a group of illnesses involving pain, tenderness, and stiffness. It may affect not only joints (rheumatoid arthritis) but also muscles and adjacent structures.

Many drugs that are highly effective for the control of arthritis have been developed during recent years. Aspirin is often used to control the pain and inflammation of rheumatoid arthritis; the average daily dose is 4.5 grams (g), 14 tablets. Enteric-coated tablets may be taken by patients with stomach or duodenal ulcers to avoid the exacerbation of the ulcers by the aspirin. The problem of serious dysfunction of a joint can sometimes be handled by surgery. Total hip replacement is often successful.

Nutritional factors are important in both causing and controlling some kinds of arthritis. An attack of gout may occur from overeating, especially eating too much meat, and from drinking too much alcohol and not enough water. Eating a large amount of meat, especially certain organ meats, increases the level of uric acid in the blood, and increasing the amount of alcohol and decreasing the amount of water in the body fluids make it easier for the crystals of sodium hydrogen urate to deposit in the joints. To prevent an attack of gout the intake of meat should be kept low and a large amount of water should be drunk, at least three quarts per day.

Also, the urine should be kept alkaline, because sodium hydrogen urate is more soluble in alkaline urine than in acidic urine. Alkaline urine can be achieved by taking sodium bicarbonate, trisodium citrate, or sodium ascorbate. I recommend the last.

As with other diseases, the question of the value of supplementary vitamins for the control of arthritis has been confused by misleading statements. Not long ago I read a brief report by a professor in a leading medical school about his trial of the value of unconventional treatments for arthritis. He stated that vitamin supplements were found to have no value. I wrote to him, asking how many patients he had studied, and how much vitamin supplement he had given them. His answer was that he had given an ordinary multivitamin tablet every day to a half-dozen patients, who seemed not to improve. The patients described later in this chapter took between one hundred and five hundred times the amounts in these tablets; it is these optimum intakes that have value in helping to control arthritis.

The pioneer in vitamin therapy for rheumatism and arthritis was a young physician in New England, Dr. William Kaufman. To secure objective assessment of the state and progress of his patients he built a set of goniometers (angle-measuring devices) with which he could measure the angles through which different joints of the human body could move. By measuring one thousand people in ordinary good health he obtained a standard curve showing the average joint mobility index as a function of age—it falls off slowly with increasing age. He also measured the joint mobility for patients with joint dysfunction and found that the index fell far below the standard curve. In addition, he verified that the patients had much larger values of the rate of sedimentation of the red corpuscles of the blood than did the healthy controls. Thus he had two objective ways of assessing the state of health of the patients.

In 1937 vitamin $B_3$, niacin or niacinamide, was identified. Kaufman decided to find out whether it could help his patients. Upon administering it to his arthritic patients, he found that most of them responded rapidly by feeling better and by an increase in the joint mobility index to nearly the normal curve and a decrease in the red-cell sedimentation rate. Stopping the niacinamide caused a return to the abnormal state within a day or two.

Kaufman published an account of his study of 150 arthritic patients in 1943 in *The Common Form of Niacin Amide Deficiency Disease, Aniacinamidosis,* and in 1949 he published his study of 450 patients in *The Common Form of Joint Dysfunction: Its Incidence and Treatment.* In 1955 in a report to the American Geriatric Society he stated that most of the patients improved greatly on a regimen of 1 to 5 g of niacinamide per day in divided doses (six to sixteen per day), continuing for as long as nine years. He observed no untoward reactions from niacinamide in several thousand patient-years of continuous use. His recommended intake for treatment of restricted mobility of joints and other manifestations of deficiency of vitamin $B_3$ (aniacinamidosis) is 4 to 5 g per day.

Even before the work of Abram Hoffer and Humphry Osmond on acute schizophrenia, Kaufman had written that many of his patients showed striking improvement in mental health as well as physical health on this niacinamide regimen. I have had the opportunity to check the effectiveness of niacinamide, together with vitamin C, in controlling arthritis in a few patients, with results that support the conclusions stated by Kaufman. So far as I know, no group of researchers in the field of arthritis has attempted to repeat Kaufman's work. This lack of interest may be the result in part, again, of the general bias of the medical profession against vitamins and in part of the fact that no one can make money from niacinamide, which is just as cheap as vitamin C.

Another vitamin that brings relief to the sufferers from rheumatism is vitamin $B_6$, pyridoxine. Vitamin $B_6$ shrinks the synovial membranes that line the bearing surfaces of the joints. It thus helps to control pain and to restore mobility in the elbows, shoulders, knees, and other joints, as was observed by Dr. John M. Ellis, a physician in Mt. Pleasant, Texas.

In his 1983 book *Free of Pain* Ellis has reported that the vitamin is effective at high intakes. There is now little doubt that the optimum intake of vitamin $B_6$ is somewhere in the region of 50 to 100 milligrams (mg) per day, and probably more for some people. There is an upper limit, however, to the intake of this vitamin. A daily intake of 2000 mg or more of vitamin $B_6$ continued for months or years leads to a temporary peripheral neuropathy, a feeling of numbness in the toes. The optimum intake of this vitamin is accordingly less than one thousand times the Recommended Daily Allowance but somewhat greater than the RDA.†

Because of its shrinking effect on the synovial membranes, vitamin $B_6$ has found another use; in the relief of a nerve disorder called carpal tunnel syndrome. This is a painful and crippling disease of the hands and wrists that results from compression of a principal nerve to the hand as it passes through a tunnel lined with synovial membrane between the tendons and ligaments in the wrist. It occurs about three times as frequently in women as in men and has a higher incidence during pregnancy and at the time of the menopause than at other times. Until recently the principal treatment was surgery.

In 1962 Ellis began giving vitamin $B_6$ in large doses to pregnant women to control the edema and some other problems from which they tend to suffer. He noticed that the large doses, 50 to 100 mg per day (twenty-five to five hundred times the RDA) also controlled the tingling in the fingers, cramps, weakness of grip, and lack of feeling in the hands. Around 1970 he noticed that these large doses of vitamin $B_6$ provided good control of the carpal tunnel syndrome (Ellis, 1966; Ellis and Presley, 1973), usually such that surgery was not needed.

An interesting aspect of Ellis' work is the discovery that the abnormality in the metabolism of the amino acid tryptophan that is caused by the steroidal birth-control pills is prevented by the daily intake of about 50 mg of vitamin $B_6$.

Many of the vitamins serve as coenzymes in various enzyme systems in the human body. Vitamin $B_6$, for example, is known to serve in this way for more than one hundred different enzymes. In the past it has been said that the intake of the RDAs of vitamins provided enough for the enzyme systems to function at nearly their maximum effectiveness, but it has now been learned that this statement is not true.

Karl Folkers† is a distinguished organic chemist and biochemist who is now a professor at the University of Texas in Austin, and who earlier was for twenty years director of research for Merck and Company. He decided to study the enzymes for which vitamin $B_6$ is a coenzyme and selected the easily available glutamic oxaloacetic transaminase of erythrocytes (EGOT), which is in the red cells of the blood. By 1975 he and his collaborators had shown that in their Texan subjects on an ordinary diet the EGOT enzymatic activity was far less than the maximum value that could be achieved by a high intake of vitamin $B_6$. This observation supported the conclusion already reached by Ellis that many people suffer from a deficiency of this vitamin.

Ellis and Folkers then collaborated in a double-blind study in which the effectiveness of vitamin $B_6$ was compared with that of a placebo in patients with the carpal tunnel syndrome. The result, with high statistical significance ($P = 0.0078$), was that the $B_6$ patients improved and the placebo patients did not (Ellis, Folkers, et al., 1982). The authors conclude that "Clinical improvement of the syndrome with pyridoxine therapy may frequently obviate hand surgery." The mechanism of control of the disease is the action of the vitamin in reducing the swelling of the synovial membrane that lines the tunnel.

It is not surprising that $B_6$ has been found also to be helpful in controlling arthritis. Its action as an antihistaminic agent and regulator of the rate of synthesis of prostaglandins (Chapter 26) makes it to some extent a substitute for aspirin in controlling pain and inflammation.

The best known example of the effectiveness of vitamin C in controlling an arthritic disorder is the experience of Norman Cousins, the former editor of the *Saturday Review,* who was suffering intensely from an ailment diagnosed as ankylosing spondylitis, a progressive form of arthritis characterized by inflammation and then the fusing together of adjacent bones, especially of the spine. As described by him in his book, *Anatomy of an Illness as Perceived by the Patient,* Cousins decided to try the effect of vitamin C and persuaded his physician to give him intravenous infusions of 35 g of sodium ascorbate per day. This treatment, together with the psychosomatic aid of his determination to remain cheerful and to enjoy himself, achieved partially by leaving the hospital and receiving the treatment in a hotel room, led to his recovery. He now holds a special professorship in the University of California Medical School in Los Angeles.†

There is evidence that arthritis, rheumatism, and related diseases often are the result of nutritional deficiencies. Sufferers from these diseases would be wise to try to improve their nutritional status by regulating their diet and taking supplementary vitamins and minerals, perhaps approximating the intake described in the table on page 10, possibly with additional niacinamide, vitamin C, and vitamin $B_6$. There is also the possibility that an increased intake of some other vitamin, such as pantothenic acid, would be helpful. These nutritional measures should serve as an adjunct to appropriate conventional treatment, if there is such a treatment, but sometimes, as with carpal tunnel syndrome, the need for the conventional treatment (surgery) disappears.

# 23

## *The Eye, the Ear, and the Mouth*

From the larger concerns about health and illness that have engaged our attention in the last chapters let us turn now to consider what the optimum use of vitamins may do for certain afflictions that bring pain and disability even though they do not threaten life. Some of the observations and recommendations I shall make are as solidly based on reliable and repeated observations as are most of the things I have had to say in the earlier chapters. Some are based, however, on only a small amount of evidence. If I were recommending drugs I should have to be far more cautious in mentioning some of their reported uses. Fortunately, however, the vitamins are astonishingly low in toxicity, and few people need to limit their intake. The optimum intake of vitamins improves the general health and strengthens the body's natural protective mechanisms. Vitamin D, however, should not be taken in excess, and too much vitamin A may cause headache.

The eye is an important organ and a delicate one. It is sensitive to the environment, including the molecules provided to it by the blood. Toxic substances can cause cataracts. Too high partial pressure of oxygen given to premature infants can cause restriction and obliteration of the arteries to the retina (retrolental fibroplasia) resulting in blindness. Chronic use of topical corticosteroids leads to glaucoma, cataracts, and other eye problems in some persons.

The value of a proper intake of vitamins to achieve good health of the eyes is well known. In some countries in southern and eastern Asia and in Brazil, blindness is often caused by vitamin-A deficiency. Xerophthalmia (abnormal dryness of the eyeball) resulting from lack of vitamin A is the principal cause of blindness in young children. Blindness from retinitis pigmentosa caused by the Bassen-Kornzweig syndrome can be prevented by massive doses of vitamins E and A.

The importance of vitamin C for good eye health is suggested by the fact that the concentration of this vitamin in the aqueous humor is very high, twenty-five times that in the blood plasma.

There is much evidence linking a low intake of vitamin C to cataract formation. Cataracts are opacities in the lens of the eye caused by the aggregation of protein molecules into particles large enough to scatter light. Early cataracts are caused by exposure of the pregnant mother or the child to toxic substances, by malnutrition, and by certain diseases, such as rubella and galactosemia. Senile cataracts may be caused by sunlight, high-energy radiation (X rays, neutrons), infections, diabetes, and poor nutrition.

Many investigators, beginning as long ago as 1935 with Monjukowa and Fradkin, have reported that there is very little vitamin C in the aqueous humor of cataractous eyes and that patients with cataracts often have a low level of vitamin C in the blood plasma (Lee, Lam, and Lai, 1977; Varma, Kumar, and Richards, 1979; Varma, Srivastava, and Richards, 1982; Varma et al., 1984). Monjukowa and Fradkin reported that the low concentration of vitamin C in the lens preceded the formation of the cataract and concluded that low vitamin C is the cause, not the consequence, of cataract formation. They suggested that in old age there is a decreased permeability of the eye to vitamin C and suggested that it might be overcome by a high intake of the vitamin. Varma et al. (1984) concluded from their studies that vitamins C and E are important for the prevention of senile cataracts.

There are also reports that the regular intake of high doses of vitamin $B_2$, 200 to 600 milligrams (mg) per day, slows down the development of cataracts. It is possible that the regimen described in Chapter 2, faithfully followed, would lead to a significant control over the development of senile cataracts.

A number of physicians have reported favorable experience with vitamin C for control of glaucoma. This painful affliction, so often terminating in blindness, is evidenced by increased intraocular pressure, causing swelling of the eyeball. The normal pressure is less than 20 millimeters of mercury (mm Hg). Mild glaucoma involves pressures 22 to 30 mm Hg, more severe 30 to 45 mm Hg, and very severe as much as 70 mm Hg. It sometimes has a hereditary cause, or it may result from an eye infection or other injury or from emotional stress. It can often be controlled by drugs.

Cheraskin, Ringsdorf, and Sisley (1983) in their discussion of glaucoma mention that Lane (1980) studied sixty subjects aged twenty-six to seventy-four and found an average intraocular pressure of 22.33 mm Hg when their average vitamin C intake was 75 mg per day, decreasing to 15.15 mm Hg when vitamin C intake was increased to 1200 mg per day. Other investigators have reported similar results. Most striking are the observations of Bietti (1967) and Virno et al. (1967), who gave doses of vitamin C of 30 to 40 grams (g) per day (0.5 g per kilogram body weight) to patients for as long as seven months. The intraocular pressure, initially 30 to 70 mm Hg, usually decreased to about half the value. High doses of vitamin C for some patients might control the glaucoma and for others decrease the amount of drugs needed for control.

The value of vitamin C in the healing of burns has been mentioned in Chapter 15. This vitamin also has been reported to have much value in the treatment of burns of the cornea of the eye. Many thousands of these burns are caused by industrial accidents in which the eye is exposed to an alkali solution or some other chemical. In 1978 the U.S. Consumer Protection Safety Commission reported 22,429 cases of chemical burns of the eye sustained in the home.

If such an accident occurs, the eye should be immediately irrigated with water, continuing for as long as two hours. Treatment by an ophthalmologist may be needed to save the sight. Ulceration of the cornea and perforation of the eyeball may result from the burns.

The injury may interfere with the transport of vitamin C into the eye, causing its concentration in the aqueous humor to drop to one-third of its normal value. It was reported long ago that vitamin C taken orally and applied topically as sodium ascorbate solution has much value in the treatment of these burns (Boyd and Campbell, 1950; Krueger, 1960; Stellamor-Peskir, 1961).

A thorough study of the nature of the action of vitamin C has been carried out over the last decade by Professor Roswell R. Pfister and his colleagues at the University of Alabama in Birmingham. In addition to conventional treatment, oral ascorbate and topical application of 10 percent sodium ascorbate solution may prevent ulceration.

Conjunctivitis is inflammation of the conjunctiva, the mucous membrane covering the inner surface of the eyelid and extending over the forward point of the eyeball. It may be caused by viral infections, allergies, intense light, or other sources of irritation. Pinkeye is a highly contagious variety of conjunctivitis. Iriditis and uveitis are inflammations of parts of the iris. All of these conditions may be benefitted by eyedrops of a freshly made isotonic solution (3.1 percent) of sodium ascorbate, as an adjunct to appropriate conventional treatment.

Acute otitis media, a bacterial or viral infection of the middle ear, causes much suffering for many people. It is usually the result of an upper respiratory infection. A good way to prevent this problem is to stop or control the respiratory infection, which can be done by the proper intake of vitamin C.

A correspondent has written to me that he has had success with infection of the middle ear by introducing some drops of a solution of sodium ascorbate into the ear. Although no thorough study of this treatment has been made, it seems to me to be sensible and worth trying.

The health of the mouth—the teeth, the gums, and the mucous membranes—depends upon the intake of vitamin C. A very low intake is disastrous. A moderate intake, such as is provided by an ordinary balanced diet, leads to moderately good health. For really good health of the mouth the optimum intake, provided by supplementary vitamin C in amounts of several grams per day, is required.

The effects of such a low intake as to lead to scurvy were described by Jacques De Vitry, bishop of Acre, speaking of the scurvy that afflicted Crusaders in the Holy Lands: ". . . their teeth and gums were soon tainted with a kind of gangrene and the sick could no longer eat." (Quoted by Fullmer, Martin, and Burns, 1961.)

A low intake of vitamin C affects the teeth directly. The cells that produce teeth deteriorate, and production of new dentin ceases and the dentin becomes porous. Good supplies of vitamin C, calcium, and fluoride are essential for healthy teeth.

Vitamin-C deficiency leads to capillary fragility. When the capillaries in the gums break down and bleed, the flow of blood to the gum tissues is interrupted and the tissues break down. The gums become swollen, violet colored, and soft, and are easily damaged. Infection and gangrene then follow, with danger of losing the teeth. The inflammation of the gums is called gingivitis, which becomes pyorrhea (periodontal disease) as it worsens.

The conclusion reached by Fullmer, Martin, and Burns (1961) and other investigators is that vitamin C is required for the formation and maintenance of normal dentin, bone, gums, and other connective tissues of the periodontium.

The usual treatment of periodontal disease is removal of plaque and sometimes selective grinding of teeth, changes in fillings and prostheses, and surgical excision of some gum tissue. This treatment is painful and expensive. The need for it can often be averted by increasing the intake of vitamin C.

For the foregoing statement there has been no extensive controlled clinical demonstration; so far as I know, no such trial has been carried out. It is instead supported by some individual cases, which, combined with our knowledge about the properties of vitamin C, commend the use of the vitamin for this purpose. I shall quote one case, that of Joshua M. Rabach, as told in his book on vitamin C (1972):

> I was introduced to vitamin C in 1966 by a dentist—not my regular dentist, but a new man whom I had consulted in desperation. The cause of my desperation was $900, the fee a periodontist wanted to get my gums in "better" shape. . . . The periodontist's prognosis was *really* grim. Bad enough that the fee would be $900; worse, he couldn't promise that his work would keep me from losing my teeth prematurely. . . . I saw the second dentist—now "my" dentist—a week later. After poking in my mouth and asking many questions, he agreed that my gums were receding and the problem shouldn't be ignored. He did not agree that periodontal work was necessary "for the time being." He prescribed a course of treatment as follows: I was to have my teeth cleaned then and every three months thereafter; I was to brush my teeth and massage my gums as instructed; morning and evening I was to take one of the white tablets he gave me.
>
> Six months passed before I learned that the white tablets were vitamin C (500 mg) and that, in certain kinds of gum disease, my dentist employs vitamin C therapy before other, more radical, kinds of treatment. . . . That was six years ago. I still have all my teeth, and my gums are healthy."

For Rabach 1000 mg of vitamin C per day was enough to prevent periodontal disease, but for some other people much more may be needed.

There is no doubt, as pointed out by Cheraskin and Ringsdorf in their book *Predictive Medicine* (1973), that your general health is affected to some extent by the health of your mouth and that the health of your mouth serves as an indicator of your general health. If you have trouble with your gums or teeth, increase your regular daily supplement of vitamin C and other vitamins to see if the problem cannot be solved in this simple way. Also, keep in touch with your dentist—and be sure that he or she knows about the value of proper nutrition.

# 24

## *Aging: Its Moderation and Delay*

Aging is the process of growing old and approaching normal death. It is accompanied by a gradual deterioration in the biochemical and physiological functions, such as the activity of enzymes, beginning at about age thirty-five years and continuing at an increasing rate thereafter.

The death rate increases with age, in consequence of the aging process. Death may be caused at any age by illness, accident, suicide, or murder. Accidents cause about 4.5 percent of all deaths in the United States, suicide about 1.4 percent, homicide about 1.0 percent, and illness about 93 percent. The mortality (death rate) from illness is a measure of the change in health caused by aging.

A valuable contribution to the study of aging was made in 1825 by an English scholar, Benjamin Gompertz, in a paper titled, "On the Nature of the Function Expressive of the Law of Human Mortality," published in the *Philosophical Proceedings of the Royal Society of London.* He studied the death records from four areas and noticed that the probability of death increases from year to year after age thirty or thirty-five by a constant factor. This means that the death rate after this age increases exponentially with increase in age. A useful way of checking the Gompertz relationship is to plot the logarithm of the mortality as a function of age; the Gompertz function is then a straight line.

In the illustration on page 234 I have plotted the logarithm of the number of deaths per one thousand persons per year in the United States as a function of the age. We see that a straight line fits the points from age thirty-five to age eighty-five. The slope of the line is such that we can say that for the average American the chance of death increases by 8.8 percent with each birthday after the thirty-fifth. His or her chance of dying during the year doubles with every increase of 8.2 years in age.

Over the range from thirty-five to seventy-five years of age the death rate for women remains close to one half that for men. From birth to age five the ratio for girls to boys is about 80 percent, but then it drops rapidly

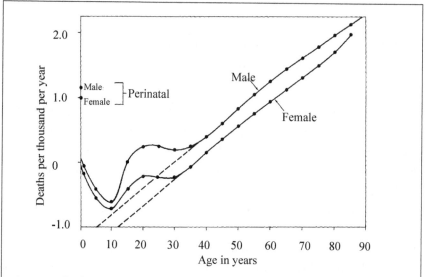

*Age-specific death rates. Gompertz diagram shows the logarithm of the annual death rate (per thousand living at each age) for white males and white females in the United States, 1979.*

to about 30 percent from age seventeen to twenty-five, rising to 50 percent at thirty-five. After age seventy-five it increases to about 65 percent.

The values in infancy are attributed to genetic defects and childhood diseases. The best health is seen to come at age ten. The high death rate from ages seventeen to thirty can be attributed mainly to automobile accidents. These accidents cause about forty thousand deaths per year, at the average age of twenty-two. The hump in the curve is higher for young men than for young women, who have a smaller chance of being killed at this age in an automobile accident.

The human female in the United States starts life with somewhat better health than the male, and by age thirty-five she is twice as healthy, as shown by the difference in the death rates. (Part of this difference is the result of more cigarette smoking by men than by women.) From then on, however, she ages at the same rate, as shown by the parallelism of the Gompertz lines.

People who smoke cigarettes have poor health. This poor health is made evident not only by the greater incidence of minor and major ailments but also by a striking increase in the death rate from all causes.

Cigarette smokers lead miserable lives. They are the captives of their drug addiction.

Scores of careful studies have been made in which the death rate of a population of cigarette smokers is compared with that of a similar population of nonsmokers. The smokers die faster than the nonsmokers, at every age and with every larger number of cigarettes smoked, and they die at a greater rate from every disease. Their natural protective mechanisms are damaged to such an extent as to make them vulnerable to every assault. Even the nonsmoking wives or husbands of cigarette smokers are damaged to such an extent by living in a smoky atmosphere as to have decreased life expectancy.

One-pack-a-day smokers have twice the chance of nonsmokers of dying at age fifty to sixty (somewhat smaller at higher ages), and two-pack-a-day smokers have three times the chance. Average smokers die about eight years younger than nonsmokers. Cigar smokers are not damaged so much, perhaps because they do not inhale the smoke. They die a year or two earlier than nonsmokers, however, often of cancer of the mouth or throat.

Twenty-five years ago I calculated that life expectancy is decreased by fifteen minutes for each cigarette smoked. Since smoking a cigarette takes about five minutes, I concluded that it is not worthwhile to smoke unless the smoker is more than four times as happy when smoking as when not smoking (Pauling, 1960).

Lung cancer is an unpleasant disease. A smoker living in the city has three hundred times greater chance of dying of lung cancer than a nonsmoker living in the country. There used to be a striking difference between the death rate of men from lung cancer and that of women, but now many more women are smoking, and they are catching up with the men, as shown in the top illustration on page 236.

The major cause of the decreased life expectancy as a result of smoking cigarettes is not cancer; it is heart disease. The bottom illustration on page 236 shows the logarithm of the death rate for coronary heart disease plotted against age, as found from a statistical study of 187,783 men by Hammond and Horn (1958). The slopes of the lines correspond to a doubling time of seven years. The curve for one-pack-a-day smokers is shifted to lower ages by seven years; that is, a one-pack-a-day smoker dies of coronary heart disease seven years earlier than a nonsmoker.

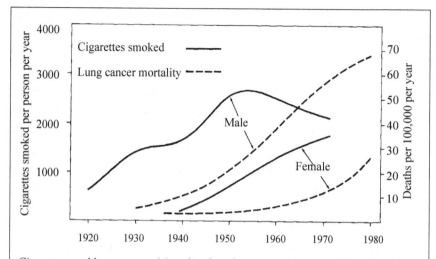

*Cigarettes and lung cancer. Mortality from lung cancer increased sharply about twenty-five years after cigarette smoking became popular, first among men and then among women. (From Cameron and Pauling, 1979.)*

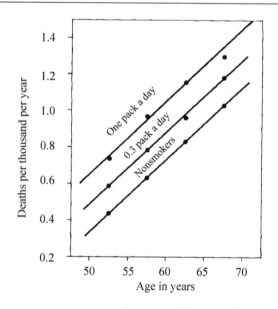

*Cigarettes and heart disease. Gompertz lines show the logarithm of the age-specific death rate (deaths per year per thousand persons) from coronary heart disease from a study of 187,783 men for one-pack-a-day cigarette smokers, 0.3-pack-a-day cigarette smokers, and nonsmokers.*

It was discovered many years ago that the level of vitamin C is lower in the blood of smokers than of nonsmokers (Strauss and Scheer, 1939), and scores of investigators have verified this observation. At one recent international conference on vitamin C four of the twenty papers presented were on this subject, with discussion of populations in Brazil, Canada, Switzerland, and the United States (Hoefel, 1977; Pelletier, 1977; Ritzel and Bruppacher, 1977; Sprince, Parker, and Smith, 1977).

The investigators agree that the vitamin-C level in the plasma in smokers is usually only half or two-thirds that of nonsmokers. McCormick in 1952 estimated that each cigarette smoked can destroy 25 milligrams (mg) of vitamin C, and Irwin Stone (1972) wrote that smokers suffer from a chronic subacute stage of scurvy.

A part of the poor health of cigarette smokers can be attributed to their deficiency in vitamin C. This deficiency can be rectified by the regular intake of a few grams of the vitamin each day. In this way some, but not all, of the harmful effects of smoking can be prevented. The smoker taking supplementary vitamin C will not catch up with the nonsmoker taking vitamin C until he or she stops smoking.

During the last few decades many people have stopped smoking, but others have not been able to escape from the addiction. For them there is the possibility of stopping in two stages. First, replace the cigarettes by chewing gum that contains nicotine (a prescription is needed), and after some time stop the gum.

With respect to alcohol, people may be divided into three classes: nondrinkers, moderate drinkers (one to four drinks per day), and heavy drinkers (more than four drinks per day). Many epidemiological studies have agreed that moderate drinkers on the average have slightly better health than nondrinkers, living about two years longer (Jones, 1956; Chope and Breslow, 1955). This effect of a moderate intake of alcohol may be the result of its acting as a tranquilizer. For this purpose it is less harmful than the tranquilizing drugs.

A high intake of alcohol can lead to great misery: interference with the ability of the person to get along with his or her spouse and children and with friends and business associates, destruction of the marriage, loss of the job, injury to himself or herself and others by drunk driving, arrest for drunkenness, and deterioration in physical and mental health. The effects of alcoholism are often compounded by the effects of cigarette smoking—heavy drinkers tend also to be heavy smokers.

The problem of alcoholism is hard to control. For many sufferers psychosocial support such as is provided by Alcoholics Anonymous has been helpful. The drug disulfiram has been effective for some alcoholics. It blocks the further oxidation of acetaldehyde, which is an oxidation product of alcohol. If a patient drinks alcohol after taking disulfiram he or she flushes, has a throbbing headache, and becomes nauseated and generally miserable. Such an experience may help him or her to give up drinking.

Roger J. Williams, the discoverer of pantothenic acid, has written about the value of vitamins in controlling alcoholism (Williams, 1951). Many investigators have found that the B vitamins and vitamin C have value. Abram Hoffer (1962) reported the control of acute alcoholism and delirium tremens by giving 9 grams (g) of niacin and 9 g of vitamin C per day. Niacin and vitamin C in relation to alcoholism are discussed by several authors, especially Hawkins, in the book *Orthomolecular Psychiatry.* Hawkins mentions one study in which 507 alcoholic patients on megavitamin treatment had been carefully followed for five years. All were long-time treatment failures before beginning to take the vitamins. Four hundred of the 507 had then remained sober for two years or more.

Sprince, Parker, and Smith (1977) have pointed out that heavy smoking and heavy drinking introduce into the body not only nicotine and ethanol but also other toxic substances, including acetaldehyde, N-nitroso compounds, polynuclear hydrocarbons, cadmium, and carbon monoxide. They also stimulate the release of catecholamines and corticosteroids, which are associated with adverse cardiovascular, respiratory, and nervous-system effects. They discuss the evidence that large doses of vitamin C have value in decreasing the toxic effects of acetaldehyde and some of the other substances.

In sum, cigarette smoking and excessive drinking are important factors leading to unhappiness, poor health, and early death.

Unavoidably, aging is accompanied by the slowing down of the physiological and biochemical processes that go on in the body, by decreasing strength, and by increasing incidence of illness and probability of death. The molecules of deoxyribonucleic acid (DNA) that control the synthesis of enzymes and other proteins undergo changes (somatic mutations) that lead to decreased production of these important substances or to changes in the molecules that decrease their activity. These changes in enzymes throughout the body are compounded by poor nutrition resulting from poor appetite, failure to take supplementary vitamins, and decreased activity of the digestive enzymes. The increase in the number of cells containing chromosomal abnormality contributes to these effects.

One theory of aging is that many molecular changes that build up in the human body with the passage of time are caused by free radicals, atoms or molecules that are especially reactive because they contain an unpaired electron (Harman, 1981). They can cause changes in the structure and function of important molecules, such as enzymes, and these changes can produce somatic mutations, mutations in the cells of the body as distinguished from mutations in the egg or sperm that may result in the birth of defective infants or in stillbirths or prevent the development of the fetus.

One characteristic of aging is the decrease in the elasticity of the skin and the production of wrinkles, especially in the areas exposed to sunlight—the hands, face, and neck. Bjorksten (1951) developed a theory of aging that explains these changes in the skin. In the process of the tanning of leather, molecules are introduced into the animal hide that form chemical bonds with the skin molecules and cross-link them into large aggregates, making the skin insoluble and tough. Bjorksten pointed out that in the course of increasing age the molecules in the human skin become cross-linked, and the skin becomes leathery.

This process can be slowed down by restricting the exposure of the skin to strong sunlight and by protecting it against the ultraviolet rays in the sunlight by using a lotion or salve that contains a substance that absorbs ultraviolet light. In the same way the chance of developing skin cancer is decreased.

A common accompaniment of old age is the formation of yellow deposits of cholesterol in the skin below the eyes. It has been observed that after such a deposit has been removed another does not appear if the blood level of cholesterol is decreased by the regular intake of high-dose vitamin C and by cutting down the intake of sucrose.

Ultraviolet light, X rays, cosmic rays, natural radioactivity, radioactive fallout from nuclear explosions, and mutagenic and carcinogenic chemicals produce their effects in part by forming free radicals, which then attack other molecules by changing them or cross-linking them. Part of the aging process may be the production of insoluble cross-linked sludge in cells throughout the body. The oxidation-reduction power of vitamin C and vitamin E provides protection against cancer and against aging by causing these molecules to combine with, reduce, and so destroy free radicals.

I do not recommend that drugs be taken in the effort to control aging. In a large (and, to me, rather confusing) popular book on aging and life extension by Pearson and Shaw (1982), the authors list thirty-one substances in their personal experimental life-extension formula. The list includes vitamins and other orthomolecular substances but also a number of drugs, including several that they describe as antioxidants: dilauryl thiopropionate, thiodipropionic acid, butylated hydroxytoluene, and hydrogenated ergot alkaloids (dihydroergocornine methanesulfonate, dihydroergocristine methanesulfonate, dihydroergocryptine methanesulfonate). I do not recommend taking these substances.

It is generally agreed that physical activity is important for the preservation of good health. Cheraskin and Ringsdorf in their book *Predictive Medicine* conclude that "the addition of physical activity discourages disease; the absence of exercise invites disease."

One early study is that of Hammond (1964), who reported on more than a million men and women who were enrolled in the study and then followed for two years. The death rates for 461,440 men between forty-five and ninety years of age are shown in the illustration on the facing page. It is seen that the men who did not exercise had death rates much larger than those of the men who did. The ratios correspond to between ten and twenty years difference in life expectancy. Other investigators have reported about a five-year difference between people who have little or no exercise and those who exercise moderately, with no advantage to strenuous exercise. People who exercise probably also follow other good health practices. Regular exercise benefits the heart and lungs, improves the blood vessels, increases muscular strength, tightens the ligaments, and helps to control the body weight.

The word *aerobic,* which means pertaining to the presence or use of the oxygen of the air, has been used in recent years to describe exercising vigorously enough to require more rapid breathing and an increased rate of the heartbeat. Aerobic exercise can be carried out by walking rapidly, jogging, bicycling, or swimming. There is no doubt that it is beneficial when it is practiced regularly and not excessively.

Every insult to the body, every illness, every stress increases the physiological age of a person and decreases his or her life expectancy. The amounts by which life expectancy is decreased by episodes of illness have been reported by Dr. Hardin Jones of the Donner Laboratory of Medical Physics of the University of California in Berkeley. He pointed out that there is evidence that aging results from episodes that damage the bodily functions. Among these damaging episodes are illnesses; each illness leaves the body with decreased ability to function in the optimum way. One disease experience tends to lead to another and to decrease life expectancy. This effect has been described by saying that each person is born with a certain amount of vitality, that some vitality is used up by each episode of illness or other cause of stress, and that death comes when the quota of vitality has been exhausted (Jones, 1955).

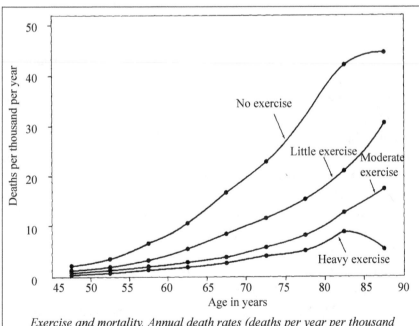

*Exercise and mortality. Annual death rates (deaths per year per thousand persons) differ significantly for men who exercise and men who do not. The ratios correspond to between ten and twenty years difference in life expectancy. (From Hammond, 1964.)*

Jones concludes that the way to avoid disease is by not having earlier diseases: ". . . we may be able to achieve an even greater preservation of physiologic health by the elimination of our more trivial diseases; the successful removal of such 'benign' diseases as the common cold, chicken pox, measles, etc., may be more effective in lessening the disease tendency of later life than anything else we may attempt to do."

By controlling the common cold, the flu, and other ailments through the intake of supplementary vitamin C and other health practices, we not only avoid the discomfort of these diseases but also slow down the rate at which our bodies deteriorate and at which our stores of vitality are used up. Old people and sick people often move rapidly toward death because they do not eat enough food. Their malnutrition is often the result of poverty, but it may also come about because the food does not taste good or smell good to them. The deterioration in the senses of taste and olfaction may itself be the result of malnutrition, but it is often exacerbated by the toxic products of illnesses, especially cancer, by the changes accompanying the aging process, and by poor health habits, such as constipation.

Good nutrition can decrease the number of these episodes and prevent the onslaught on the physiological age by improving the general health, strengthening the body's natural protective mechanisms, and helping to control illness. To all these ends, the optimum intake of supplementary vitamins contributes heavily. It is possible, as Lewis Thomas has said, for us all to die healthy!

Even if the aging person is not healthy, the last days can be made more comfortable by good nutrition. Dr. Ewan Cameron has reported that patients with advanced cancer who began taking 10 grams of vitamin C per day quickly responded by having better appetite and eating more, probably in part because the food smelled better and tasted better. The resulting improved nutrition may be part of the explanation of the effect of the vitamin on the health of the patients.

At the present time the average age at death in the United States is about seventy-five years. The slope of the Gompertz curve begins to decrease beyond age eighty-five; that is, the death rate does not increase quite so rapidly with increasing age as in earlier years. This effect is probably the result of the selection of the survivors as generally healthier people than those who have died. At age 100 the annual death rate is 0.30, and this rate increases by about 0.012 for each succeeding year. A calculation on this basis indicates that in the U.S. population there should be one person who has survived to age 125.

My estimate, made on the basis of the results of epidemiological studies and other observations, is that through the optimum use of vitamin supplements and other health measures, the length of the period of well-being and the length of life could be increased by twenty-five to thirty-five years. For the subpopulation following this regimen the life expectancy would be 100 to 110 years, and in the course of time the maximum age, reached by a few, might be 150 years.

# IV

## *VITAMINS AND DRUGS*

# 25

## *Organized Medicine and the Vitamins*

Fifteen years ago I was writing *Vitamin C and the Common Cold*. I was pleased with myself. I had made many discoveries in chemistry and other fields of science and had even made some contributions to medicine, although it was not clear that these contributions would have much effect in decreasing the amount of suffering caused by disease. Now, I thought, I have learned about something that can decrease somewhat the amount of suffering for tens of millions or even hundreds of millions of people, something that had been noticed by other scientists and by some physicians but for some reason had been ignored.

I thought that all that I needed to do was to present the facts in a simple, straightforward, and logical way in order that physicians and people generally would accept them. I was right, in this expectation, about the people but wrong about the physicians, or perhaps not about the physicians as individuals but about organized medicine.

A modest number of all U.S. physicians, perhaps 1 percent, are now practicing orthomolecular medicine and calling themselves orthomolecular physicians. They make use of conventional prophylactic and therapeutic measures and in addition supplement these measures by the proper recommendations about the optimum intake of vitamins and other nutrients, together with the use of other orthomolecular substances. The American Orthomolecular Medical Association, of which I have been honorary president since its formation ten years ago, today has five hundred members.

It is not easy to be an orthomolecular physician. This field has not yet been recognized as a medical specialty. Orthomolecular medicine for some reason seems to be considered a threat to conventional medicine. Orthomolecular physicians are harassed by the medical establishment. One of my friends, in fact the present president of the Orthomolecular Medical Association, had his California medical license revoked in 1984 and has had to move to another state in order to continue his practice of medicine. I testified at his hearing, where I was asked some rather silly questions by the assistant attorney general of the State of California. None of his patients presented charges against him; instead, the charges were brought by another physician, who may have felt that orthomolecular medicine constituted unfair competition, in that the patients are benefitted too much and at too low a cost (vitamins are much cheaper than drugs). My understanding is that the principal charge against my friend is that "He did not try hard enough to get his cancer patient who had decided against chemotherapy to change her mind." This sort of excuse seems to me to be about as flagrant as the one used thirty-three years ago by the U.S. Department of State for not giving me my passport to permit me to attend a two-day international symposium in London arranged by the Royal Society of London to discuss my discoveries about the structure of proteins. I was to have been the first speaker. The State Department said that my "anti-Communist statements had not been strong enough."

In Chapter 13 I mentioned that whereas many people believe that vitamin C helps prevent colds, most physicians deny that this vitamin has much value. My experiences after the publication of *Vitamin C and the Common Cold* (1970) substantiated this idea and have stimulated me to attempt to explain the fact.

Many physicians have written me that they find vitamin C to be effective in controlling the common cold and other infections of the respiratory tract and use it in treating themselves, members of their families, and patients. Some hundreds of nonphysicians also have written me about their successful use of vitamin C, usually over a period of years. I have received only three or four letters from physicians who are convinced that vitamin C has no such effectiveness. It is likely, however, that this small number is misleading: skeptics do not write to me.

Cortez F. Enloe, Jr., M.D., editor *of Nutrition Today,* in an editorial (1971) on my book, mentioned that he had not found one physician among his friends or among those attending a meeting of a state medical society who "would admit to having even read the book." I surmise that most physicians have read neither this book nor any of the articles describing the controlled studies that have been made of vitamin C in relation to the common cold. I estimate that one American physician in a thousand has read the 1942 article by Cowan, Diehl, and Baker, and that one in ten thousand has read the 1961 article by Ritzel. The opinions of all but a handful are secondhand.

Almost all physicians rely upon the statements made by authorities. This situation is inevitable. The practicing physician is too busy to make a thorough study of the complex and often voluminous original literature on every medical topic. For example, a physician in Albuquerque, New Mexico, wrote a letter to the local newspaper, saying that it had been shown that vitamin C has no value at all in protecting against the common cold and other respiratory diseases. I wrote to him, asking him on which published accounts of investigations he had based his statement. He replied that he was a gynecologist and knew little about the infectious diseases; he had based his statement in the newspaper on information given to him by his old professor, Dr. F. J. Stare, by telephone. This physician had relied upon an authority who, like many members of the medical establishment, has ignored the mounting evidence in favor of the treatment of the common cold with vitamin C.

Some of the medical investigators themselves have failed to analyze their own observations in a sound way and to act in accordance with these results. Cowan, Diehl, and Baker (1942) provide an example. In their careful study these three physicians observed a decreased incidence of colds for the ascorbic-acid group (relative to the placebo group) by 15 percent and a decreased severity by 19 percent (Chapter 13). These decreases are statistically significant, according to the rules generally accepted by statisticians, and they should not be ignored. Nevertheless, Cowan, Diehl, and Baker did ignore the results. In the summary of their paper, which is the only part that would be read by most readers of the *Journal of the American Medical Association,* they omitted mention of these facts. Their summary consists of a single sentence: "This controlled study yields no indication that either large doses of vitamin C or large doses of vitamins A, $B_1$, $B_2$, C, D, and nicotinic acid have any important effect on the number or severity of infections of the upper respiratory tract when administered to young adults who presumably are already on a reasonably adequate diet."

In my opinion this statement is incorrect. The vitamin-C subjects had only 69 percent as much illness with the common cold (as measured by days of illness per subject, the product of the number of colds per subject and the days of illness per cold) as the placebo subjects. This surely is an important effect, the result of a 15 percent decrease in incidence and a 19 percent decrease in severity. The only explanation of the action of Cowan, Diehl, and Baker in writing the summary in this way is that they did not consider the observed effect important; but surely most people would consider it important to be able to cut their amount of illness with the common cold by nearly one-third. In a letter to *The New York Times* in 1970, Diehl indicated that he still thought that he and his collaborators had not obtained positive results. In a reply to that letter I pointed out that Dr. Diehl and I agreed about the facts but disagreed about the word *important,* and that Cowan, Diehl, and Baker had made an error of judgment in omitting from their summary mention of the fact that they had observed a statistically significant protective effect of ascorbic acid against the common cold.

Glazebrook and Thomson (1942) also misconstrued their own observations in the summary of their paper. It is mentioned in Chapter 13 that in their main study, with 435 subjects, they found the incidence of colds and tonsillitis in the ascorbic-acid group to be 13 percent less than for the controls. The incidence of colds alone was 17 percent less in this main study and 12 percent less in a second study, with 150 subjects, in which they also observed a 15 percent smaller incidence of colds and tonsillitis. These facts, presented in the body of the paper, are not repeated in the summary. Instead, the statement is made, contrary to the facts, that "the incidences of common cold and tonsillitis were the same in the two groups." Similar failure to present in the summaries of their papers a correct account of the results of their work can be found also in the reports of other investigators.

The actions of these investigators in understating their observations in the summaries of their papers may have been the result of a sort of conservatism and restraint, the feeling that one should not claim that a therapeutic or preventive effect has been observed unless it is a large and obvious one. It is my opinion that feelings of this sort, admirable though they may be, do not justify an incorrect description of one's observations. The authors of a scientific or medical article should always strive for accuracy. It is just as wrong to understate one's findings as to overstate them. There is no doubt that the original investigators themselves have been partly responsible for the failure of the medical establishment to recognize the significance of the observations.

The attitude of the medical authorities is illustrated by the statement in the unsigned editorial in *Nutrition Reviews* (1967), quoted in Chapter 3, that there is no conclusive evidence that ascorbic acid has any protective or therapeutic effect on the course of the common cold in healthy people. The study of the evidence made by the anonymous author was clearly a careless and superficial one, in that, as is mentioned in Chapter 13, he erroneously reported that Ritzel (1961) had observed only a 39 percent reduction in the number of days of illness and a 36 percent reduction in the incidence of symptoms, the correct values being nearly twice as great (61 percent and 65 percent, respectively). There is no indication in the editorial that its author made any attempt to analyze the evidence in the published papers to find out whether the statement could be made that the evidence shows with statistical significance that ascorbic acid either has or has not a protective or therapeutic effect (of a given assumed magnitude). It seems not unlikely that the author was misled by the incorrect summary statements of some investigators, as mentioned above, and by the prevailing medical opinion, and that this bias led to the superficiality of his editorial.

Even after the appearance of *Vitamin C and the Common Cold* (7 December 1970), when the evidence was clearly brought to the attention of the medical authorities, they continued to deny the existence of the evidence. This denial was sometimes accompanied by statements that contradicted or misconstrued the facts.

Among the authorities who denied this evidence was Dr. Charles C. Edwards, the chief of the U.S. Food and Drug Administration (FDA). On 18 December 1970 Commissioner Edwards telephoned me and asked me to come to Washington for a conference about this matter with the Food and Drug Administration. I agreed and suggested that some questions be clarified by correspondence before the meeting. On the very next day, as reported in a United Press International dispatch under the byline of Craig A. Palmer, printed in many newspapers, he summoned reporters to tell them that the run on drugstores for vitamin C since publication of my book was "ridiculous" and stated that "There is no scientific evidence and [there] never have been any meaningful studies indicating that vitamin C is capable of preventing or curing colds." I wrote several letters to Commissioner Edwards, asking him to explain how he could reconcile this statement with the existence of the evidence summarized in my book, especially the results obtained by Ritzel. In his replies, which included material by Allan L. Forbes, M.D., deputy director of the Division of

Nutrition of the FDA, he made several critical comments about the work of Ritzel and of other investigators quoted in my book. He concluded, however, that Ritzel "does present what seem to be meaningful data." With "clarification" carried as far as it could go by correspondence, I wrote Commissioner Edwards in June 1971 that I would come to Washington for the conference immediately or at a date convenient to him. He then withdrew his invitation, and the conference has never taken place.

Despite the repeated findings that an increased intake of vitamin C does provide some protection against respiratory illnesses and other diseases, the federal medical agencies continue to deny that it has any value. In August 1975 the National Institutes of Health issued a pamphlet (566-AMDD-975-B) containing many incorrect statements: "The body uses only the amount of ascorbic acid it needs and excretes the rest in the urine!" "Other questions about the safety of high doses of ascorbic acid include its possible effect on fertility and the fetus, interference with the treatment of patients whose urine must be kept alkaline. . . ." "Recent reports further demonstrate that high doses of vitamin C destroy substantial amounts of the vitamin $B_{12}$ in food." It is stated in the pamphlet that it is reasonable to assume that 45 milligrams (mg) per day is sufficient to prevent disease and maintain health. The only mention of the evidence is the assertion that the studies are unconvincing.

The authors of the authoritative reference books and textbooks have failed to assess properly the evidence about vitamin C. For example, in the sixth edition of the textbook *Human Nutrition and Dietetics* by Davidson, Passmore, Brock, and Truswell (1975), the authors write: "The claim by Pauling (1970) that the consumption of 1 or 2 g per day promotes optimum health and protects against the common cold rests on slender evidence." In support of this statement they cite the conclusions of Cowan et al. and of Glazebrook and Thomson but say nothing about their data. They make no mention of the work by Ritzel, even though they knew about Ritzel's study. One of the authors, Passmore, wrote a review of *Vitamin C and the Common Cold,* in which I discussed that work (Passmore, 1971). Why these authorities in the field of nutrition should misinterpret and ignore the evidence is not clear.

The *Medical Letter,* a nonprofit publication on drugs and therapeutics for physicians put out by Drug and Therapeutic Information Inc., published an unsigned, unfavorable review of *Vitamin C and the Common Cold* on 25 December 1970. The anonymous author said that I had relied on uncontrolled studies and went on to say, "A controlled trial of the effectiveness of vitamin C against upper respiratory infections must be conducted over a long period and include many hundreds of persons to give meaningful results. No such trial has been performed." I wrote a letter pointing out the falsity of this statement and showing the writer of the article how the Cowan, Diehl, and Baker study, for one, surely met all of his specifications. I concluded by asking the *Medical Letter* to publish my letter.

This was not done; instead, on 28 May 1971 the *Medical Letter* published a second article with the title "Vitamin C—Were the Trials Well Controlled and Are Large Doses Safe?" This article argued that the Cowan, Diehl, and Baker study had to be rejected because it was not double-blind (although Cowan himself said in a letter to me that it could be so described) and the allocation of subjects to the ascorbic-acid group and the placebo group was not randomized (although the investigators describe their method of randomization in their paper). The study by Ritzel was attacked on the trivial ground that Ritzel had not given the ages and sex of the subjects. In fact, his paper indicated that the subjects were all schoolboys (in a letter to me Ritzel verified that they were all boys and said that they were fifteen to seventeen years old). The article also raised the question, without offering any evidence, of the possible formation of kidney stones.

The weakness of the arguments advanced by the *Medical Letter* and some other critics caused a Canadian physician, Dr. Abram Hoffer, to make the following comment (1971): "[These critics] use two sets of logic. Before they are prepared to look at Dr. Pauling's hypothesis, they demand proof of the most rigorous kind. But when arguing against his views, they refer to evidence of the flimsiest sort for the toxicity of ascorbic acid."

Popular writers are, of course, misled by such authoritative misstatements. In a thoroughly unreliable article in *Reader's Digest* (Ross, 1971) there is the sentence, "But some of these patients [who had taken 4000 to 10,000 mg of vitamin C a day] have developed kidney stones." My request to *Reader's Digest* and the author of the article to give me the references to the medical literature about these patients was unsuccessful. The *Medical Letter* did not mention any patients in whom ascorbic acid had caused kidney stones to form but mentioned only such a possibility.

For many years the stand of the American Medical Association, as expressed especially by Dr. Philip L. White, its principal spokesman on nutrition and health, was that vitamin C has no value in preventing or treating the common cold or other diseases (White, 1975). On 10 March 1975 the AMA issued a statement to the press with the heading "Vitamin C will not prevent or cure the common cold." The basis for this quite negative statement was said to be two papers published on that day in the *Journal of the American Medical Association* (Karlowski et al., 1975; Dykes and Meier, 1975). Karlowski and his associates had made a study of ascorbic acid in relation to the common cold, with employees of the National Institutes of Health as the subjects. The paper by Dykes and Meier was a review of some other studies. The results observed by Ritzel (1961), Sabiston and Radomski (1974), and some other investigators were not, however, presented. Despite their incomplete coverage of the evidence, Dykes and Meier concluded that the studies seemed to show that vitamin C decreases the amount of illness accompanying the common cold, although in their opinion its protective effect might not be large enough to be clinically important. Thus their review of the evidence did not provide any basis for the AMA statement that vitamin C will not prevent or cure the common cold.

In order to present to the readers of the *Journal of the American Medical Association (JAMA)* an account of all of the evidence, I at once prepared a thorough but brief analysis of thirteen controlled trials and submitted it to the editor on 19 March. He returned it to me twice, with suggestions for minor revisions, which I made. Finally on 24 September, six months after I had submitted the article to him, he wrote me that it was not wholly convincing and that he had decided to reject the article and not publish it in *JAMA*. It was later published in *Medical Tribune* (Pauling, 1976b).

It is my opinion that it is quite improper for the editor of *JAMA* (or of any other journal) to follow the policy of publishing only those papers that support only one side of a scientific or medical question and also to interfere with the proper discussion of the question by holding a paper that had been submitted to him for half a year, during which period, according to accepted custom, the paper could not be submitted to another journal.

This is not the only example of this sort of action by the editor of *JAMA*. The paper by Herbert and Jacob, which makes the claim that vitamin C taken with a meal destroys the vitamin $B_{12}$ in the food and may cause a serious disease similar to pernicious anemia, was published in *JAMA*. When Newmark and his coworkers found that the claim could not be substantiated, and that in fact vitamin C does not destroy the vitamin $B_{12}$ in the food, they sent their paper to the editor *of JAMA,* which seems clearly to be the place where the correction should be published. He held it for half a year, and then refused to publish it, thus delaying its publication in another journal and preventing many of the readers of the original article by Herbert and Jacob from learning that their results were incorrect. These actions suggest that the AMA works to protect American physicians from information that runs counter to its own prejudices. The evidence indicates that the AMA is prejudiced against vitamin C.

The editor of *JAMA* and his advisers have a hard task to handle. Medicine is an extremely complicated subject. It is to a large extent based on the sciences—physics, physical chemistry, organic chemistry, biochemistry, molecular biology, bacteriology, virology, genetics, pharmacology, and others—but it has not yet become a science. No one can know thoroughly more than a small part of medicine. Moreover, many physicians are limited in their scientific knowledge and have not had experience in the field of scientific discovery. They do not know how to greet and how to assess new ideas.

The literature of science and medicine has now become so extensive that an editor may form his or her opinions on the basis of only a small part of the existing evidence. The editor of *JAMA* may have been too busy to look thoroughly into the vitamin-C question. The distinguished editor of another medical journal, *Modern Medicine,* Dr. Irvine H. Page, was on unsure ground when he wrote an editorial entitled "Are Truth and Plain Dealing Going Out of Style?" for his 15 January 1976 issue. Page had this to say: "When even responsible investigators use shady tactics to promote their 'discoveries,' it is no wonder that the public loses confidence in the scientific establishment." He went on to say: "To me, the most tragic example of self-deception was that in which Dr. Linus Pauling—twice a Nobel prize winner—proposed and exploited the use of huge doses of vitamin C for the common cold."

After an exchange of correspondence with me, Page retracted his statements about me in the 1 July 1976 issue of *Modern Medicine.* There he wrote:

> I withdraw this statement and regret the unjustified use of the pejorative words that because of a misunderstanding I improperly claimed that Dr. Pauling demanded that his critics prove him wrong. Dr. Pauling in fact presented in his 1970 book *Vitamin C and the Common Cold* and in his articles a reasonable summary of the published reports of the several controlled studies that had been made, together with his own discussion and conclusions. He has not demanded that his critics prove him wrong, although he has urged them to examine the evidence. . . . The high opinion that this magazine has of Dr. Pauling is indicated by our action in giving him the Modern Medicine Award for Distinguished Achievement in 1963 for his discovery that sickle cell anemia is a molecular disease.

Page also said that physicians should provide reliable information about such major public-health topics as nutrition (including the use of vitamin C), drugs, immunizations, and life-styles and by their own deportment should earn and keep the respect and confidence of those they hope to benefit by preventive medicine. In addition, *Modern Medicine* published in the 1 July 1976 issue a paper by me on the argument for vitamin C in maintaining health and preventing disease.

*Modern Medicine* seems to be developing a more open-minded attitude toward the recent progress in nutrition and preventive medicine, following the lead of another medical magazine, *Medical Tribune,* which over the years has continually been free from bias of this sort. I hope that in the course of time some improvement will become discernible in the publications of the American Medical Association.

Physicians must be conservative in the practice of medicine, but the medical profession needs to be open to new ideas, if medicine is to progress. A new idea, that large amounts of vitamins might help in controlling disease, was discussed about fifty years ago but was not property developed. Claus W. Jungeblut, the physician who first showed that ascorbic acid can inactivate viruses and provide some protection against viral diseases (Chapter 14) became discouraged by the poor reception given his idea and went into another field of medicine.

The most recent and the most outrageous action by organized medicine against the new science of nutrition and the well-being of the American people has been perpetrated by the Mayo Clinic. This action, the publication of a fraudulent paper in the 17 January 1985 issue of *The New England Journal of Medicine,* has been mentioned in Chapter 19. The principal author of the paper, Dr. Charles G. Moertel, and his five collaborators, deliberately misrepresented their investigation of the value of high doses of vitamin C for patients with metastatic cancer of the colon or rectum as a repetition of and check on the work by Dr. Ewan Cameron and his collaborators (of whom I was one). They concluded that high doses of vitamin C have no value for patients with advanced cancer. In fact (although they suppressed this information), they supplied vitamin C to the patients in a way completely different from that followed by Cameron.†Cameron's patients received high doses of vitamin C from the beginning of their treatment until the end of their lives or the present time, as much as twelve or thirteen years, whereas the Mayo Clinic patients received a smaller amount for a short time. Cameron and I had warned that suddenly stopping the high doses of vitamin C could be dangerous. This warning was ignored by the Mayo Clinic doctors.

The National Cancer Institute was also a victim of the Mayo Clinic fraud. Its officers were misled into thinking that the Mayo Clinic had repeated Cameron's work. By making a public statement to this effect, they loaned their authority to this bogus effort and compounded its error.

The Mayo Clinic doctors have refused to discuss this matter with me. I conclude that they are not scientists, devoted to the search for the truth. I surmise that they are so ashamed of themselves that they would prefer that the matter be forgotten. The Mayo Clinic used to have a great reputation. This episode indicates to me that it is no longer deserved. I shall refer to the Mayo Clinic again in the next chapter, comparing vitamins and drugs.

In 1985 the American Medical Association, the American Cancer Society, and the editors of the leading medical journals have not yet recognized that vitamin supplements in the optimum amounts have value. There are indications, however, that a change in their attitude may come

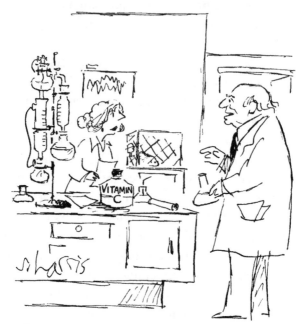

"ACTUALLY I STARTED OUT IN QUANTUM MECHANICS, BUT SOMEWHERE ALONG THE WAY I TOOK A WRONG TURN."

during the next few years. Individual physicians in large numbers have changed from being antagonistic to high intakes of vitamins to being willing to consider the idea that they have value. I am impressed by the number of them who write or telephone me or one of my associates, especially Dr. Ewan Cameron, for additional information. Also, many people have written me about the response of their physician when he (or, rarely, she) learned that the patient had been taking 5 or 10 grams (g) of vitamin C per day. A decade ago the patients often refrained from telling the physician about this intake. When the physician learned about it, he would say, "You've been listening to Linus Pauling—that quack!" or sometimes would make a stronger, more vulgar statement. During the last three or four years, patients have been reporting to me that the physician has said, "It may not be the vitamin C, but keep on taking it!" or, if the patient had not divulged his or her intake, "I don't know what you have been doing, but keep on doing it."

A dozen years ago I was persona non grata in medical schools. During the last few years I have spoken many times about vitamins in medical schools and at medical meetings—ten times in 1984. On 14 November 1984, for example, I spoke on the value of nutritional science in medicine to a large audience in Jefferson Medical College, Philadelphia, at the invitation of the Division of Gastroenterology and the Jefferson Nutrition Program. After my lecture one of the professors of medicine said to me, "Up to two hours ago I believed that vitamins in amounts greater than the RDAs had no value. I have now changed my mind, because of the facts that you presented."

Also during 1984 I gave twenty-five talks to health groups or other groups of laymen or on television or radio programs. There is no doubt that the public has great interest in improving health by the optimum intake of vitamin C and other nutrients. In November I appeared on the Toronto evening television program called Speaking Out. The viewers could telephone the station and vote on a question about vitamins. The station received 25,229 telephone calls during the program. I was told that this was the largest popular response of any program in the history of the station.

This great popular interest in improved nutrition is now having an influence on the medical establishment. I believe that the time has come not only for orthomolecular medicine to be recognized as a field of specialization but also for all physicians and surgeons to incorporate improvements of nutrition into their procedures for helping their patients.

# 26

## Vitamins and Drugs Compared

If you have a serious problem with your health you should see your physician. He or she probably will prescribe a drug for you. Often the drug is effective in controlling the disease. Also, the drug may have harmful side effects. Sometimes a second drug is prescribed to control the side effects of the first drug.

The reason that most drugs are available only through a doctor's prescription is that they are dangerous. They are still dangerous even though a doctor prescribes them.

In case of serious illness the drug may be essential. Before taking it, you should understand why it should be taken and what the likely consequences will be, and you should combine your own judgment with that of the doctor.

In the book *Matters of Life and Death,* cited in Chapter 1, Dr. Eugene D. Robin says:

> The doctor's opinion is not infallible and you need not be passive. It is your future that is being decided. Remember that you, the patient, have the highest stake in the decision—the most to gain and the most to lose. You, the patient, if you are capable of making the decision, are the one to decide what constitutes a happy and productive life. Don't let your doctor, however well intentioned, usurp this right.

This advice may be especially important with respect to vitamins and to nutrition in general. Even the specialists in nutrition tend to be unreliable because education in nutrition has not changed very much during the last thirty years and there is a bias against the new knowledge about the value of megavitamins.

Also, you should not consider that the over-the-counter nonprescription drugs, even aspirin, are safe. Your health is apt to be better if you do not take any of them. Be leery of the statements made on television commercials. For example, hemorrhoids are probably more effectively controlled by taking vitamin C in large enough amounts to keep the stools soft and liquid and by applying vitamin E topically than by using Preparation H.

Drugs are dangerous; vitamins are safe. The vitamins are *foods*—essential foods, required by human beings for life and good health. They are safe, even when taken in large amounts. Side effects occur only infrequently and are rarely serious (Chapter 27). Also, vitamins are inexpensive, compared with most drugs.

In this chapter I shall use vitamin C as my main example, comparing it, for example, with the over-the-counter drugs that are sold as remedies for the common cold.

The drugs that are used in tremendous amounts for treating the common cold are very different from vitamin C in that they are harmful and dangerous and are themselves responsible for much illness and many deaths. They do not control the viral infection but only the symptoms, to some extent, whereas vitamin C controls the infection itself, as well as the symptoms.

Aspirin is an example of a drug that is said to have low toxicity and few side effects. This drug, which is the chemical substance acetylsalicylic acid, is present in most cold medicines. The fatal dose for an adult is 20 grams (g) to 30 g. The ordinary aspirin tablet contains 324 milligrams (mg) (5 grains); hence sixty to ninety tablets can kill an adult, and a smaller amount can kill a child. Aspirin is the most common single poison used by suicides (it is second only to the group of substances used in sleeping pills). About 15 percent of accidental poisoning deaths of young children are caused by aspirin. Many lives would be saved if the medicine chest contained vitamin C in place of aspirin and the other cold medicines.

Some people show a severe sensitivity to aspirin, such that a decrease in circulation of the blood and difficulty in breathing follow the ingestion of 0.3 g to 1 g (one to three tablets).

The symptoms of mild aspirin poisoning arc burning pain in the mouth, throat, and abdomen, difficulty in breathing, lethargy, vomiting, ringing in the ears, and dizziness. More severe poisoning leads to delirium, fever, sweating, incoordination, coma, convulsions, cyanosis (blueness of the skin), failure of kidney function, respiratory failure, and death.

Aspirin, like other salicylates, has the property that in concentrated solution it can attack and dissolve tissues. An aspirin tablet in the stomach may attack the stomach wall and cause the development of a bleeding ulcer.

The U.S. Centers for Disease Control have reported that if children and teenagers suffering from influenza or chicken pox are given aspirin they have fifteen to twenty-five times greater chance of developing Reye's syndrome, an acute encephalopathy and fatty degeneration of the viscera, causing death in about 40 percent of the patients. In 1982 the Department of Health and Human Services announced that it would require labels on aspirin warning against its use for childhood diseases, but it withdrew the proposal after the drug industry lobbied heavily against it. In 1985, however, the firms voluntarily agreed to use those warnings. Then in October 1985 the Subcommittee on Health of the House of Representatives Energy and Commerce Committee stated that the voluntary agreement was not effective and voted to require explicit messages on all aspirin bottles warning of the association between the drug and the often fatal Reye's syndrome in children and teenagers.

Aspirin had been in use as a nonprescription drug, sold casually over the counter, for more than a century before the physiological basis of its pain-killing and fever-reducing action was discovered in 1971. Then it was found that aspirin acts upon a central hormonal control system in the body. If it were now coming on to the market from a pharmaceutical laboratory, it would be surely placed under the constraint of prescription. The story of how its potency came to be understood is a roundabout one.

In 1930 Kurzrok and Lieb in the Department of Obstetrics and Gynecology of Columbia University in New York reported that women receiving artificial insemination sometimes showed violent contraction or relaxation of the uterus. In 1933 Goldblatt in England reported that human semen contains a substance that reduces blood pressure and stimulates smooth muscle. At about the same time the Swedish investigator U. S. von Euler isolated a similar factor from the prostate glands of humans, monkeys, sheep, and goats (von Euler, 1937). He gave the name prostaglandin to the factor. Since then many prostaglandins have been found. They are called PGE1, PGE2, PGE3, PGA1, PGB1, and so on. Intensive study of these substances has since been carried out by many researchers; about thirty-five thousand scientific and medical papers on the prostaglandins had been published by 1980.

The prostaglandins are hormones, serving as messengers to control the biochemical and physiological activity in the body. They are rather simple compounds, the formula of PGE1, for example, being $C_{20}H_{34}O_5$. The molecule consists of a five-member ring of atoms with two chains attached, one being a fatty acid and the other a hydrocarbon chain with an attached hydroxyl group. They are fat-soluble lipids. They are found in many tissues in addition to the male reproductive organs and have many functions.

There was evidence that prostaglandins are involved in the processes that cause inflammation, fever, and pain. In 1971 John R. Vane, a British pharmacologist working in the University of London, made the important discovery that the action of aspirin as an anti-inflammatory, antipyretic, and analgesic agent depends upon its power to inhibit the synthesis of the prostaglandins PGE2 and PGE2-alpha. Aspirin thus reduces the redness, pain, and swelling associated with inflammation of tissues. It is one of the few drugs for which we know the mechanism of its action in the human body.

Such is the nature of this "harmless" household remedy, prescribed by the physician on the telephone in lieu of a house call. Vitamin C has been found to act in a way similar to aspirin in inhibiting the synthesis of some prostaglandins (Pugh, Sharma, and Wilson, 1975; Sharma, 1982). This may be the mechanism of the effectiveness of large doses of vitamin C in controlling inflammation, fever, and pain. It differs from aspirin, however, in that it increases the rate of synthesis of PGE1 (Horrobin, Oka, and Manku, 1979). Horrobin, Manku et al. (1979) have pointed out that this prostaglandin is involved in lymphocyte function and other aspects of the immune system, in rheumatoid arthritis, in various autoimmune diseases, in multiple sclerosis, and in cancer. Further studies of the relations between vitamin C and the several prostaglandins may throw additional light on the complex problem of the remarkable properties of this vitamin. At the present time it is worth while to keep in mind that an increased intake of vitamin C may act in such a way as to obviate the need to take aspirin or any similar drug. Its power to control pain in cancer patients was reported by Cameron and Baird in 1973 and has been reported also for headache, arthritis, toothache, and earache. As distinguished from aspirin, vitamin C is a substance naturally and necessarily present in the tissues of the body.

Several other substances closely related to aspirin have analgesic properties (the ability to decrease the sensitivity to pain) and antipyretic properties (the ability to lower increased body temperature) and are present in some of the popular cold medicines. One of these is salicylamide (the amide of salicylic acid). It has about the same toxicity as aspirin: 20 g to 30 g is the lethal dose for an adult.

The closely related analgesic substances acetanilide (N-phenylacetamide), phenacetin (acetophenetidin), and acetaminophen (p-hydroxyacetanilide) are used alone or in combination with other drugs in a number of cold medicines, in amounts of 150 to 200 mg per tablet. These substances damage the liver and kidneys. A single dose of 0.5 g to 5 g may cause fall of blood pressure, failure of kidney function, and death by respiratory failure.

Many of the cold medicines available without prescription contain not only aspirin or some other analgesic but also an antihistamine and an antitussive (to control severe coughing). For example, one preparation, recommended on the box for "Fast temporary relief of cold symptoms and accompanying coughs, sinus congestion, headache, the symptoms of hay fever," contains in each tablet 12 mg of the antihistamine methapyrilene hydrochloride and 5 mg of the antitussive dextromethorphan hydrobromide, as well as some phenacetin, salicylamide, and other substances. In the *Handbook of Poisoning* (Dreisbach, 1969) it is reported that the death of a small child was caused by an estimated 100 mg of methapyrilene (114 mg of the hydrochloride). At least twenty deaths of children have resulted from accidental poisoning by antihistamines. The estimated fatal dose for these reported poisonings lies in the range of 10 mg to 50 mg per kilogram body-weight for phenindamine, methapyrilene, diphenhydramine, and pyrilamine and is probably about the same for many other antihistamines. These substances are more toxic than aspirin; one or two grams might cause the death of an adult.

These medicines often cause side effects, such as drowsiness and dizziness, even when taken in the recommended amounts. On the package there is usually a warning about the possibility of poisoning, for example, "Keep this and all medicines out of children's reach. In case of accidental overdose, contact a physician immediately."

Moreover, there is often a more extensive warning, such as the following:

> CAUTION: Children under 12 should use only as directed
> by a physician. If symptoms persist or are unusually severe,
> see a physician. Do not exceed recommended dosage. Not
> for frequent or prolonged use. If excessive dryness of the
> mouth occurs, decrease dosage. Discontinue use if rapid
> pulse, dizziness, skin rash, or blurring of vision occurs. Do
> not drive or operate machinery as this preparation may cause
> drowsiness in some persons. Individuals with high blood
> pressure, heart disease, diabetes, thyroid disease, glaucoma or
> excessive pressure within the eye, and elderly persons (where
> undiagnosed glaucoma or excessive pressure within the eye
> may be present) should use only as directed by physician.
> Persons with undiagnosed glaucoma may experience eye pain;
> if this occurs discontinue use and see physician immediately.

The substance dextromethorphan hydrobromide, mentioned above as an antitussive, controls severe coughing by exerting a depressant effect on the brain. Also, the related substance codeine (as codeine phosphate) in amounts of 15 mg to 60 mg every three or four hours is often prescribed by physicians for severe coughing. In most states of the United States codeine is not present in the medicines sold without prescription, but many of these medicines contain some other antitussive, such as dextromethorphan. The minimum fatal doses of these substances range from 100 mg to 1 g for an adult; much less for infants and more for narcotic addicts.

Some nonprescription cold medicines also contain belladonna alkaloids (atropine sulfate, hyoscyamine sulfate, scopolamine hydrobromide) in amounts as great as 0.2 mg per capsule. These drugs serve to dilate the bronchi and prevent spasms. They are intensely poisonous; the fatal dose in children may be as low as 10 mg. Side effects that may occur from ordinary doses are abnormal dryness of the mouth, blurred vision, slow beating of the heart, and retention of the urine.

Phenylpropanolamine hydrochloride (25 mg per tablet in some cold medicines) and phenylephrine hydrochloride (5 mg per tablet) serve to decrease nasal congestion and dilate the bronchi. These and related drugs, such as epinephrine and amphetamine, are also used in nose drops. It is estimated that 1 to 10 percent of users of such nose drops have reactions from overdosage, such as chronic nasal congestion or personality changes with a psychic craving to continue the use of the drug. Fatalities are rare. The estimated fatal dose for children ranges from 10 mg for epinephrine to 200 mg for phenylpropanolamine.

The prescriptions of physicians for treating colds and other respiratory ailments contain these drugs and other drugs that are equally toxic or more toxic and have a similar incidence of side reactions.

Instead of the warning "KEEP THIS MEDICINE OUT OF REACH OF CHILDREN" carried by cold medicines, I think that they should say "KEEP THIS MEDICINE OUT OF REACH OF EVERYBODY! USE VITAMIN C INSTEAD!"

The people of the United States spend about $2 billion per year on cold medicines. These medicines do not prevent the colds. They may decrease somewhat the misery of the cold, but they also do harm, because of their toxicity and their side effects.

The natural, essential food, vitamin C, taken in the right amounts at the right time, would prevent most of these colds from developing and would in most cases greatly decrease the intensity of the symptoms in those that do develop. Vitamin C is nontoxic, whereas all the cold drugs are toxic, and some of them cause severe side reactions in many people. In every respect, vitamin C is to be preferred to the dangerous and only partially effective analgesics, antipyretics, antihistamines, antitussives, bronchodilators, antispasmodics, and central-nervous-system depressants that constitute most medicines sold for relief of the common cold.

The drugs used to control other diseases may have even more serious side effects. I have mentioned in Chapter 22 that Dr. William Kaufman has reported success in treating patients with rheumatoid arthritis, osteoarthritis, and milder joint dysfunction by administering large amounts (about 5 g per day) of niacinamide, sometimes with other vitamins. The conventional treatment now, however, is with aspirin or stronger drugs. Here are the warnings about one of these drugs, which I call Drug X, instead of its correct name, because it is not much different from the others:

*Contraindications:* Drug X should not be used in patients who have previously exhibited hypersensitivity to it or in individuals with the syndrome comprised of bronchospasm, nasal polyps and angioedema precipitated by aspirin or other nonsteroidal anti-inflammatory drugs.

*Warnings:* Peptic ulceration, perforation, and gastrointestinal bleeding—sometimes severe, and in some instances, fatal—have been reported with patients receiving Drug X. If Drug X must be given to patients with a history of upper gastrointestinal tract disease the patient should be under close supervision (see *Adverse Reactions).*

*Precautions:* As with other anti-inflammatory agents, long-term administration to animals results in renal papillary necrosis and related pathology in rats, mice, and dogs.

Acute renal failure and hyperkalemia as well as reversible elevations of BUN and serum creatinine have been reported with Drug X. In addition to reversible changes in renal function, interstitial nephritis, glomerulitis, papillary necrosis, and the nephrotic syndrome have been reported with Drug X.

Although other nonsteroidal anti-inflammatory drugs do not have the same direct effect on platelets that aspirin does, all drugs inhibiting prostaglandin biosyntheses do interfere with platelet function to some degree.

Because of reports of adverse eye findings with non-steroidal anti-inflammatory agents, it is recommended that patients who develop visual complaints during treatment with Drug X have ophthalmic evaluation.

As with other nonsteroidal anti-inflammatory drugs, borderline elevations of one or more liver tests may occur in up to 15% of patients. A patient with symptoms and/or signs suggesting liver dysfunction or in whom abnormal liver tests have occurred should be evaluated for evidence of the development of more severe hepatic reaction while on therapy with Drug X.

Severe hepatic reactions, including jaundice and cases of fatal hepatitis, have been reported with Drug X. Although such reactions are rare, if abnormal liver tests persist or worsen, if clinical signs and symptoms consistent with liver disease develop, or if systemic manifestations occur (e.g., eosinophilia, rash, etc.), Drug X should be discontinued (see also *Adverse Reactions).*

Although at the recommended dose of 20 mg/day of Drug X, increased fecal blood loss due to gastrointestinal irritation did not occur, in about 4% of the patients treated with Drug X alone or concomitantly with aspirin, reductions in hemoglobin and hematocrit values were observed.

Peripheral edema has been observed in approximately 2% of the patients treated with Drug X. Therefore Drug X should be used with caution in patients with heart failure, hypertension, or other conditions predisposing to fluid retention.

A combination of dermatological and/or allergic signs and symptoms suggestive of serum sickness have occasionally occurred in conjunction with the use of Drug X. These include arthralgias, pruritus, fever, fatigue, and rash including vesiculobullous reactions and exfoliative dermatitis.

*Adverse Reactions,* with incidence 20% to less than 1%: stomatitis, anorexia, gastric distress, nausea, constipation, abdominal pain, indigestion, pruritus, rash, dizziness, drowsiness, vertigo, headache, malaise, tinnitus, jaundice, hepatitis, vomiting, hematemesis, melena, gastrointestinal bleeding, bone marrow depression, aplastic anemia, colic, fever, swollen eyes, blurred vision, bronchospasm, urticaria, angioedema.

The warning has here been printed in readable book type, not the small print of the flyer in the box.

Drug X is recommended for rheumatoid arthritis and osteoarthritis and is said to have been administered to millions of patients in eighty different countries. How many of these patients suffered from the side effects? How many read the foregoing contraindications before beginning to take the drug? And how many knew that the easy, harmless, and cheap vitamin niacinamide might have controlled their arthritis?

Kaufman's work and the observations of many persons show that a gram or more of niacinamide per day has value in controlling arthritis, and Dr. Ellis has reported good results with vitamin $B_6$. Even if I had very severe arthritis, I doubt that I would take Drug X. Instead, I would try niacinamide, 5 g or more per day, if necessary, and I would increase my intake of vitamin $B_6$.

Warnings similar to those quoted above for Drug X are made also for the drugs used in the effort to control diseases other than joint dysfunction. Patients often are helped by these drugs, but sometimes a drug is administered by the physician even when the physician has doubts about its probable value.

For example, in Europe chemotherapy is administered to only a small percentage of patients with advanced cancer, those with the kinds of cancer that have been found to respond to this treatment, but in the United States most advanced-cancer patients receive chemotherapy, with its disagreeable side effects. In our book *Cancer and Vitamin C,* Cameron and I mention that Dr. Charles G. Moertel of the Mayo Clinic, the well-known cancer authority, had made a valuable comment on the important question of whether or not an adult patient with a solid malignant tumor that had not been controlled by other treatments should, as the last resort, receive chemotherapy. In a summary of current opinion on the use of chemotherapy in the treatment of gastrointestinal cancer published in *The New England Journal of Medicine* in 1978, Moertel pointed out that twenty-five years ago the fluorinated pyrimidines 5-fluorouracil (5-FU) and 5-fluoro-2'-deoxyuridine were found to be capable of producing a transient decrease of tumor size in patients with metastatic cancer of intestinal origin. An intravenous treatment in amount that produces toxic reactions is the most effective, but the effect is not great:

> Even when administered in most ideal regimens, the
> fluorinated pyrimidines, in a large experience, will produce
> objective response in only about 15 to 20 percent of treated
> patients. In this context, objective response is usually defined
> as a reduction of more than 50 percent in the product of
> longest perpendicular diameters of a measurable tumor mass.

These responses are usually only partial and very transient, persisting for a median time of only about five months. This minor gain for a small minority of patients is probably more than counterbalanced by the deleterious influence of toxicity for other patients and by the cost and inconvenience experienced by all patients. There is no solid evidence that treatment with fluorinated pyrimidines contributes to the overall survival of patients with gastrointestinal cancer regardless of the stage of the disease at which they are applied.

Moertel also discussed the clinical trials of 5-FU and other chemotherapeutic agents singly and in various combinations in relations to colorectal cancer, gastric carcinoma, squamous-cell carcinoma of the esophagus, and others, with essentially the same conclusion, except that adriamycin seems to have significant value for the treatment of primary liver cancer. He then states that "In 1978 it must be concluded that there is no chemotherapy approach to gastrointestinal carcinoma valuable enough to justify application as standard clinical treatment."

We would interpret this conclusion as sound reason for not subjecting these patients to the misery, trouble, and expense of chemotherapy. Moertel continues, however, as follows:

By no means, however, should this conclusion imply that these efforts should be abandoned. Patients with advanced gastrointestinal cancer and their families have a compelling need for a basis of hope. If such hope is not offered, they will quickly seek it from the hands of quacks and charlatans. Enough progress has been made in chemotherapy of gastrointestinal cancer so that realistic hope can be generated by entry of those patients into well designed clinical research studies. . . . If we can channel our efforts and resources into constructive research programs of sound scientific design, we shall offer the most hopeful treatment for the patient with gastrointestinal cancer today and lay a sound foundation for chemotherapy approaches of substantive value for the patient of tomorrow.

In diametric contrast with this prescription and the practice at the Mayo Clinic and other U.S. medical centers, it has been the rather general practice in most hospitals in Britain, for more than a decade, not to subject patients with advanced gastrointestinal cancer and similar cancers to the misery of chemotherapy, experience having shown that this treatment has little value. Instead, these "hopeless" patients were given only palliative treatment, including morphine and heroin as needed to control pain. Cameron improved upon these procedures at the Vale of Leven Hospital by administering vitamin C. As discussed in Chapter 19, he thereby eased the suffering and increased the number of "good days" in the last days of the lives of terminal-cancer patients.

It was the same Moertel who misrepresented Cameron's work in Moertel's poorly designed experiments with patients at the Mayo Clinic. Compare Cameron's procedure with the Moertel strategy of subjecting such patients to the misery of chemotherapy for the sake of their families and their physicians' morale! If Moertel had followed the Vale of Leven procedure, he would have seen that there is now a real reason for these patients and their families to have hope. These "untreatable" patients can be given supplemental ascorbate as their only form of treatment and can derive some benefit, and just occasionally the degree of benefit obtained might be quite remarkable.

The average increase in survival time of patients with advanced gastrointestinal cancer treated with 10 g of ascorbate per day is greater than that reported by Moertel for those treated with chemotherapy, and the ascorbate-treated patients have the advantages of feeling well under the treatment and of not having the financial burden of chemotherapy. Moreover, little effort has been made as yet to determine the most effective dosages of vitamin C and the possible supplementary value of vitamin A, the B vitamins, minerals, and a diet high in fruits, vegetables, and their juices. This nutritional treatment of cancer, with emphasis on vitamin C, is probably far more effective at earlier stages of cancer than in the terminal stage, and if it is instituted at the first sign of cancer and in the most effective amounts it may well decrease the cancer mortality by much more than our earlier estimate of 10 percent.

The message of this chapter is that you should be wary of drugs—over-the-counter drugs and drugs prescribed by a physician. You should, of course, also be wary of the claims for vitamins and other nutrients, even though for the most part they are not so dangerous as drugs. Find out what the facts are and make the best decisions that you can, using the best advice that you can obtain.

The older books about nutrition and health are, of course, unreliable, because it is only during the last two decades that we have gathered reliable information about the optimum intakes of vitamins. Some of the recent books are also unreliable. For example, Nathan Pritikin in his book *The Pritikin Promise: 28 Days to a Longer, Healthier Life* discusses his program of exercise and rigorously restricted diet, which, without doubt, improves the health of persons who follow it. He states, however, that

> When a varied diet, as recommended in the Pritikin Program,
> is eaten, you will get all the vitamins your body can use and
> then some. Many persons, however, believe that taking extra
> vitamins, especially B, C, and E, in the form of supplements
> will provide additional health benefits. This, however, is
> simply not the case. . . . Vitamin supplements not only are
> uncalled for, but are potentially hazardous to your health . . .
> There are many salesmen in this country and many gullible
> people who are victimized financially by vitamin "pushers."
> Americans excrete the most expensive urine in the world
> because it is loaded with so many vitamins.

I think that Pritikin received poor advice from his medical and nutritional advisers. His clients no doubt benefit from his regimen, so long as they follow it. They would benefit more with supplementary nutrients, and the diet could be made less restrictive, giving better client compliance.

A modern authority on nutrition, Dr. Brian Leibovitz, agrees with me. In his sensible discussion of dieting and diets (1984) he states, "One may not be in danger of vitamin deficiency on the Pritikin plan, but neither will one be able to achieve a state of optimum health."

In another popular book, *Life Extension: A Practical Scientific Approach* (1982), the authors, Durk Pearson and Sandy Shaw, recommend a high intake of vitamins, often far more than I recommend. In addition, however, they discuss many drugs as beneficial to health and conducive to life extension. One of these drugs, a mixture of hydrogenated ergot alkaloids, which blocks the functioning of the adrenal glands, is mentioned about 150 times under one of its trademarked names. Leibovitz (1984), after mentioning the high doses of vitamins, comments that "Of greater concern, however, is the inclusion of hormones, drugs, and other potentially dangerous substances in the Pearson-Shaw formula. While the list of compounds with potential toxicity is too extensive to discuss in detail, it should be noted that some of the substances recommended have known toxicities. Vasopressin, also called antidiuretic hormone, is one such compound."

In sum, try to keep your intake of drugs low and your intake of vitamins and other nutrients at the optimum level.

# 27

## *The Low Toxicity of Vitamins*

Physicians, these days, are armed with increasingly potent drugs, which they must prescribe and administer with great care, keeping their patients under alert surveillance. In extension of this chary attitude, I think, they are cautious about vitamins. It is easy to develop an exaggerated and unjustified fear of the toxicity of vitamins. During recent years it has become the practice of writers on medical matters and on health to warn their readers that large doses of vitamins may have serious side effects. For example, in *The Book of Health, a Complete Guide to Making Health Last a Lifetime* (1981), edited by Dr. Ernst L. Wynder, president of the American Health Foundation, it is said that "So-called megavitamin treatment—taking massive doses of a particular vitamin—should be avoided. Vitamins are essential nutrients, but high dosages become drugs and should only be taken to treat a specific condition. Large doses of the fat-soluble vitamins A and D have well-recognized ill effects, and this must be true of others, too. Large doses of vitamin C are mainly excreted in the urine. In the absence of certainty that 'megavitamins' are safe, they are better avoided."

The authors of this book on health are depriving their readers of the benefit of the optimum intakes of these important nutrients, the vitamins, by creating in them the fear that any intake greater than the usually Recommended Daily Allowances (RDA) may cause serious harm.

I believe that the main reason for this poor advice is that the authors are ignorant. They make the false statement that large doses of vitamin C are mainly excreted in the urine. They give no indication that they know that the RDAs of the vitamins are the intakes that probably would prevent most people in "ordinary good health" from dying of scurvy, beriberi, pellagra, or other deficiency disease but are not the intakes that put people in the best of health. They seem not to know that there is a great span between the RDAs and the toxic amounts of those that exhibit any toxicity and that for several vitamins there is no known upper limit to the amount that can be taken. These authorities on health should show greater concern about the health of the American people.

The *Reader's Digest Family Health Guide and Medical Encyclopedia* (1976) in its section on vitamins states that "A well-balanced, varied diet contains all the vitamins normally needed for health. Vitamins in excess of what the body needs do not increase health or well-being and may actually produce disease. A poor diet cannot be corrected simply by taking vitamins in concentrated form."

The first sentence, which seems to express the belief of nearly all nutritionists and physicians, may be true or false, depending on what is meant by "normally needed for health." If we mean needed for the average health of "healthy" people in the United States, who presumably eat a well-balanced, varied diet, then the statement is no more than a truism, a self-evident, obvious truth; but if by "health" we mean that state of health that can be achieved by the optimum intakes of vitamins, as discussed in this book, the statement is false.

Moreover, the second sentence is clearly false. There is overwhelming evidence, only a small part of which I am able to include in this book, that supplementary vitamins (beyond what the body "needs" by the criterion of the preceding sentence) improve health and well-being in many ways. The last words, "may actually produce disease," refer to possible side effects in such a way as to deter the reader from improving his or her health by increasing intake of these important nutrients.

The last sentence is seriously misleading, because of the omission of the adverb *completely*. A true statement is, "A poor diet cannot be completely corrected simply by taking vitamins in concentrated form, but taking the vitamins can do a lot of good."

The writers of the *Reader's Digest* book on health should have known enough by 1976 to make better statements about the value of supplementary vitamins. I am reminded of an experience I had in 1984 on a radio medical program (on station KQED) in San Francisco. There was another guest on the program, a retired professor of nutrition from the University of California in Berkeley. I made a statement about the value of a high intake of vitamin C (such as my own 18,000 milligrams [mg] per day) and mentioned some evidence to support it, giving the references to papers published in medical and scientific journals. The retired professor of nutrition said simply, "No one needs more than 60 mg of vitamin C per day," without giving any evidence to support his flat statement. I then presented some more evidence for my large intake, and he responded by saying, "Sixty mg of vitamin C per day is adequate for any person." After I had presented some more evidence, this retired professor said, "For fifty years I and other leading authorities in nutrition have been saying that 60 mg of vitamin C per day is all that any person needs!" There was just time enough left on the live radio program for me to say "Yes—that's just the trouble: you are fifty years behind the times."

We are surrounded by toxic substances. In our buildings and in the countryside we may be exposed to asbestos or other siliceous materials that cause dyspnea (difficulty in breathing) and pneumoconiosis (fibrous hardening of the lungs). In the neighborhood of a farm we may be exposed to one or more of the fifty organic phosphate insecticides or twenty chlorobenzene-derivative insecticides or thirty pesticides of other kinds. At home we may be exposed to several household chemicals and to drugs.

It is drugs, especially the analgesics and antipyretics, such as aspirin, that are responsible for most of the five thousand deaths by poisoning that occur each year in the United States. Of that mournful total about twenty-five hundred are children. About four hundred of these children die each year of poisoning by aspirin (acetylsalicylic acid) or some other salicylate. Aspirin and similar drugs are sold openly, without a prescription. They are considered to be exceptionally safe substances. The fatal dose is 0.4 to 0.5 grams per kilogram body weight; that is 5 to 10 g for a child, 20 to 30 g for an adult.

Nobody dies of poisoning by an overdose of vitamins.

I have credited the physician with caution for the patient, even though the caution is entirely misplaced. Several people have suggested another possible explanation to me. It is that the drug manufacturers and the people involved in the so-called health industry do not want the American people to learn that they can improve their health and cut down on their medical expenses simply by taking vitamins in the optimum amounts.

The bias against vitamins may be illustrated by an episode that occurred a few years ago. A small child swallowed all the vitamin-A tablets that he found in a bottle. He became nauseated and complained of a headache. His mother took him to an East Coast medical-school hospital, where he was treated and then sent home. The professors of medicine then wrote an article about this case of vitamin poisoning. The article was published in *The New England Journal of Medicine*, the same journal that had rejected a paper by Ewan Cameron and me on observations of cancer patients who received large intakes of vitamin C. *The New York Times* and many other newspapers published stories about this child and about how dangerous the vitamins are.

Some child in the United States dies of aspirin poisoning every day. These poisonings are ignored by the medical-school doctors, the medical journals, and *The New York Times*.

There are seven thousand entries in the index of the *Handbook of Poisoning* by Dr. Robert H. Dreisbach, professor of pharmacology at Stanford University School of Medicine. Only five of these seven thousand are about vitamins. These five entries refer to vitamins A, D, K, $K_1$ (a form of K), and the B vitamins.

You do not need to worry about vitamin K. It is the vitamin that prevents hemorrhage by promoting coagulation of the blood. It is not often put into vitamin tablets. Adults and children usually receive a proper amount, which is normally supplied by intestinal bacteria. The physician may prescribe vitamin K to newborn infants, to women in labor, or to people with an overdose of an anticoagulant. The toxicity of vitamin K is a problem of interest to the physician who administers it to a patient.

Vitamin D is the fat-soluble vitamin that prevents rickets. It is required, together with calcium and phosphorus, for normal bone growth. The RDA is 400 International Units (IU) per day.† It is probably wise not to exceed this intake very much. Dreisbach gives 158,000 IU as the toxic dose, with many manifestations of toxicity: weakness, nausea, vomiting, diarrhea, anemia, decreased renal functions, acidosis, proteinuria, elevated blood pressure, calcium deposition, and others. Kutsky *(Handbook of Vitamins and Hormones,* 1973) states that 4000 IU per day leads to anorexia, nausea, thirst, diarrhea, muscular weakness, joint pains, and other problems.

Vitamin A is usually mentioned as a prime example in any discussion of the toxicity of vitamins. Thus in her 1984 *New York Times* article "Vitamin Therapy: The Toxic Side Effects of Massive Doses," the writer about foods, Jane E. Brody, stated that "Vitamin A has been the cause of the largest number of vitamin poisoning cases." She did not mention that the patients did not die (as do many of those poisoned by aspirin and other drugs), but she did give two case histories, presumably the worst that she could find:

A 3-year-old girl was hospitalized with confusion,
dehydration, hyperirritability, headache, pains in the abdomen
and legs, and vomiting, the result of daily ingestion of
200,000 I.U. of vitamin A a day for three months (2,500 is
the amount recommended for a child her age, theoretically to
prevent respiratory infections).

A 16-year-old boy who took 50,000 I.U. daily for two
and a half years to counter acne developed a stiff neck, dry
skin, cracked lips, swelling of the optic nerves, and increased
pressure in the skull.

These reports indicate that the long-continued daily intake of doses
of vitamin A ten to eighty times the RDA may cause moderately severe
effects. Dreisbach in his book on poisons says that twenty to one hundred
times the RDA may in time cause painful nodular periosteal swelling,
osteoporosis, itching, skin eruptions and ulcerations, anorexia, increased
intracranial pressure, irritability, drowsiness, alopecia, liver enlargement
(occasionally), diplopia, and papilledema.

The RDA for vitamin A is 5000 IU (for an adult).† A single dose of
5,000,000 IU, one thousand times the RDA, causes nausea and headache.
It is reasonable to recommend that single doses approaching this size not
be taken.

On repeated regular intake of this fat-soluble vitamin the amount stored
in the body increases, and ultimately its activity may reach such a level
as to cause manifestations such as headache from increased intracranial
pressure and others mentioned above. Repeated intakes of 100,000 or
150,000 IU per day for a year or more have caused these problems in some
people but not in others. My recommendation is that in general 50,000 IU
per day be considered the upper limit for regular intake. Any person taking
large amounts of vitamin A should be on the watch for signs of toxicity.

As for the B vitamins, $B_1$ has no known fatal dose and no known dose
with serious toxicity. The RDA for an adult male is 1.4 mg.† The regular
daily intake of 50 or 100 mg is tolerated by most people and may be
beneficial.

$B_2$ has no known fatal dose and no known dose with serious toxicity.
The RDA for an adult is about 1.6 mg.† Regular daily intakes of 50 or 100
mg per day are tolerated by most people and may be beneficial.

$B_3$, niacin (nicotinic acid, nicotinamide, niacinamide), has no known fatal dose. Intakes of nicotinic acid of 100 mg or more (different for different people) cause flushing, itching, vasodilation, increased cerebral blood flow, and decreased blood pressure. This flushing reaction usually stops after four days with daily intake of 400 mg or more. Large doses of nicotinamide cause nausea in some people. The RDA is about 18 mg for an adult.† The low toxicity of niacin (either nicotinic acid or nicotinamide) is shown by the fact that daily amounts from 5000 to 30,000 mg have been taken for years by schizophrenic patients without toxic effects (Hawkins and Pauling, 1973).

Vitamin $B_6$, pyridoxine, has no known fatal dose. When this vitamin is taken regularly in very large daily doses, it causes a significant neurological damage in some people. Vitamin $B_6$ is the only water-soluble vitamin that has significant toxicity.

There are several substances (pyridoxol, pyridoxal, pyridoxamine, pyridoxal phosphate, and pyridoxamine phosphate) with $B_6$ activity (protection against convulsions, irritability, skin lesions, decreased production of lymphocytes). Pyridoxine is the name used for all the forms of $B_6$. Converted in the body to pyridoxal phosphate, vitamin $B_6$ serves as the coenzyme for many enzyme systems. A good intake of this vitamin is needed in order that the many essential biochemical reactions in the human body proceed at the rate that leads to the best health.

Until 1983 it was thought that none of the water-soluble vitamins had significant toxicity even at very high intakes. Then a report was made that seven persons who had been taking 2000 to 5000 mg per day (one thousand to three thousand times the RDA) of vitamin $B_6$ for between four months and two years had developed a loss of feeling in the toes and a tendency to stumble (Schaumberg et al., 1983). This peripheral neuropathy disappeared when the high intake of the vitamin was stopped, and the patients showed no damage to the central nervous system.

We may conclude that there is an upper limit, one thousand times the RDA, to the daily intake of vitamin $B_6$. The authors of the report were far more cautious, however; they recommended that no one take more than the RDA of this vitamin, 1.8 to 2.2 mg per day.† To follow this recommendation would deprive many people of a means for improving their health by taking 50 or 100 mg or more every day, as I have recommended in Chapter 2. Many orthomolecular psychiatrists recommend 200 mg per day to their patients, with some patients taking 400 to 600 mg per day (Pauling, 1984). Hawkins reported that "In more than 5,000 patients we have not observed a single side effect from pyridoxine administration of 200 mg of vitamin $B_6$ daily" (Hawkins and Pauling, 1973).

Single doses of 50,000 mg of vitamin $B_6$ are given without serious side effects. These large doses are given as the antidote to patients suffering from poisoning with an overdose of the antituberculosis drug isoniazid (Sievers and Herrier, 1984).

No fatal doses are known for folacin (folic acid), pantothenic acid, vitamin $B_{12}$, and biotin. These four water-soluble vitamins are described as lacking in toxicity, even at very high intakes. The values of the RDA for adult males are 400 micrograms (μg) for folacin,† 7 mg for pantothenic acid,† 3 μg for vitamin $B_{12}$,† and 200 μg for biotin.†

There is an odd situation involving folacin. In 1960 the U.S. Food and Drug Administration (FDA) ordered that no vitamin tablet or one-day supply of vitamins contain more than 250 μg of folacin, later increased to 400 μg. These cautious orders were not issued because of evidence that folacin is toxic in larger doses. Folacin is not toxic. Indeed, the FDA limit of 400 μg is less than the amount considered necessary for good health. Professor Roger J. Williams, who discovered pantothenic acid and carried out some of the early work on folacin, has written that "More than the specified amount (about 2000 micrograms, instead of 400 micrograms) would be recommended if it were not for the conflicting FDA regulations" (Williams, 1975).

Why, then, does the FDA prevent all of us from obtaining the proper amount of this important vitamin? The action was taken by the FDA to make it easier for physicians to diagnose a disease, pernicious anemia. This disease results from the failure to transport vitamin $B_{12}$ from the stomach into the bloodstream. The resulting deficiency of vitamin $B_{12}$ is characterized by anemia and by neurological damage leading to psychosis. Both vitamin $B_{12}$ and folacin are required for the production of red blood cells in the bone marrow, and a deficiency in $B_{12}$ is in part compensated for by increasing the intake of folacin. Accordingly a high intake of folacin may prevent the anemia from developing, but it does not control the neurological damage resulting from $B_{12}$ deficiency and may possibly exacerbate it by helping to use up the limited supply of $B_{12}$ by increasing the red-cell production.

In 1960 spokesmen for the medical profession argued that physicians relied on the development of anemia to recognize the disease and that if folacin prevented the anemia they would not know that a patient beginning to show signs of psychosis was in fact suffering from pernicious anemia. The FDA then announced its order limiting the amount of folacin in vitamin preparations. This action was, therefore, not to protect the public against folacin toxicity but to help physicians to recognize pernicious anemia in a few patients who might be receiving larger amounts of folacin.

Now, a quarter of a century later, physicians know more about pernicious anemia, vitamin $B_{12}$, and folacin. It is easy to test any patient with neurological problems for $B_{12}$ deficiency. There is no longer any need for the FDA regulation that limits the amount of folacin in vitamin preparation. This regulation should be revoked.

There is no known fatal dose of vitamin C. As much as 200 grams (g) has been taken by mouth over a period of a few hours without harmful effects. Between 100 and 150 g of sodium ascorbate has been given by intravenous infusion without harm.

There is little evidence of long-term toxicity. I know a man who has taken over 400 kilograms (kg) of this vitamin during the last nine years. He is a chemist, working in California. When he developed metastatic cancer, he found that he could control his pain by taking 130 g of vitamin C per day, and he has taken this amount, over a quarter of a pound per day, for nine years. Except that he has not succeeded in ridding himself completely of his cancer, his health is reasonably good, with no indication of harmful side effects of the vitamin.

There has been extensive discussion of possible side effects of high intakes of vitamin C. This subject is treated in the following chapter.

There is no known fatal intake of the several closely related substances, called tocopherols, that have vitamin E activity. Different mixtures of these tocopherols are available, with their activity, determined by a standard test, expressed as international units. For example, 1 mg of D-alpha-tocopherol equals 1.49 IU and 1 mg of D, L-alpha-tocopheryl acetate (a mixture of D and L) equals 1 IU.†

Vitamin E is valuable in many ways, including the treatment of cardiac and muscular disorders. It acts both as a general antioxidant, in collaboration with vitamin C, and in some specific ways involving interactions with proteins and lipids not yet well understood.

The RDA of vitamin E is 10 IU per day.† Many people have taken much larger amounts over long periods of time. Dr. Evan V. Shute and Dr. Wilfrid E. Shute in Canada reported on thousands of persons who received between 50 and 3200 IU of vitamin E per day for long periods with no signs of significant toxicity (Shute and Taub, 1969; Shute, 1978). Vitamin E as the fat-soluble antioxidant is a valuable companion to vitamin C, the main water-soluble antioxidant.

# 28

## *The Side Effects of Vitamins*

During recent years, as more and more people have recognized the value of an increased intake of vitamin C, there has developed a lively interest in the question of possible side effects of this vitamin taken over long periods of time. This concern in the public mind has been amplified by physicians who carry over to vitamins the caution about side effects that they quite properly attach to drugs. In publication and in consultation with their patients, they have spread misinformation and false alarm.

The problem is complicated by the biochemical individuality (Chapter 10) that gives rise to the heterogeneity of the American population. The fact (Chapter 27) that one man has taken 130 grams (g) of vitamin C per day for nine years without developing any signs of harmful side effects does not mean that every person would do well with this intake. More pertinent is the report by Dr. Fred R. Klenner that hundreds of persons he observed ingested 10 g of vitamin C per day for years and remained in good health with no problems that could be attributed to their high intake of the vitamin.

In a review of toxic effects of vitamin C, Dr. L. A. Barness of the University of South Florida College of Medicine listed fourteen (Barness, 1977). I shall discuss all of them. He said that many toxic effects are insignificant or rare or troublesome but of little consequence. Among these are sterility caused by vitamin C, of which there is a single doubtful case. About reports of fatigue the author is skeptical; many people report an increase in vigor with increased intake of the vitamin. Reports of hyperglycemia following intake of vitamin C may be unreliable because of interference with the test for sugar in the urine, as discussed below. It seems unlikely that the allergic reactions occasionally attributed to vitamin C are caused by the ascorbic acid or sodium ascorbate, because these crystalline substances are subjected to so many processes of purification in their synthesis from glucose that allergens are not expected to remain; I do not know of any careful study that showed vitamin C itself to be allergenic.

Some of the side effects of large doses of vitamin C have been subjected to careful study and analysis during the last ten or twelve years, and much of the misunderstanding about their significance has been corrected (Pauling, 1976b). Many popular writers about nutrition, however, have only incomplete knowledge and continue to write scare stories about the dangers of megavitamins and to recommend that no one take more than the Recommended Daily Allowance (RDA) without first asking the advice of a physician (who may also be ignorant about vitamins). An example is the 1984 *New York Times* article by Jane E. Brody (mentioned in Chapter 27), which is outstanding for the large number of false or misleading statements in it. When I called the attention of the publisher of the *Times* to these errors, a correction was published but of only one error (May 7, 1984). Nearly all of the "dangers" mentioned in the article are discussed in this chapter or the preceding chapter.

One effect of vitamin C in large doses has been reported by many people. This is its effect as a laxative, its action in causing looseness of the bowels. For some people a single dose of 3 g taken on an empty stomach exerts too strong a laxative action, whereas the same amount taken at the end of a meal does not. One physician who treats patients with infectious diseases by having them take as much ascorbic acid as they can without discomfort has reported that most of them take between 15 and 30 g per day (Cathcart, 1975). Virno et al. (1967) and Bietti (1967) have written that glaucoma patients taking 30 to 40 g of ascorbic acid per day suffer from "diarrhea" for three or four days but not thereafter.

Constipation can usually be controlled by adjusting the intake of vitamin C (Hoffer, 1971). To be in the best of health it is wise to evacuate the contents of the lower bowel regularly every day. To carry the waste matter around for a longer time than necessary might do harm. On the other hand, moderately irritant laxatives, such as milk of magnesia, cascara sagrada, or sodium sulfate, might themselves cause some harm. Physicians often advise patients suffering from constipation to eat a good diet, including plenty of fruit and vegetables. This is good orthomolecular treatment, but the use of vitamin C, in addition to that in the fruit and vegetables, is also good orthomolecular treatment.

One well-known medical treatise says that no real harm is done if the bowel does not move for three or four days and that the bowel itself must be given a chance to function. I think that this opinion is wrong, for several reasons. We know from the work of Dr. Robert Bruce, director of the Toronto branch of the Ludwig Cancer Research Institute, that there are presumptive carcinogens in human fecal material. Continued exposure of the lower bowel to these substances increases the probability of developing cancer of the rectum and colon. There is also an increase in the amount of bile acids reabsorbed from the fecal material into the bloodstream, which takes them to the liver for reconversion to cholesterol, thus raising the cholesterol level and increasing the chance of developing heart disease. Other toxic substances that the body should get rid of as fast as possible are also reabsorbed. Sometimes they can be detected on a person's breath. This should give special incentive to people interested in the opposite sex for taking care of their waste material expeditiously.

This goal can be achieved through the laxative action of a natural substance, vitamin C. You can take a good amount, 3, 5, 8, or 10 g, of vitamin C when you rise in the morning. It should be the amount, which you determine for yourself by trial, that causes a loose bowel movement immediately after breakfast. This should put you right for the day.

From my observations I make the rough estimate that this procedure speeds up the elimination of the waste materials by about twenty-four hours, or even more for those people who pay attention to the medical authority quoted above.

A large intake of vitamin C has also been reported to increase the production of intestinal gas (methane) in many people. To minimize these effects, to the extent that they are undesirable, one might try various kinds of vitamin C and various ways of taking it (after meals, for example, as mentioned earlier). Some people say that they can handle the salt sodium ascorbate better than ascorbic acid, and for some a mixture of the two may be best; people in the latter group may obtain both sodium ascorbate and ascorbic acid or a fifty:fifty mixture from Bronson Pharmaceuticals and other suppliers. Some undesirable effects might be attributable to the filler or binder or the coloring or flavoring additives in tablets, making it desirable to change the brand or to use the pure substances. For some people the time-release tablets may solve the problem.

It should not surprise us that our intestinal tracts cause some temporary trouble for us when we ingest 5 or 10 g of ascorbic acid per day, even though this quantity is indicated to be the optimum by the fact that animals manufacture this amount for themselves. The animals make it inside their bodies, in the liver or kidney. It does not pass into the stomach and intestines, except for the smaller amount obtained from their food. After we lost the ability to synthesize this nutrient and began eating foods that provided us with only a small amount, 1 or 2 g per day, our digestive systems were not under any evolutionary pressure to adapt to the reception of larger amounts. We may have adapted to some extent to get along with smaller amounts, but there are indications, discussed elsewhere in this book, that our optimum intake is not less than the amount synthesized by other animals for their own benefit.

Some people have asked me if ascorbic acid, by acting as an acid, might not cause stomach ulcers. In fact, the gastric juice in the stomach contains a strong acid, and ascorbic acid, which is a weak acid, does not increase its acidity. Aspirin tablets and potassium chloride tablets can corrode the wall of the stomach and cause ulcers. Vitamin C keeps them from forming and helps to heal them (for references and additional discussion see Stone, 1972).

In the review of my book *Vitamin C and the Common Cold* in the *Medical Letter,* referred to in the last chapter, it was alleged that vitamin C might have the adverse effect of causing kidney stones to form. The author of this unsigned review wrote, "When 4 to 12 grams of vitamin C are taken daily for acidification of the urine, however, as in the management of some chronic urinary tract infections, precipitation of urate and cystine stones in the urinary tract can occur. Very large doses of vitamin C, therefore, should be avoided in patients with a tendency to gout, a formation of urate stones, or to cystinuria."

This statement is wrong. The editors might quite properly have written that very large doses of ascorbic acid should be avoided in these patients, but there is no reason for the patients to refrain from taking vitamin C in large doses, because it can be taken as sodium ascorbate, which does not acidify the urine. The statement made in the *Medical Letter* shows that the editors of the publication simply did not understand what they were writing about.

Vitamin C is in fact the ascorbate ion. This ion carries a negative electric charge, and we are accordingly not able to take vitamin C without taking an equivalent amount of some atom that carries a positive electric charge. In ascorbic acid this atom is a hydrogen ion, $H^+$; in sodium ascorbate it is the sodium ion, $Na^+$; and in calcium ascorbate it is half of a calcium ion, 1/2 $Ca^{++}$. All of these substances contain vitamin C, the ascorbate ion, and each of them also contains something else. The effects of the "something else," the hydrogen ion, sodium ion, or calcium ion, should not be confused with the effects of the ascorbate ion, as was done by the editors of the *Medical Letter* and continues to be done by writers whose understanding is incomplete.

It is well known that there are two classes of kidney stones, and that a tendency to form them should be controlled in two quite different ways. The stones of one class, comprising nearly one half of all urinary calculi, are composed of calcium phosphate, magnesium ammonium phosphate, calcium carbonate, or mixtures of these substances. They tend to form in alkaline urine, and persons with a tendency to form them are advised to keep their urine acidic. A good way, probably the best way, to acidify the urine is to take 1 g or more of ascorbic acid each day. Ascorbic acid is used by many physicians for this purpose and for preventing infections of the urinary tract, especially infection by organisms that hydrolyze urea to form ammonia and in this way alkalize the urine and promote the formation of kidney stones of this class.

The kidney stones of the other class, which tend to form in acidic urine, are composed of calcium oxalate, uric acid, or cystine. Persons with a tendency to form these stones are advised to keep their urine alkaline. This can be achieved by their taking vitamin C as sodium ascorbate or by taking ascorbic acid with just enough sodium hydrogen carbonate (ordinary baking soda) or other alkalizer to neutralize it.

Not a single case has been reported in the medical literature of a person who formed kidney stones because of a large intake of vitamin C.† There is the possibility, however, that some people might have an increased tendency to form calcium oxalate kidney stones while taking a large amount of vitamin C. It is known that ascorbic acid can be oxidized to oxalic acid in the body. Lamden and Chrystowski (1954) studied fifty-one healthy male subjects with an ordinary intake of vitamin C (only that in their food) and found the average amount of oxalic acid excreted in the urine to be 38 milligrams (in a range of 16 to 64 mg). The average increased by only 3 mg for 2 g per day additional ascorbic acid and by only 12 mg per day for 4 g. Additional intake of 8 g per day, increased the excretion of oxalic acid by 45 mg, and of 9 g by 68 mg (average—as much as 150 mg was excreted by one subject). It seems likely that most people would not have trouble with oxalic acid while taking large doses of vitamin C, but a few might have to be careful, just as they have to refrain from eating spinach and rhubarb, which have a high oxalate content. A few people have a rare genetic disease that leads to the increased production of oxalic acid in their own cells (largely from the amino acid glycine), and one young man is known who converts about 15 percent of ingested ascorbic acid into oxalic acid, fifty times more than is converted by other people (Briggs, Garcia-Webb, and Davis, 1973). This man, and others who have the same genetic defect, must limit their intake of vitamin C.

During recent years I have received many letters from people who were troubled by a report that large doses of vitamin C taken with food destroyed the vitamin $B_{12}$ in the food, leading to a deficiency resembling pernicious anemia. I replied that the report was not reliable, because the conditions under which the food had been investigated in the laboratory were not closely similar to those for food that is swallowed and kept in the stomach. It has now been shown that the original report, by Herbert and Jacob (1974), was wrong, because of their use of an unreliable method of analysis, and that in fact vitamin C does not destroy the vitamin $B_{12}$ in food to any significant extent.

Herbert and Jacob studied a meal with modest vitamin $B_{12}$ content and a meal with high $B_{12}$ content, the latter containing 90 g of grilled beef liver, which is known to be rich in $B_{12}$. Some of the meals had 100 mg, 250 mg, or 500 mg of ascorbic acid added. The meals were homogenized in a blender, held for thirty minutes at body temperature (37°C), and then analyzed for vitamin $B_{12}$ by a radioactive-isotope method. The investigators reported that 500 mg of ascorbic acid added to the meal destroyed 95 percent of the vitamin $B_{12}$ in the modest-$B_{12}$ meal and nearly 50 percent in the high-$B_{12}$ meal. They concluded that "High doses of vitamin C, popularly used as a home remedy against the common cold, destroy substantial amounts of vitamin $B_{12}$ when ingested with foods. . . . Daily ingestion of 500 mg or more of ascorbic acid without regular evaluation of vitamin $B_{12}$ status is probably unwise." This statement has been repeated in many articles on nutrition and health in newspapers and magazines during recent years.

It is known that pure hydroxycobalamin and pure cyanocobalamin (forms of vitamin $B_{12}$) are attacked and destroyed (cyanocobalamin less rapidly) by ascorbic acid in the presence of oxygen and copper ions, but the amount of destruction reported by Herbert and Jacob was surprisingly high. Moreover, there was evidence in the account of their results given by Herbert and Jacob that something was wrong in their work. The amount of vitamin $B_{12}$ reported by them from their analysis of the meals (without added ascorbic acid) was only about one-eighth of that known to be present in the foods comprising the meals. It is known that some of the vitamin $B_{12}$ in foods is tightly bound to proteins and other constituents of the foods. Biochemists developed some special procedures to release the bound vitamin. If these procedures are not used, only the amount of loosely bound $B_{12}$ is determined in the analysis. Investigators in two different laboratories then repeated the work, using reliable analytical methods (Newmark, Scheiner, Marcus, and Prabhudesai, 1976). They found amounts of $B_{12}$ in the two meals equal, to within 5 percent, to the amounts calculated from the food tables. Their amounts were six to eight times those reported by Herbert and Jacob, and, moreover, they found that addition of 100 mg, 250 mg, or 500 mg of ascorbic acid led to no change in the amount of $B_{12}$ in the meal.

The allegation that vitamin $B_{12}$ is destroyed in meals consumed with vitamin C has also been considered by two other studies (Marcus, Prabhudesai, and Wassef, 1980; Ekvall and Bozian, 1979). We may conclude that the hazard ascribed to the intake with meals of moderately large amounts of vitamin C, 500 mg or more, by Herbert and Jacob does not exist. They were led to draw an incorrect conclusion by having used a poor method of chemical analysis for vitamin $B_{12}$. Writers who write articles on vitamins and physicians who give advice about health should now stop quoting destruction of vitamin $B_{12}$ as a reason for not taking the optimum amounts of vitamin C.

One of the reasons proposed by the *Medical Letter* for not taking an increased amount of vitamin C is that the presence of that vitamin in the urine might cause the ordinary tests for glucose in the urine, a sign of diabetes, to give a false positive result. This fact is hardly an argument against taking the valuable substance vitamin C. It is instead an argument for developing reliable tests for glucose in the urine.

Brandt, Guyer, and Banks (1974) have shown how the test for glucose in the urine can be modified to prevent interference by ascorbic acid. An even simpler way is to refrain from taking vitamin C for a few hours on the day when the urine sample is obtained.

Another common test that is interfered with by ascorbic acid is that for blood in the stool, an indication of internal bleeding (Jaffe et al., 1975). Dr. Russell M. Jaffe of the National Institutes of Health, who discovered this effect, is now developing a more reliable test.

When a person ingests an ordinary quantity of vitamin C each day the concentration of ascorbate in his or her blood remains constant at about 15 mg per liter. Spero and Anderson (1973) studied twenty-nine subjects who were put on an intake of 1, 2, or 4 g per day. Their blood levels rose at first to over 20 mg per liter but after some days decreased. A similar effect was also noticed by Harris, Robinson, and Pauling (1973), and was attributed by them to increased metabolic utilization of the vitamin C in response to the increase in intake.

This phenomenon is well known in bacteria. The ordinary intestinal bacterium *E. coli* usually uses the simple sugar glucose as its source of carbon. It can also live on the disaccharide lactose (milk sugar). When a culture of *E. coli* is transferred from glucose to lactose it grows very slowly for a while and then rapidly. In order to live on lactose the organism must contain an enzyme that splits lactose into two halves. *E. coli* is able to manufacture this enzyme, betagalactosidase, because it has the corresponding gene in its genetic material, but when it is living on glucose each cell in the culture contains only a dozen molecules of this enzyme. When it is transferred to a medium containing lactose each cell synthesizes several thousand molecules of the enzyme, permitting it to use the lactose more effectively.

This process is called induced enzyme formation. It was discovered in 1900, and was carefully investigated by the French biologist Jacques Monod, who received a Nobel Prize in medicine, shared with François Jacob and Andrew Lwoff, in 1965. Monod and his associates demonstrated that the rate of manufacture of the enzyme under the control of its specific gene is itself controlled by another gene, called a regulatory gene. When there is little or no lactose in the medium the regulatory gene stops the synthesis of the enzyme. This decreases the unnecessary burden on the bacterium of manufacturing a useless enzyme. When lactose is present the regulatory gene starts the process of synthesizing the enzyme, in order that the lactose can be used as food.

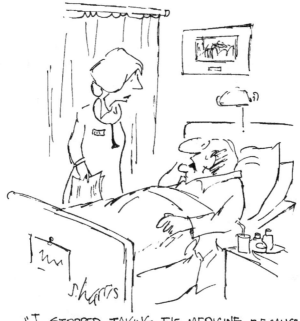

"I STOPPED TAKING THE MEDICINE BECAUSE
I PREFER THE ORIGINAL DISEASE TO
THE SIDE EFFECTS."

The evidence indicates that human beings have similar regulatory genes that control the synthesis of the enzymes involved in the conversion of ascorbic acid into other substances. These other substances, oxidation products, are valuable; it is known, for example, that they are more effective in the control of cancer in animals than is ascorbic acid (Omura et al., 1974 and 1975). But ascorbic acid itself is also an important substance, directly involved in the synthesis of collagen and in other reactions in the human body. It would be catastrophic if the enzymes were to operate so efficiently as to convert all of the ascorbic acid and dehydroascorbic acid into oxidation products that do not have the same biochemical properties as the vitamin. For this reason the regulatory genes stop or slow down the manufacture of the enzymes when the intake of vitamin C is small. When the intake is large the enzymes are produced in larger amounts, permitting more of the ascorbic acid to be converted into the other useful substances.

When a person has been receiving a large amount of vitamin C for a few days or longer the amount of these enzymes is so large that if he or she reverts to a small amount most of the ascorbic acid in the blood is rapidly converted into other substances, and the concentration of ascorbic acid and dehydroascorbic acid in the blood becomes abnormally low. The person's resistance to disease may be decreased. This is the discontinuation effect (also called the rebound effect).†

The discontinuation effect lasts for a week or two. By that time the amount of the enzymes has decreased to the normal value for a low intake, and the concentration of ascorbic acid in the blood has risen to its normal value. It is accordingly wise for people who have been taking a large amount of vitamin C and who decide to revert to a small intake to decrease the intake gradually, over a week or two, rather than suddenly.

The discontinuation effect may not be very important for most people. Anderson, Suryani, and Beaton (1974) checked the amount of winter illness (mainly colds) in their subjects during the month just after they had stopped taking their tablets of ascorbic acid or placebo. During this month the subjects who had been receiving 1 or 2 g of vitamin C each day and those who had been receiving the placebo had nearly the same number of episodes of illness per person, 0.304 and 0.309, respectively. The mean values of number of days indoors per person, 0.384 and 0.409, and number of days off work, 0.221 and 0.268, were a little smaller for the first group than for the second, rather than the reverse, which would be expected if the effect were important. Also, there was no greater amount of illness during the first half than the second half of the month.

Some people might suffer from an abnormality involving these regulatory genes. The presence of an excess of the enzymes that catalyze the oxidation of vitamin C might be responsible for the abnormality in metabolizing the vitamin that is observed for some schizophrenic subjects.

Dr. Ewan Cameron and I, however, pointed out in our book *Cancer and Vitamin C* (1979) that the discontinuation effect might be dangerous for cancer patients and recommended that the intake not be stopped for these patients, even for a single day. This question is discussed further in Chapter 19.

It has been known for more than thirty years that pregnant women need more vitamin C than other women. Part of the reason for this extra need is that the developing fetus needs a good supply of this vitamin, and there is a mechanism in the placenta for pumping vitamin C from the blood of the mother into that of the fetus. In one early study by Javert and Stander (1943) the ascorbate concentration in the blood of the umbilical cord was found to be 14.3 mg per liter, four times that of the blood of the mother. Depletion of the maternal blood for the benefit of the infant continues even after parturition, as ascorbate is secreted in the mother's milk. Cow's milk is much less rich in vitamin C than human milk; the calf does not need extra vitamin C, because it manufactures its own in the cells of its liver.

In normal pregnancy women with the usual low intake of vitamin C have been reported to show a steady decrease in blood plasma concentration from 11 mg per liter (average for 246 women) to 5 mg per liter at four months and then to 3.5 mg at full term (Javert and Stander, 1943). These low values correspond to poor health not only for the mother but also for the infant. A low value of the concentration of vitamin C in the blood has been shown to be correlated with incidence of hemorrhagic disease of the newborn. Javert and Stander concluded that for good health an intake of 200 mg per day is needed by the pregnant woman, and it is likely that for most pregnant women the optimum intake is still greater, 1 g or more per day. Other nutritional needs must, of course, also be satisfied. Brewer (1966) has emphasized that a good intake of protein and other nutrients is essential to prevent puerperal eclampsia and that the diuretics and diet restrictions that are used to control the increase in weight during pregnancy are harmful.

A good intake of vitamin C has great value in controlling threatened, spontaneous, and habitual abortion. In their study of seventy-nine women with threatened, previous spontaneous, or habitual abortion Javert and Stander had 91 percent success with thirty-three patients who received vitamin C, together with bioflavonoids and vitamin K (only three abortions), whereas all of the forty-six patients who did not receive the vitamin aborted. In his analysis of the management of habitual abortion Greenblatt (1955) concluded that vitamin C with bioflavonoids and vitamin K is the best treatment, the next best being progesterone, vitamin E, and thyroid extract.

During the last seven years various authorities in the field of nutrition who write newspaper columns have repeatedly stated that high intake of vitamin C can cause abortions. The basis for this statement seems to be a brief paper by two physicians in the Soviet Union, Samborskaya and

Ferdman (1966). They reported that twenty women in the age range of twenty to forty years whose menstruation was delayed by ten to fifteen days were given 6 g of ascorbic acid by mouth on each of three successive days, and that sixteen of them then menstruated. I wrote to Samborskaya and Ferdman, asking if any test of pregnancy had been carried out. In reply they sent me only another copy of their paper.

Abram Hoffer (1971) has stated that he has used megadoses of ascorbic acid, 3 to 30 g per day, with more than a thousand patients since 1953 and has not seen one case of kidney-stone formation, miscarriage, excessive dehydration, or any other serious toxicity.

It seems unlikely that ascorbic acid causes abortions, although it may help to control difficulties with menstruation. Lahann (1970) has reviewed the literature, especially that in German and Austrian journals. He concluded that noticeable improvement in menstruation had been observed through the oral intake of 200 to 1000 mg of ascorbic acid per day. Moreover, the utilization of ascorbic acid increases sharply in the course of the menstrual cycle, especially at the time of ovulation, and measurement of this utilization can be used for determining the end of ovulation and accordingly for determining the time of optimum conception in relation to the problem of overcoming sterility (Paeschke and Vasterling, 1968).

The prophylactic value of vitamin supplements, even in the small amounts recommended by the Food and Nutrition Board, is indicated by a report from England of a study of vitamin supplements as a way of preventing the development of neural tube defects, such as *spina bifida,* in the developing embryo (Smithells, Sheppard, and Schorah, 1976). Neural tube defects occur in the North American white population with an incidence of about two per thousand live births. The incidence is much higher for a second child of parents whose preceding child has such a defect. The study in England was made with women who had given birth to a child with neural tube defect, by involving 448 such mothers, of whom about half received a multiple vitamin and iron preparation and the other half received a placebo. There was nearly complete prevention of neural tube defects, in that the incidence was only 0.6 percent for the infants of mothers who received the supplement, as compared with 5.0 percent for the infants of unsupplemented mothers.

# V
## *HOW TO LIVE LONGER AND FEEL BETTER*

# 29

## *A Happy Life and a Better World*

From understanding developed during the last twenty years by the new science of nutrition, this book has shown how you can live longer and feel better. For this reward you need not follow a burdensome and disagreeable regimen. On the contrary, the regimen you are to follow is the sensible and pleasant one specified in the second chapter of this book, on which contemporaries of yours are already leading longer and healthier lives. You will multiply the benefits of that regimen by making a habit of the most important recommendation from the new science of nutrition; that is,

TAKE THE OPTIMUM SUPPLEMENTARY AMOUNT OF
EACH OF THE ESSENTIAL VITAMINS EVERY DAY.

No matter what your present age is, you can achieve significant benefits by starting the regimen now. Older people can benefit greatly, because they have special need for optimum nutrition. Steadfast adherence is essential. It is fortunate that the regimen imposes few restrictions on the diet, so that for the most part you can add to the quality of your life by eating foods that you enjoy. What is more, you can, and it is even recommended that you do, enjoy the moderate intake of alcoholic beverages.

In fact, as to eating and drinking there is in this book only one real *don't;* that is sugar. Like the cigarette, the sugar sucrose is a novelty of industrial civilization. Together, they have brought pandemics of cancer and cardiovascular disease to the otherwise fortunate populations of the developed countries. Sugar in breakfast foods (as much, sometimes, as the cereal) is especially harmful to infants and children, and the problem of a good beverage, free of sugar or of the chemical sweeteners that are substituted for it, remains to be solved. The cigarette hazard can be eliminated by quitting the smoking habit. Sucrose cannot be avoided, but a large decrease in the intake of this sugar is essential.

This book has explained the necessity for the supplementary vitamins in human nutrition. It was a significant evolutionary advantage of the early vertebrates that they could leave to the plants they ate the task of synthesizing the vitamins and even some of the amino acids. As the new understanding of life at its molecular level has shown, the latest genetic deletion of this kind deprived the primates of the capacity to manufacture their own vitamin C. Thanks in part to the adaptive advantage conferred by that deletion, the primate line gave rise to humans. The new science of nutrition now instructs us to take advantage of the rational faculty that is the supreme adaptive advantage of the human species to circumvent whatever disadvantage we suffer from those genetic deletions. We can and we must do so by supplementary intakes of the vitamins, especially vitamin C.

In this book we have seen, further, that by keeping in the best of health, in particular by maintaining optimum intake of the vitamins, we can resist the entire long list of illnesses that afflict mankind. The list begins with the afflictions laid upon us by deficiencies of the vitamins, deficiencies so easily cured by restoring the functions in the biochemistry of the body; the vitamins help us to fend off infection and fortify our tissues against the self-assault of cancer and the autoimmune diseases. With the best understood vitamin, vitamin C, as our example, we have been able to envision a new kind of medicine, the orthomolecular medicine that uses substances natural to the body both to protect it from, and to cure, illness. Already, orthomolecular medicine has shown how vitamin C can prevent and cure and may yet eliminate from human experience the illness most familiar and most baffling to the old medicine, the common cold.

At the end, I have given space in this book to the arguments against its thesis that come from many physicians and from old-fashioned nutritionists. I have had to do so because I have not always been able to answer them in the publications and other forums where they have made their criticisms. It is more likely that you have heard from them than from me. In these pages you have heard both sides.

So you see that I shall have a second reason to rejoice in knowing that you are living longer and feeling better.

During the last twenty years we have been experiencing a revolution in our lives, a revolution that permits us to have greater freedom to be productive, to exercise our creativity, and to enjoy life.

Animals in the wild devote most of their time and energy to obtaining enough food to keep alive. Primitive men, women, and children also had to devote most of their time and energy to hunting and to food gathering, searching for fruits, berries, nuts, seeds, and succulent plants. Then, around ten thousand years ago, there occurred a revolution, when agriculture was discovered and animals were domesticated. Obtaining enough food to stay alive did not require all of the time and energy of everyone. Some people were able to think about new ways of doing things, about new tools made from stone or metals, about the motion of the heavenly bodies, about language, even about the meaning of life. Civilization was beginning to develop.

Another step came with the industrial revolution, when machines powered by waterfalls and the combustion of coal and other fuels liberated human beings still more from the drudgery of routine work.

The revolution that has been occurring during the last two decades involves liberation from the great effort that has been required to obtain the proper foods, those that confer the best of health and the best opportunity to lead a good and long life, as free as possible from the suffering caused by illness. This revolution is occurring through the discovery of vitamins and other essential nutrients and the recognition that the optimum intakes, the intakes that provide the best of health, are often far larger than the usually recommended intakes, so large that they can be obtained only as nutritional supplements, not in any diet involving ordinary foods.

The physicians and the old-fashioned professors of nutrition have for fifty years been urging that everyone adopt a diet that is described as healthful. For two or three decades we were all urged to eat a well-balanced diet, with servings of the four categories of food: meat or fish or fowl; cereals; fruits and red or yellow vegetables; and dairy products. This dietary regimen was urged on us whether or not we liked all these foods. Recently much of the enjoyment of life has been taken away from many of us by additional strong recommendations by these authorities. We are told that we should not eat a succulent steak, because of the animal fat. We are told that we should not eat eggs, because of the cholesterol they contain; instead, we are urged to eat a sort of factory product, a preparation, probably not very appealing to the taste, that is made by treating eggs with some chemical solvent to remove some of the cholesterol. We are told not to eat butter. Going to a fine restaurant then is not a pleasure, but a source of worry and a cause of a feeling of guilt.

Why are these recommendations being made to us? A part of the reason is that good health depends on a good supply of vitamins. In the past, to obtain even a passable supply of vitamins, leading to even ordinary poor health, required a moderately large intake of fruits and vegetables. In every culture in countries other than the tropical ones some special foods, such as sauerkraut and pickles, had to be eaten in order for us to survive the winter. Even with the best selection of foods the health of most people has in the past not been very good.

The revolution that is taking place now liberates us from this obsession to restrict our diet, to refrain from eating those foods that we like. The only limitations that I suggest are that you not eat large amounts of food and that you limit your intake of the sugar sucrose. This nutritional freedom has become possible because of the availability of vitamin and mineral supplements.

Moreover, it is now possible to take these important nutrients in the optimum amounts, far larger than can be obtained in foods, and in this way to achieve a sort of superhealth, far beyond what was possible in earlier times. We can be grateful to the organic chemists and biochemists of the past 140 years who laboriously solved the riddles of the nature of the compounds of carbon and the way that they interact with one another in the human body. Because of their efforts, we are now able to get greater enjoyment of life.

Finally, I cannot refrain from mentioning that the greatest threat to your health and that of your children, grandchildren, and others is the possibility of nuclear war. The real possibility that the American people, and everyone else, would be killed in a nuclear war between the United States and the Soviet Union might seem to make it a waste of effort for me to suggest ways for you to live longer and be happier. I believe, however, that the catastrophe can be averted, and that it is worthwhile to work to improve the quality of life. You can contribute to improving not only the quality of your own life but also that of your fellow human beings by working for sanity in international relations. The criterion of success is a decrease in the military budgets of the great nations.

Do not let either the medical authorities or the politicians mislead you. Find out what the facts are, and make your own decisions about how to live a happy life and how to work for a better world.

# Bibliography

ABBOTT, P.; SEVENTY-SEVEN OTHERS (1968). Ineffectiveness of Vitamin C in Treating Coryza. *The Practitioner* 200:442-445.

ABRAHAM, S., LOWENSTEIN. F. W.; JOHNSON, C. L. (1976). Dietary Intake and Biochemical Findings (preliminary). *First Health and Nutrition Examination Survey, United States, 1971-1972.* Department of Health, Education, and Welfare Publication No. (HRA) 76-1219-1.

ADAMS, J. M. (1976). *Viruses and Colds: The Modern Plague.* American Elsevier, New York.

AFZELIUS, B. A. (1976). A Human Syndrome Caused by Immotile Cilia. *Science* 193:317-319.

ALTMAN, P. L.; DITTMER, D. S. (1968). Metabolism. *Federation of American Societies for Experimental Biology.* Bethesda, Md.

ALTSCHUL, R. (1964). *Niacin in Vascular Disorders and Hyperlipemia.* Charles C. Thomas, Springfield, Ill.

ALTSCHULE, M. D. (1976). Is It True What They Say about Cholesterol? *Executive Health* 12: no.11.

AMERICAN PSYCHIATRIC ASSOCIATION (1973). Megavitamin and Orthomolecular Therapy in Psychiatry. *Task Force Report 7.* American Psychiatric Association. Washington, D.C.

ANAH, C. O.; JARIKE, L. N.; BAIG, H. A. (1980). High Dose Ascorbic Acid in Nigerian Asthmatics. *Tropical and Geographical Medicine* 32:132-137.

ANDERSON, R. (1981a). Ascorbate-Mediated Stimulation of Neutrophil Motility and Lymphocyte Transformation by Inhibition of the Peroxidase-$H_2O_2$-Halide System in Vitro and in Vivo. *American Journal of Clinical Nutrition* 34:1906-1911.

ANDERSON, R. (1981b). Assessment of Oral Ascorbate in Three Children with Chronic Granulomatous Disease and Defective Neutrophil Motility over a Two-Year Period. *Clinical and Experimental Immunology* 43:180-188.

ANDERSON, R. (1982). Effects of Ascorbate on Normal and Abnormal Leukocyte Functions, in *Vitamin C: New Clinical Applications in Immunology, Lipid Metabolism, and Cancer,* ed. A. Hanck. Hans Huber, Bern, pp. 23-34.

ANDERSON, R.; HAY, I.; VAN WYK, H.; OOSTHUIZEN, R.; THERON, A. (1980). The Effect of Ascorbate on Cellular Humoral Immunity in Asthmatic Children. *South African Medical Journal* 58:974-977.

ANDERSON, T. W.; BEATON, G. H.; COREY, P. N.; SPERO, L. (1975). Winter Illness and Vitamin C: The Effect of Relatively Low Doses. *Canadian Medical Association Journal* 112:823-826.

ANDERSON, T. W.; REID, D. B. W.; BEATON, G. H. (1972). Vitamin C and the Common Cold: A Double Blind Trial. *Canadian Medical Association Journal* 107:503-508.

ANDERSON, T. W ; SURYANI, G.; BEATON, G. H. (1974). The Effect on Winter Illness of Large Doses of Vitamin C. *Canadian Medical Association Journal* 11:31-36.

ANDREWES, C. (1965). *The Common Cold.* W. W. Norton, New York.

ANONYMOUS (1911). Scurvy. *The Encyclopedia Britannica,* 11th ed., vol. XXIV, p. 517. University of Cambridge, England.

ASFORA, J. (1977). Vitamin C in High Doses in the Treatment of the Common Cold, in *Re-evaluation of Vitamin C,* eds. A. Hanck and G. Ritzel. Hans Huber, Bern, pp. 219-234.

ATKINS, G. I.; BELLER, G. A.; PAINE. L. S.; THORUP, O. A., JR. (1985). High Tech Cardiology—Issues and Costs. *The Pharos* 48. no. 3:31-37.

BANKS, H. S. (1965). Common Cold: Controlled Trials. *The Lancet* 2:790.

BANKS, H. S. (1968). Controlled Trials in the Early Antibiotic Treatment of Colds. *The Medical Officer* 119:7-10.

BARNES, F. E., JR. (1961). Vitamin Supplements and the Incidence of Colds in High School Basketball Players. *North Carolina Medical Journal* 22:22-26.

BARNESS, L. A. (1977). Some Toxic Effects of Vitamin C, in *Re-evaluation of Vitamin C,* eds., A. Hanck and G. Ritzel. Hans Huber, Bern, pp. 23-29.

BARR, D. P.; RUSS, E. M.; EDER, H. A. (1951). Protein-Lipid Relationships in Human Plasma. II. In Atherosclerosis and Related Conditions. *American Journal of Medicine* 11:480-493.

BARTLETT, M. K.; JONES, C. M.; RYAN, A. E. (1942). Vitamin C and Wound Healing. II. Ascorbic Acid Content and Tensile Strength of Healing Wounds in Human Beings. *New England Journal of Medicine* 226:474-481.

BARTLEY, W.; KREBS, H. A.; O'BRIEN, J. R. P. (1953). *Medical Research Council Special Report Series* No. 280. Her Majesty's Stationery Office, London.

BATES, C. J.; MANDAL, A. R.; COLE, T. J. (1977). HDL-Cholesterol and Vitamin-C Status. *The Lancet* 3:611.

BELFIELD, W. O.; STONE, I. (1975). Megascorbic Prophylaxis and Megascorbic Therapy: A New Orthomolecular Modality in Veterinary Medicine. *Journal of the International Academy of Preventive Medicine* 2:10-26.

BELFIELD, W. O.; ZUCKER, M. (1983). *The Very Healthy Cat Book.* McGraw-Hill, New York.

BELFIELD, W. O; ZUCKER, M. (1981). *How to Have a Healthier Dog: The Benefits of Vitamins and Minerals for Your Dog's Life Cycles.* Doubleday, New York.

BELLOC, N. B.; BRESLOW, L. (1972). The Relation of Physical Health Status and Health Practices. *Preventive Medicine* 1:409-421.

BELLOC, N. B.; BRESLOW, L. (1973). Relationship of Health Practices and Mortality. *Preventive Medicine* 2:67-81.

BESSEL-LORCK, C. (1959). Erkältungsprophylaxe bei Jugendlichen im Skilager. *Medizinische Welt* 44:2126-2127.

BIETTI, G. B. (1967). Further Contributions on the Value of Osmotic Substances as Means to Reduce Intra-Ocular Pressure. *Ophthalmological Society of Australia* 26:61-71.

BJELKE, E. (1973). Epidemiologic Studies of Cancer of the Stomach, Colon, and Rectum. Dissertation, University of Minnesota.

BJELKE, E. (1974). Epidemiologic Studies of Cancer of the Stomach, Colon, and Rectum with Special Emphasis on the Role of Diet. *Scandinavian Journal of Gastroenterology* 9 (Suppl. 31): 1-235.

BJORKSTEN, J. (1951). Crosslinkages in Protein Chemistry. *Advances in Protein Chemistry* 6:343-381.

BOISSEVIN, C. H.; SPILLANE, J. H. (1937). Effect of Synthetic Ascorbic Acid on the Growth of Tuberculosis Bacillus. *American Review of Tuberculosis* 35:661-662.

BORDEN, E. C. (1984). Progress toward Therapeutic Application of Interferons. *Cancer* 54:2770-2776.

BOURNE, G. H. (1946). The Effect of Vitamin C on the Healing of Wounds. *Proceedings of the Nutrition Society* 4:204-211.

BOURNE, G. H. (1949). Vitamin C and Immunity. *British Journal of Nutrition* 2:346-356.

BOXER, L. A.; WATANABE, A. M.; RISTER, M.; BESCH, H. R., JR.; ALLEN, J.; BACHNER, R. L. (1976). Correction of Leukocyte Function in Chediak-Higashi Syndrome by Ascorbate. *New England Journal of Medicine* 295:1041-1045.

BOXER, L. A.; VANDERBILT, B.; BONSIB, S.; JERSILD, R.; YANG, H. H.; BACHNER, R. L. (1979). Enhancement of Chemotactic Response and Microtubule Assembly in Human Leukocytes by Ascorbic Acid. *Journal of Cellular Physiology* 100:119-126.

BOYD, A. M.; MARKS, J. (1963). Treatment of Intermittent Claudication: A Reappraisal of the Value of Alphatocopherol. *Angiology* 14:198-208.

BOYD, T. A. S.; CAMPBELL, F. W. (1950). Influence of Ascorbic Acid on the Healing of Corneal Ulcers in Man. *British Medical Journal* 2:1145-1148.

BRAENDEN, O. J. (1973). The Common Cold: A New Approach. *International Research Communications System* 7:12.

BRANDT, R.; GUYER, K. E.; BANKS, W. L., JR. (1974). A Simple Method to Prevent Vitamin C Interference with Urinary Glucose Determinations. *Clinica Chimica Acta* 51:103-104.

BREWER, T. H. (1966). *Metabolic Toxemia of Late Pregnancy: A Disease of Malnutrition.* Charles C. Thomas, Springfield, Ill.

BRIGGS, M. H.; GARCIA-WEBB, P.; DAVIS, F. (1973). Urinary oxalate and vitamin-C supplements. *Lancet* 2(7822):201 passim.

BRODY, JANE E. (1984). Vitamin Therapy: The Toxic Side Effects of Massive Doses. *New York Times,* New York, 14 March; correction 7 May.

BROWN, E. A.; RUSKIN, S. (1949). The Use of Cevitamic Acid in the Symptomatic and Coseasonal Treatment of Pollinosis. *Annals of Allergy* 7:65-70.

BROWN, W. A.; FARMER, A. W.; FRANKS, W. R. (1948). Local Application of Aluminum Foil and Other Substances in Burn Therapy. *American Journal of Surgery* 76:594-604.

BRUCE, R.; EYSSEN, G. M.; CIAMPI, A.; DION, P. W.; BOYD, N. (1981). Strategies for Dietary Intervention Studies in Colon Cancer. *Cancer* 47: 1121-1125.

BRUCE, W. R.; VARGHESE, A. J.; WANG, S.; DION, P. (1979). *Naturally Occurring Carcinogens-Mutagens and Modulators of Carcinogenesis,* eds. E. C. Miller et al. Japan Sci. Soc. Press, Tokyo/University Park Press, Baltimore, pp. 177-184.

BURNS, J. J.; MOSBACH, E. H.; SCHULENBERG, S. (1954). Ascorbic acid synthesis in normal and drug-treated rats, studied with L-ascorbic-1-C14 acid. *J. Biol. Chem.* Apr., 207(2):679-87.

BURR, R. G.; RAJAN, K. T. (1972). Leukocyte Ascorbic Acid and Pressure Sores in Paraplegia. *British Journal of Nutrition* 28:275-281.

BUZZARD, I. M.; MC ROBERTS, M. R.; DRISCOLL, D. L.; BOWERING, J. (1982). Effect of Dietary Eggs and Ascorbic Acid on Plasma Lipid and Lipoprotein Cholesterol Levels in Healthy Young Men. *American Journal of Clinical Nutrition* 36:94-105.

CAMERON, E. (1966). *Hyaluronidase and Cancer.* Pergamon Press, New York.

CAMERON, E. (1975). Vitamin C. *British Journal of Hospital Medicine.* 13:511-514.

CAMERON, E. (1976). Biological Function of Ascorbic Acid and the Pathogenesis of Scurvy. *Medical Hypotheses* 2:154-163.

CAMERON, E.; BAIRD, G. (1973). Ascorbic Acid and Dependence on Opiates in Patients with Advanced Disseminated Cancer. *IRCS* Letter to the Editor, August.

CAMERON, E.; CAMPBELL, A. (1974). The Orthomolecular Treatment of Cancer. II. Clinical Trial of High-dose Ascorbic Supplements in Advanced Human Cancer. *Chemical-Biological Interactions* 9:285-315.

CAMERON, E.; CAMPBELL, A.; JACK, T. (1975). The Orthomolecular Treatment of Cancer. III. Reticulum Cell Sarcoma: Double Complete Regression Induced by High-dose Ascorbic Acid Therapy. *Chemical-Biological Interactions* 11:387-393.

CAMERON, E.; PAULING, L. (1973). Ascorbic Acid and the Glycosaminoglycans: An Orthomolecular Approach to Cancer and Other Diseases. *Oncology* 27:181-192.

CAMERON, E.; PAULING, L. (1974). The Orthomolecular Treatment of Cancer. I. The Role of Ascorbic Acid in Host Resistance. *Chemical-Biological Interactions* 9:273-283.

CAMERON, E.; PAULING, L. (1976). Supplemental Ascorbate in the Supportive Treatment of Cancer: Prolongation of Survival Times in Terminal Human Cancer. *Proceedings of the National Academy of Sciences USA* 73:3685-3689.

CAMERON, E.: PAULING, L. (1978a). Supplemental Ascorbate in the Supportive Treatment of Cancer: Reevaluation of Prolongation of Survival Times in Terminal Human Cancer. *Proceedings of the National Academy of Sciences USA* 75:4538-4542.

CAMERON, E.; PAULING, L. (1978b). Experimental Studies Designed to Evaluate the Management of Patients with Incurable Cancer. *Proceedings of the National Academy of Sciences USA* 75:6252.

CAMERON, E.; PAULING, L. (1979). Ascorbate and Cancer. *Proceedings of the American Philosophical Society* 123:117-123.

CAMERON, E.; PAULING, L. (1979). *Cancer and Vitamin C.* Linus Pauling Institute of Science and Medicine. Palo Alto, Cal.

CAMERON, E.; PAULING, L.; LEIBOVITZ, B. (1979). Ascorbic Acid and Cancer: A Review. *Cancer Research* 39:663-681.

CAMERON, E.; ROTMAN, D. (1972). Ascorbic Acid, Cell Proliferation, and Cancer. *The Lancet* 1:542.

CARDINALE, G. J.; UDENFRIEND, S. (1974). Prolyl Hydroxylase. *Advances in Enzymology* 41:245-300.

CARR, A. B.; EINSTEIN, R.; LAI, L. Y.; MARTIN, N. G.; STARMER, G. A. (1981a). Vitamin C and the Common Cold, Using Identical Twins as Controls. *Medical Journal of Australia* 2:411-412.

CARR, A. B.; EINSTEIN, R.; LAI, L. Y.; MARTIN, N. G.; STARMER, G. A. (1981b). Vitamin C and the Common Cold: A Second MZ Cotwin Control Study. *Acta Geneticae Medicae et Gemellologiae* 30:249-255.

CATHCART, R. F. (1975). Clinical Trial of Vitamin C. *Medical Tribune,* June 25.

CATHCART, R. F. (1981). Vitamin C, Titrating to Bowel Tolerance, Anascorbemia, and Acute Induced Scurvy. *Medical Hypotheses* 7:1359-1376.

CATHCART, R. F. (1984). Vitamin C in the Treatment of Acquired Immune Deficiency Syndrome (AIDS). *Medical Hypotheses* 14:423-433.

CEDERBLAD, G.; LINSTEDT, S. (1976). Metabolism of Labeled Carnitine in the Rat. *Archives of Biochemistry and Biophysics* 175:173-182.

CHARLESTON, S. S.; CLEGG, K. M. (1972). Ascorbic Acid and the Common Cold. *The Lancet* 1:1401.

CHATTERJEE, I. B.; DAS GUPTA, S.; MAJUMDER, A. K.; NANDI, B. K., SUBRAMANIAN, N. (1975a). Effect of Ascorbic Acid on Histamine Metabolism in  Scorbutic Guinea Pigs. *Journal of Physiology* (London) 251:271-279.

CHATTERJEE, I. B.; MAJUMDER, A. K.; NANDI, B. K.; SUBRAMANIAN, N. (1975b). Synthesis and Some Major Functions of Vitamin C in Animals. *Annals of the New York Academy of Sciences* 258:24-47.

CHERASKIN, E.; RINGSDORF, W. M., JR.; HUTCHINS, K.; SETYAADMADJA, A. T. S. H.; WIDEMAN, G. L. (1968). Effect of Diet Upon Radiation Response in Cervical Carcinoma of the Uterus: A Preliminary Report. *Acta Cytologica* 12:433-438.

CHERASKIN, E.; RINGSDORF, W. M., JR. (1971). *New Hope for Incurable Disease.* Arco, New York.

CHERASKIN, E.; RINGSDORF, W. M., JR. (1973). *Predictive Medicine, A Study in Strategy.* Pacific Press, Mountain View, Cal.

CHERASKIN, E.; RINGSDORF, W. M., JR. (1974). *Psychodietetics: Food as the Key to Emotional Health.* Stein and Day, New York.

CHERASKIN, E.; RINGSDORF, W. M., JR.; SISLEY, E. L. (1983). *The Vitamin C Connection.* Harper and Row, New York.

CHERKIN, A. (1967). Parnassus Revisited. *Science* 155:266-268.

CHOPE, H. D.; BRESLOW, L. (1955). Nutritional Status of the Aging. *American Journal of Public Health* 46:61-67.

CLEAVE, T. L. (1975). *The Saccharine Disease.* Keats Publishing, New Canaan, Conn.

CLECKLEY, H. M.; SYDENSTRICKER, V. P.; GEESLIN, L. E. (1939). Nicotinic Acid in the Treatment of Atypical Psychotic States. *Journal of the American Medical Association* 112:2107-2110.

CLEGG, K. M.; MAC DONALD, J. M. (1975). L-Ascorbic Acid and D-Isoascorbic Acid in a Common Cold Survey. *The American Journal of Clinical Nutrition* 28:973-976.

CLEMETSON, C. A. B. (1980). Histamine and Ascorbic Acid in Human Blood. *Journal of Nutrition* 110:662-668.

COHEN, A. M (1960). Effect of Change in Environment on the Prevalence of Diabetes among Yemenite and Kurdish Communities. *Israel Medical Journal* 19:137-142.

COHEN, A. M.; BAVLY, S.; POZNANSKI, R. (1961). Change of Diet of Yemenite Jews in Relation to Diabetes and Ischaemic Heart-Disease. *The Lancet* 2:1399-1401.

COLLIER, R. (1974). *The Plague of the Spanish Lady.* Atheneum, New York.

COLLINS, C. K.; LEWIS, A. E.; RINGSDORF, W. M., JR.; CHERASKIN, E. (1967). Effect of Ascorbic Acid on Oral Healing in Guinea Pigs. *Internationale Zeitschrift für Vitaminforschung* 37:492-495.

COMMITTEE ON ANIMAL NUTRITION (1972). *Nutrient Requirements of Laboratory Animals: Cat, Guinea Pig, Hamster, Monkey, Mouse, Rat.* National Academy of Sciences, Washington, D.C.

*Consumer Reports* (1971). Vitamin C, Linus Pauling, and the Common Cold. February issue.

*Consumer Reports* (1973). Vitamin E: What's Behind All Those Claims for It? January issue.

COOKE, W. L.; MILLIGAN, R. S. (1977). Recurrent Hemoperitoneum Reversed by Ascorbic Acid. *Journal of the American Medical Association* 237:1358-1359.

COON, W. W. (1962). Ascorbic Acid Metabolism in Postoperative Patients. *Surgery, Gynecology, and Obstetrics* 114:522-534.

CORONARY DRUG PROJECT RESEARCH GROUP (1975) Clofibrate and Niacin in Coronary Heart Disease. *Journal of the American Medical Association* 231:360-381.

COTTINGHAM, E.; MILLS, C. A. (1943). Influence of Temperature and Vitamin Deficiency upon Phagocytic Functions. *Journal of Immunology* 47:493-502.

COULEHAN, J. L.; REISINGER, K. S.; ROGERS, K. D.; BRADLEY, D. W. (1974). Vitamin C Prophylaxis in a Boarding School. *The New England Journal of Medicine* 290:6-10.

COUSINS, N. (1979). *Anatomy of an Illness as Perceived by the Patient: Reflections on Healing and Regeneration.* W. W. Norton, New York.

COWAN, D. W.; DIEHL, H. S. (1950). Antihistamine Agents and Ascorbic Acid in the Early Treatment of the Common Cold. *Journal of the American Medical Association* 143:421-424.

COWAN, D. W.; DIEHL, H. S.; BAKER, A. B. (1942). Vitamins for the Prevention of Colds. *Journal of the American Medical Association* 120:1268-1271.

CRANDON, J. H.; LENNIHAN, R., JR.; MIKAL, S.; REIF, A. E. (1961). Ascorbic Acid Economy in Surgical Patients. *Annals of the New York Academy of Sciences* 92:246-267.

CREAGAN, E. T.; MOERTEL, C. G.; O'FALLON, J. R.; SCHUTT, A. J.; O'CONNELL, M. J.; RUBIN, J.; FRYTAK, S. (1979). Failure of High-Dose Vitamin C (Ascorbic Acid) Therapy to Benefit Patients with Advanced Cancer: A Controlled Trial. *The New England Journal of Medicine* 301:687-690.

DAHLBERG, G.; ENGEL, A.; RYDIN, H. (1944). *The value of ascorbic acid as a prophylactic against common colds.* Acta Medica Scandinavica 119: 540-561.

DAVIDSON, S.; PASSMORE, R.; BROCK, J. F.; TRUSWELL, A. S. (1975). *Human Nutrition and Dietetics.* Churchill Livingstone, Edinburgh, London, and New York.

DEBRÉ, R. (1918). L'anergie dans la grippe. *Comptes rendus Soc. Biol.* (Paris) 81:913-914.

DEBRÉ, R.; CELERS, J. (1970). *Clinical Virology.* W. B. Saunders, Philadelphia.

DE COSSE, J. J.; ADAMS, M. B.; KUZMA, J. F.; LO GERFO, P.; CONDON, R. E. (1975). Effect of Ascorbic on Rectal Polyps of Patients with Familial Polyposis. *Surgery* 78:608-612.

DEMOLE, V. (1934). On the Physiological Action of Ascorbic Acid and Some Related Compounds. *Biochemical Journal* 28:770-773.

DEUCHER, W. G. (1940). Observations on the Metabolism of Vitamin C in Cancer Patients (in German). *Strahlentherapie* 67:143-151.

DICE, J. F.; DANIEL, C. W. (1973). The Hypoglycemic Effect of Ascorbic Acid in a Juvenile-onset Diabetic. *International Research Communications System* 1:41.

DICKEY, L. D. (1976). *Clinical Ecology.* Charles C. Thomas, Springfield, Ill.

DOLL, R. (1977). *Origins of Human Cancer: Book A. Incidence of Cancer in Humans,* eds. H. H. Hiatt, J. D. Watson, and J. A. Winsten. Cold Spring Harbor Laboratory, Cold Spring, N. Y., pp. 1-12.

DONEGAN, C. K.; MESSER, A. L.; ORGAIN, E. S.; RUFFIN, J. M. (1949). Negative Results of Tocopherol Therapy in Cardiovascular Disease. *American Journal of the Medical Sciences* 217:294-299.

DREISBACH, R. H. (1969). *Handbook of Poisoning: Diagnosis and Treatment.* 6th edition. Lange Medical Publications, Los Altos, Cal.

DUJARRIC DE LA RIVIÈRE, R. (1918). La grippe est-elle une maladie à virus filtrant? *Comptes rendus Acad. Sci.* (Paris) 167:606.

DU VAL, M. K. (1977). The Provider, the Government, and the Consumer, in *Doing Better and Feeling Worse: Health in the United States,* ed. J. H. Knowles. W. W. Norton, New York, pp. 185-192.

DYKES, M. H. M.; MEIER, P. (1975). Ascorbic Acid and the Common Cold. *Journal of the American Medical Association* 231:1073-1079.

EATON, S. B.; KONNER, M. (1985). Paleolithic Nutrition: A Consideration of Its Nature and Current Implications. *The New England Journal of Medicine* 312:283-289.

ECKHOLM, E. P. (1977). *The Picture of Health: Environmental Sources of Disease.* W. W. Norton, New York.

EDWIN, E.; HOLTEN, K.; NORUM, K. R.; SCHRUMPF, A.; SKAUG, O. E. (1965), Vitamin $B_{12}$ Hypovitaminosis in Mental Diseases. *Acta Medica Scandinavica* 177:689-699.

EKVALL, S.; BOZIAN, R. (1979). Effect of Supplemental Ascorbic Acid on Serum Vitamin $B_{12}$ and Serum Ascorbate Levels in Myelomeningocele Patients. *Federation of American Societies of Experimental Biology* 38:452.

ELLIOTT, B. (1973). Ascorbic Acid: Efficacy in the Prevention of Symptoms of Respiratory Infection on a Polaris Submarine. *International Research Communications System.* May.

ELLIOTT, H. C. (1982). Effects of Vitamin C Loading on Serum Constituents in Man. *Proceedings of the Society for Experimental Biology and Medicine* 169:363-367.

ELLIS, J. M. (1966). *The Doctor Who Looked at Hands.* Vantage Press, New York.

ELLIS, J. M. (1983). *Free of Pain: A Proven and Inexpensive Treatment for Specific Types of Rheumatism.* Southwest Publishing, Brownsville and Dallas, Tex.

ELLIS, J. M.; PRESLEY, J. (1973). *Vitamin $B_6$, the Doctor's Report.* Harper and Row, New York.

ELLIS, J. M.; FOLKERS, K.; LEVY, M.; SHIZUKOISHI, S.; LEWANDOWSKI, J.; NISHII, S.; SHUBERT, H. A.; ULRICK, R. (1982). Response of Vitamin $B_6$ Deficiency and the Carpal Tunnel Syndrome to Pyridoxine. *Proceedings of the National Academy of Sciences USA* 79:7494-7498.

ENGEL, A.; ANGELINI, C. (1973). Carnitine Deficiency of Human Skeletal Muscle with Associated Lipid Storage Myopathy: A New Syndrome. *Science* 179:899-902.

ENLOE, C. F., JR. (1971). The Virtue of Theory. *Nutrition Today* January-February, p. 21.

ENSTROM, J. E.; PAULING, L. (1982). Mortality Among Health-Conscious Elderly Californians. *Proceedings of the National Academy of Sciences USA* 79:6023-6027.

EPSTEIN, S. S. (1978). *The Politics of Cancer.* Sierra Club Books, San Francisco.

ERICSSON, Y.; LUNDBECK, H. (1955). Antimicrobial Effect *in vitro* of the Ascorbic Acid Oxidation. I. Effect on Bacteria, Fungi and Viruses in Pure Culture. II. Influence of Various Chemical and Physical Factors. *Acta Pathologica et Microbiologica Scandinavica* 37:493-527.

ERTEL, H. (1941). Der Verlauf der Vitamin C-Prophylaxen in Frühjahr. *Die Ernährung* 6:269-273.

EULER, U. S. VON (1937). On the Specific Vasodilating and Plain Muscle Stimulating Substances from Accessory Genital Glands in Man and Certain Animals (Prostaglandin and Vesiglandin). *Journal of Physiology* 88:213-234.

EVERSON, T. C.; COLE, W. H. (1966). *Spontaneous Repression of Cancer.* W. B. Saunders, Philadelphia.

FABRICANT, N. D.; CONKLIN, G. (1965). *The Dangerous Cold.* Macmillan, New York.

FEIGEN, G. A.; SMITH, B. H.; DIX, C. E.; FLYNN, C. J.; PETERSON, N. S.; ROSENBERG, L. T.; PAVLOVIC, S.; LEIBOVITZ, B. (1982). Enhancement of Antibody Production and Protection Against Systemic Anaphylaxis by Large Doses of Vitamin C. *Research Communications in Chemical Pathology and Pharmacology* 38:313-333.

FIDANZA, A.; AUDISIO, M.; MASTROIACOVO, P. (1982). Vitamin C and Cholesterol, in *Vitamin C: New Clinical Applications in Immunology, Lipid Metabolism, and Cancer,* ed. A. Hanck. Hans Huber, Bern, pp. 153-171.

FLETCHER, J. M.; FLETCHER, I. C. (1951). Vitamin C and the Common Cold. *British Medical Journal* 1:887.

FOLKERS, K.; ELLIS, J.; WATANABE, T.; SAJI, S.; KAJI, M. (1978). Biochemical Evidence for a Deficiency of Vitamin $B_6$ in the Carpal Tunnel Syndrome Based on a Crossover Clinical Study. *Proceedings of the National Academy of Sciences USA* 75:3418-3422.

FRANZ, W. L.; SANDS, G. W.; HEYL, H. L. (1956). Blood Ascorbic Acid Level in Bioflavonoid and Ascorbic Acid Therapy of Common Cold. *Journal of the American Medical Association* 162:1224-1226.

FRIEDMAN, G. J.; SHERRY, S.; RALLI, E. P. (1940). Mechanism of Excretion of Vitamin C by Human Kidney at Low and Normal Plasma Levels of Ascorbic Acid. *Journal of Clinical Investigations* 19:685-689.

FULLMER, H. M.; MARTIN, G. R.; BURNS, J. J. (1961). Role of Ascorbic Acid in the Formation and Maintenance of Dental Structures. *Annals of the New York Academy of Sciences* 92:286-294.

FUNK, C. (1912). The Etiology of the Deficiency Diseases: Beri-Beri Polyneuritis in Birds, Epidemic Dropsy, Scurvy, Experimental Scurvy in Animals, Infantile Scurvy, Ship Beri-Beri, Pellagra. *J. St. Med.* 20:341-368.

GALLIN, J. I. (1981). Abnormal Phagocyte Chemotaxis: Pathophysiology, Clinical Manifestations, and Management of Patients. *Reviews of Infectious Diseases* 3:1196-1220.

GALLIN, J. I.; ELIN, R. J.; HUBERT, R. T.; FAUCI, A. S.; KALINER, M. A.; WOLFF, S. M. (1979). Efficacy of Ascorbic Acid in Chediak-Higashi Syndrome: Studies in Humans and Mice. *Blood* 53:226-234.

GEORGE, N. (1951). Vitamin E and Diabetic Ulceration. *Summary* (Shute Foundation, London, Canada) 3:74-75.

GERSON, M. (1958). *A Cancer Therapy: Results of Fifty Cases,* 2d edition. Totality Books, Del Mar, Cal.

GILDERSLEEVE, D. (1967). Why Organized Medicine Sneezes at the Common Cold. *Fact,* July-August, pp. 21-23.

GINTER, E. (1970). *The Role of Ascorbic Acid in Cholesterol Metabolism.* The Slovak Academy of Sciences, Bratislava, Czechoslovakia.

GINTER, E. (1973). Cholesterol: Vitamin C Controls Its Transformation into Bile Acids. *Science* 179:702.

GINTER, E. (1975). *The Role of Vitamin C in Cholesterol Catabolism and Atherogenesis.* The Slovak Academy of Sciences, Bratislava, Czechoslovakia.

GINTER, E. (1977). Vitamin C and Cholesterol, in *Re-evaluation of Vitamin C,* eds. A. Hanck and G. Ritzel. Hans Huber, Bern, pp. 53-66.

GINTER, E. (1978). Marginal Vitamin C Deficiency, Lipid Metabolism, and Atherosclerosis. *Lipid Research* 16:167-220.

GINTER, E. (1982). Vitamin C in the Control of Hypercholesteremia in Man, in *Vitamin C: New Clinical Applications in Immunology, Lipid Metabolism, and Cancer,* ed. A. Hanck. Hans Huber, Bern, pp. 137-152.

GLAZEBROOK, A. J.; THOMSON, S. (1942). The Administration of Vitamin C in a Large Institution and Its Effect on General Health and Resistance to Infection. *Journal of Hygiene* 42:1-19.

GLOVER, E.; KOH, E. T.; TROUT, D. L. (1984). Effect of Ascorbic Acid on Plasma Lipid and Lipoprotein Cholesterol in Normotensive and Hypertensive Subjects. *Federation Proceedings* 43:1057.

GOLDBLATT, M. W. (1933). A Depressor Substance in Seminal Fluid. *Journal of the Society of Chemical Industry* 52:1056-1057.

GOETZL, E. J.; WASSERMAN, S. I.; GIGLI, I.; AUSTEN, K. F. (1974). Enhancement of Random Migration and Chemotactic Response of Human Leukocytes by Ascorbic Acid. *Journal of Clinical Investigation* 53:813-818.

GOMPERTZ, B. (1820). A Sketch of the Analysis and Notation Applicable to the Value of Life Contingencies. *Philosophical Transactions of the Royal Society* 110:214-294.

GOMPERTZ, B. (1825). On the Nature of the Function Expressive of the Law of Human Mortality and on a New Mode of Determining the Value of Life Contingencies. *Philosophical Transactions of the Royal Society* 115:513-585.

GOMPERTZ, B. (1862). A Supplement to Two Papers Published in the Transactions of the Royal Society, "On the Science Connected with Human Mortality": The One Published in 1820, and the Other in 1825. *Philosophical Transactions of the Royal Society* 52:511-559.

GREENBLATT, R. B. (1955). Bioflavonoids and the Capillary: Management of Habitual Abortion. *Annals of the New York Academy of Sciences* 61:713-720.

GREENWOOD, J. (1964). Optimum Vitamin C Intake as a Factor in the Preservation of Disc Integrity. *Medical Annals of the District of Columbia* 33:274-276.

GREER, E. (1954). Alcoholic cirrhosis; complicated by polycythemia vera and then myelogenous leukemia and tolerance of large doses of vitamin C. *Medical Times* 82:865-868.

GULEWITSCH, V. S.; KRIMBERG, R. (1905). On the Nature of Substances Extracted from Muscle: A Communication about Carnitine. *Zeitschrift für Physiologische Chemie* 45:326-330.

HAEGER, K. (1968). The Treatment of Peripheral Occlusive Arterial Disease with Alpha-tocopherol as Compared with Vasodilator Agents and Antiprothrombin [Dicumarol]. *Vascular Diseases 5:*199-213.

HALSTEAD, B. W., JR. (1979). *The Scientific Basis of EDTA Therapy.* Golden Quill, Colton, Cal.

HAMMOND, E. C. (1964). Some Preliminary Findings on Physical Complaints from a Prospective Study of 1,064,004 Men and Women. *American Journal of Public Health* 54:11-22.

HAMMOND, E. C.; HORN, D. (1958). Smoking and Death Rates: Report on 44 Months of Follow-Up on 187,783 Men. I. Total Mortality. II. Death Rates by Cause. *Journal of the American Medical Association* 166:1159-1172; 1294-1308.

HARMAN, D. (1981). The Aging Process. *Proceedings of the National Academy of Sciences USA* 78:7124-7128.

HARRELL, R. F.; CAPP, R. H.; DAVIS, D. R.; PEERLESS, J.; RAVITZ, L. R. (1981). Can Nutritional Supplements Help Mentally Retarded Children? An Exploratory Study. *Proceedings of the National Academy of Sciences USA* 78:574-578.

HARRIS, A.; ROBINSON, A. B.; PAULING, L. (1973). Blood Plasma L-Ascorbic Acid Concentration for Oral L-Ascorbic Acid Dosage up to 12 Grams per Day. *International Research Communications System,* page 19, December.

HARRIS, L. J.; RAY, S. N. (1935). Diagnosis of Vitamin C-Subnutrition by Urinalysis with Note on Antiscorbutic Value of Human Milk. *The Lancet* 1:71-77.

HARTZ, S. C.; MC GANDY, R. B.; JACOB, R. A.; RUSSELL, R. M.; JACQUES, P. (1984). Relationship of Serum Ascorbic Acid and HDL Cholesterol in Elderly Non-Users of Nutrient Supplement. *Federation Proceedings* 43:393.

HAWKINS, D.; PAULING, L. (1973). *Orthomolecular Psychiatry: Treatment of Schizophrenia.* W. H. Freeman and Company, San Francisco.

HERBERT, V.; JACOB, E. (1974). Destruction of Vitamin $B_{12}$ by Ascorbic Acid. *Journal of the American Medical Association* 230:241-242.

HERJANIC, M.; MOSS-HERJANIC, B. L. (1967). Ascorbic Acid Test in Psychiatric Patients. *Journal of Schizophrenia* 1:257-260.

HINDSON, T. C. (1968). Ascorbic Acid for Prickly Heat. *The Lancet* 1:1347-1348.

HINES, K.; DANES, B. H. (1976). Microtubular Defect in Chediak-Higashi Syndrome. *The Lancet,* 145-146, 17 July.

HOEFEL, O. S. (1977). Plasma Vitamin C Levels in Smokers, in *Re-evaluation of Vitamin C.,* ed. A. Hanck. Hans Huber, Bern, pp. 127-138.

HOFFER, A. (1962). *Niacin Therapy in Psychiatry.* Charles C. Thomas, Springfield, Ill.

HOFFER, A. (1971). Ascorbic Acid and Toxicity. *The New England Journal of Medicine* 285:635-636.

HOFFER, A.; OSMOND, H. (1960). *The Chemical Basis of Clinical Psychiatry.* Charles C. Thomas, Springfield, Ill.

HOFFER, A.; OSMOND, H. (1966). *How to Live With Schizophrenia.* University Books, New Hyde Park, New York.

HOFFER, A.; WALKER, M. (1978). *Orthomolecular Nutrition: New Lifestyle for Super Good Health.* Keats Publishing, New Canaan, Conn.

HOLMES, H. N. (1943). Food Allergies and Vitamin C. *Annals of Allergy* 1:235-241.

HOLMES, H. N. (1946). The Use of Vitamin C in Traumatic Shock. *Ohio State Medical Journal* 42:1261-1264.

HOLMES, H. N.; ALEXANDER, W. (1942). Hay Fever and Vitamin C. *Science* 96:497-499.

HOPKINS, F. G. (1912). Feeding Experiments Illustrating the Importance of Accessory Factors in Normal Dietaries. *Journal of Physiology* (London) 44:425-460.

HORROBIN, D. F.; OKA, M.; MANKU, M. S. (1979). The Regulation of Prostaglandin E1 Formation: A Candidate for One of the Fundamental Mechanisms Involved in the Actions of Vitamin C. *Medical Hypotheses* 5:849-858.

HORROBIN, D. F.; MANKU, M. S.; OKA, M.; MORGAN, R. O.; CUNNANE, S. C.; ALLY, A. I.; GHAYUR, T.; SCHWEITZER, M.; KARMALI, R. A. (1979). The Nutritional Regulation of T Lymphocyte Function. *Medical Hypotheses* 5:969-985.

HUGHES, W. T. (1984). Infections in Children with Cancer. *Primary Care and Cancer,* October, 66-72.

HUME, R.; WEYERS, E. (1973). Changes in Leucocyte Ascorbic Acid during the Common Cold. *Scottish Medical Journal* 18:3-7.

INGALLS, T. H.; WARREN, H. A. (1937). Asymptotic Scurvy. Its Relation to Wound Healing and Its Incidence in Patients with Peptic Ulcer. *The New England Journal of Medicine* 217:443-446.

IRVIN, T. T.; CHATTOPADHYAY, D. K. (1978). Ascorbic Acid Requirements in Postoperative Patients. *Surgery, Gynecology, and Obstetrics* 147:49-56.

ISSACS, A.; LINDEMANN, J. (1957). Virus Interference. I. The Interferon. *Proceedings of the Royal Society of London* B147:258-267.

JAFFE, R. M.; KASTEN, B.; YOUNG, D. S.; MAC LOWRY, J. D. (1975). False-Negative Stool Occult Blood Tests Caused by Ingestion of Ascorbic Acid (Vitamin C). *Annals of Internal Medicine* 83:824-826.

JAVERT, C. T.; STANDER, H. J. (1943). Plasma Vitamin C and Prothrombin Concentration in Pregnancy and in Threatened, Spontaneous, and Habitual Abortion. *Surgery, Gynecology, and Obstetrics* 76:115-122.

JOHNSON, G. E.; OBENSHAIN, S. S. (1981). Nonresponsiveness of Serum High-Density Lipoprotein-Cholesterol to High Dose Ascorbic Acid Administration in Normal Men. *American Journal of Clinical Nutrition* 34:2088-2091.

JOHNSON, G. T. (1975). *What You Should Know about Health Care Before You Call a Doctor.* McGraw-Hill, New York.

JONES, H. (1955). *A Special Consideration of the Aging Process, Disease, and Life Expectancy.* University of California Radiation Laboratory, No. 3105.

JONES, H. B. (1956). Demographic Consideration of the Cancer Problem. *Transactions of the New York Academy of Sciences* 18:298-333.

JUNGEBLUT, C. W. (1935). Inactivation of Poliomyelitis Virus by Crystalline Vitamin C (Ascorbic Acid). *Journal of Experimental Medicine* 62:517-521.

KALDEN, J. R.; GUTHY, E. A. (1972). Prolonged skin allograft survival in vitamin C-deficient guinea-pigs. Preliminary communication. *Eur. Surg. Res.* 4(2):114-9.

KALOKERINOS, A. (1981). *Every Second Child.* Keats Publishing, New Canaan, Conn.

KARLOWSKI, T. R.; CHALMERS, T. C.; FRENKEL, L. D.; KAPIKIAN, A. Z.; LEWIS, T. L.; LYNCH, J. M. (1975). Ascorbic Acid for the Common Cold: A Prophylactic and Therapeutic Trial. *Journal of the American Medical Association* 23:1038-1042.

KAUFMAN, W. (1943). *The Common Form of Niacin Amide Deficiency Disease, Aniacinamidosis.* By author. Bridgeport, Conn.

KAUFMAN, W. (1949). *The Common Form of Joint Dysfunction: Its Incidence and Treatment.* E. L. Hildreth, Brattleboro, Vermont.

KAUFMAN, W. (1955). The Use of Vitamin Therapy to Reverse Certain Concomitants of Aging. *Journal of the American Geriatrics Society* 3:927-936.

KAUFMAN, W. (1983). Niacinamide, A Most Neglected Vitamin. *International Academy of Preventive Medicine* 8:5-25.

KEYS, A. (1956). The Diet and the Development of Coronary Heart Disease. *Journal of Chronic Diseases* 4:364-380.

KHAN, A. R.; SEEDARNEE, F. A. (1981). Effect of Ascorbic Acid on Plasma Lipids and Lipoproteins in Healthy Young Women. *Atherosclerosis* 39:89-95.

KIMOTO, E.; TANAKA, H.; GYOTOKU, J.; MORISHIGE, F.; PAULING, L. (1983). Enhancement of Antitumor Activity of Ascorbate against Ehrlich Ascites Tumor Cells by the Copper-Glycylglycylhistidine Complex. *Cancer Research* 43:824-828.

KLASSON, D. H. (1951). Ascorbic Acid in the Treatment of Burns. *New York State Journal of Medicine* 51:2388-2392.

KLENNER, F. R. (1948). Virus Pneumonia and Its Treatment with Vitamin C. *Journal of Southern Medicine and Surgery* 110:60-63.

KLENNER, F. R. (1949). The Treatment of Poliomyelitis and Other Virus Diseases with Vitamin C. *Journal of Southern Medicine iand Surgery* 113:101-107.

KLENNER, F. R. (1951). Massive Doses of Vitamin C and the Viral Diseases. *Southern Medicine and Surgery* 113:101-107.

KLENNER, F. R. (with BARTZ, F. H.) (1969) *The Key to Good Health: Vitamin C.* Graphic Arts Research Foundation. Chicago, Ill.

KLENNER, F. R. (1971) Observations on the Dose and Administration of Ascorbic Acid When Employed beyond the Range of a Vitamin in Human Pathology. *Journal of Applied Nutrition* 23:61-88.

KLENNER, F. R. (1974). Significance of High Daily Intake of Ascorbic Acid in Preventive Medicine. *Journal of the International Academy of Preventive Medicine* 1:45-69.

KNOX, E. G. (1973). Ischaemic Heart Disease Mortality and Dietary Intake of Calcium. *The Lancet* 1:1465.

KODICEK, E. H.; YOUNG, F. G. (1969). Captain Cook and Scurvy. *Notes and Records of the Royal Society* 24:43-60.

KOGAN, B. A. (1970). *Health.* Harcourt, Brace and World, New York.

KORBSCH, R. (1938). Cevitamic Acid Therapy of Allergic Inflammatory Conditions. *Medizinische Klinik* 34:1500-1505.

KORDANSKY, D. W.; ROSENTHAL, R. R.; NORMAN, P. S. (1979). The Effect of Vitamin C on Antigen-Induced Bronchospasm. *Journal of Allergy and Clinical Immunology* 63:61-64.

KROMHOUT, D.; BOSSCHIETER, E. B.; COULANDER, C. DE L. (1985). The Inverse Relation between Fish Consumption and 20-Year Mortality from Coronary Heart Disease. *The New England Journal of Medicine* 312:1205-1209.

KRUEGER, R. (1960). Experimental and Clinical Observations on the Treatment of Alkali Corneal Burns with Ascorbic Acid. *Berichte der Versammlung der deutschen ophthalmologischen Gesellschaft* 62:255-258.

KRUMDIECK, C.; BUTTERWORTH, C. E. (1974). Ascorbate-Cholesterol-Lecithin Interactions: Factors of Potential Importance in the Pathogenesis of Atherosclerosis. *American Journal of Clinical Nutrition* 27:866-876.

KUBALA, A. L.; KATZ, M. M. (1960). Nutritional Factors in Psychological Test Behavior. *Journal of Genetic Psychology* 96:343-352.

KUBLER, W.; GEHLER, J. (1970). Zur Kinetik der enteralen Ascorbinsäureresorption zur Berechnung nicht dosisproportionaler Resorptionsvorgänge. *Internationale Zeitschrift für Vitaminforschung* 40:442-453.

KURZROK, R.; LIEB, C. C. (1930). Biochemical Studies of Human Semen. II. The Action of Human Semen on the Human Uterus. *Proceedings of the Society of Experimental Biology and Medicine* 28:268-272.

KUTSKY, R. J. (1973). *Handbook of Vitamins and Hormones.* Van Nostrand Reinhold, New York.

LAHANN, H. (1970). *Vitamin C, Forschung und Praxis.* Merck, Darmstadt.

LAI, H.-Y. L.; SHIELDS, E. K.; WATNE, A. L. (1977). Effect of Ascorbic Acid on Rectal Polyps and Rectal Steroids. *Federation Proceedings* (Abs.) 35:1061.

LAMDEN, M. P.; CHRYSTOWSKI, G. A. (1954). Urinary Oxalate Excretion by Man Following Ascorbic Acid Ingestion. *Proceedings of the Society for Experimental Biology and Medicine* 85:190-192.

LANE, B. C. (1980). Evaluation of Intraocular Pressure with Daily Sustained Closework Stimulus to Accommodation to Lowered Tissue Chromium and Dietary Deficiency of Ascorbic Acid (Vitamin C). Ph.D. dissertation, New York University.

LEAKE, C. D. (1955). Drug Allergies. *Postgraduate Medicine* 17:132-139.

LEE, P.-F.; LAM, K.-W.; LAI, M.-M. (1977). Aqueous Humor Ascorbate Concentration and Open-Angle Glaucoma. *Archives of Ophthalmology* 95:308-310.

LEE, T. H.; HOOVER, R. L.; WILLIAMS, J. D.; SPERLING, R. I.; ET AL. (1985). Effects of Dietary Enrichment with Eicosapentaenoic and Decosahexaenoic Acids on In Vitro Neutrophil and Monocyte Leukotriene Generation and Neutrophile Function. *The New England Journal of Medicine* 312:1217-1224.

LEIBOVITZ, B. (1984). *Carnitine: The Vitamin $B_T$ Phenomenon.* Dell, New York.

LESSER, M. (1977). Mental Health: It's Not Just in Our Heads, in *Diet Related to Killer Diseases.* V. *Nutrition and Mental Health.* Hearing before the Select Committee on Nutrition and Human Needs of the United States Senate. Government Printing Office, Washington, D.C., pp. 13-27, 94-96.

LIEB, C. W. (1926). The Effect of an Exclusive, Long-Continued Meat Diet, Based on the History, Experiences, and Clinical Survey of Vilhjalmur Stefansson, Arctic Explorer. *Journal of the American Medical Association* 87:25-26.

LIBBY, A. F.; STONE, I. (1977). The Hypoascorbemia-Kwashiorkor Approach to Drug Addiction Therapy: A Pilot Study. *Journal of Orthomolecular Psychiatry* 6:300-308.

LIGHT, N. D.; BAILEY, A. J. (1980). Molecular Structure and Stabilization of the Collagen Fibre, in *Biology of Collagen,* eds. A. Viidik and J. Vuust. Academic Press, New York, pp. 15-38.

LIND, J. A. (1753). *A Treatise of the Scurvy.* Sands, Murray, and Cochrane. Edinburgh; reprinted (1953) Edinburgh University Press.

LUND, C. C.; CRANDON, J. H. (1941). Human Experimental Scurvy and the Relation of Vitamin C Deficiency to Postoperative Pneumonia and to Wound Healing. *Journal of the American Medical Association* 116:663-668.

LUNIN, N. (1881). Über die Bedeutung der anorganischen Salze für die Ernährung des Tieres. *Zeitschrift für physiologische Chemie* 5:31-39.

MACON, W. L. (1956). Citrus Bioflavonoids in the Treatment of the Common Cold. *Industrial Medicine and Surgery* 25:525-527.

MANN, G. V. (1977). Diet-Heart: End of an Era. *The New England Journal of Medicine* 297:644-650.

MARCKWELL. N. W. (1947). Vitamin C in the Prevention of Colds. *Medical Journal of Australia* 2:777-778.

MARCUS. M.; PRABHUDESAI, M.; WASSEF, S. (1980). Stability of Vitamin $B_{12}$ in the Presence of Ascorbic Acid in Food and Serum: Restoration by Cyanide of Apparent Loss. *American Journal of Clinical Nutrition* 33:137-143.

MARTIN, N. G.; CARR, A. B.; OAKESHOTT, J. G.; CLARK, P. (1982). Co-Twin Control Studies: Vitamin C and the Common Cold. *Progress in Clinical and Biological Research* 103A:365-373.

MASEK, J.; NERADILOVA, M.; HEJDA, S. (1972). Vitamin C and Respiratory Infections. *Review of Czechoslovak Medicine* 18:228-235.

MATSUO, E.; SKINSNES, O. K.; CHANG, P. H. C. (1975). Acid Mucopolysaccharide Metabolism in Leprosy. III. Hyaluronic Acid Mycobacterial Growth Enhancement, and Growth Suppression by Saccharic Acid and Vitamin C as Inhibitors of Betaglucuronidase. *International Journal of Leprosy* 43:1-13.

MAYER, J. (1977). *A Diet for Living.* Pocket Books, New York

MC CANN, J.; AMES, B. N. (1977). The *Salmonella/Typhimurium* Microsome Mutagenicity Test: Predictive Value for Animal Carcinogenicity, in *Origins of Human Cancer:* Book C, *Human Risk Assessment,* eds. H. H. Hiatt, J. D. Watson, and J. A. Winsten. Cold Spring Harbor Labratory, Cold Spring, N. Y., pp. 1431-1450.

MC CORMICK, W. J. (1952). Ascorbic Acid as a Chemotherapeutic Agent. *Archives of Pediatrics* 69:151-155.

MC CORMICK, W. J. (1959). Cancer, a Collagen Disease, Secondary to a Nutritional Deficiency. *Archives of Pediatrics* 76:166-171.

MC COY, E. E.; YONGE, K.; KARR, G. W. (1976). *Megavitamin Therapy: Final Report of the Joint University Megavitamin Therapy Review Committee.* Ministry of Social Services and Community Health. Alberta, Canada.

MC GINN, F. P.; HAMILTON, J. C. (1976). Ascorbic Acid Levels in Stored Blood and in Patients Undergoing Surgery after Blood Transfusion. *British Journal of Surgery* 63:505-507.

MC PHERSON, K.; FOX, M. S. (1977). Treatment of Breast Cancer, in *Costs, Risks, and Benefits of Surgery,* eds. J. P. Bunker, B. A. Barnes, and F. Mosteller. Oxford University Press, New York, pp. 308-322.

MC WHIRTER, K. (1948). The Value of Simple Mastectomy and Radiotherapy in the Treatment of Cancer of the Breast. *British Journal of Radiology* 21:252.

MILLER, J. Z.; NANCE, W. E.; NORTON, J. A.; WOLEN, R. L.; GRIFFITH, R S.; ROSE, R. J. (1977). Therapeutic Effect of Vitamin C, a Co-Twin Control Study. *Journal of the American Medical Association* 237:248-251.

MILLER, J. Z.; NANCE, W. E.; KANG, K. (1978). A Co-Twin Control Study of the Effects of Vitamin C. *Progress in Clinical and Biological Research* 24:151-156.

MILLER, N. E.; FÖRDE, O. H.; THELLE, D. S.; MJÖS, O. D. (1977). The Tromso Heart Study: High-Density Lipoprotein and Coronary Heart Disease, a Prospective Case-Control Study. *The Lancet* 1:965.

MILLER, T. E. (1969). Killing and Lysis of Gram-Negative Bacteria through the Synergistic Effect of Hydrogen Peroxide, Ascorbic Acid, and Lysozyme. *Journal of Bacteriology* 98:949-955.

MOERTEL, C. G. (1978). Current Concepts in Cancer Chemotherapy of Gastrointestinal Cancer. *The New England Journal of Medicine* 299:1049-1052.

MOERTEL, C. G.; FLEMING, T. R.; CREAGAN, E. T.; RUBIN, J.; O'CONNELL, M. J.; AMES, M. M. (1985). High-Dose Vitamin C versus Placebo in the Treatment of Patients with Advanced Cancer Who Had No Prior Chemotherapy. *The New England Journal of Medicine* 312:137-141.

MOHSENIN, V.; DU BOIS, A. B.; DOUGLAS, J. S. (1982). Ascorbic Acid Exerts its Effect on Asthmatics through Prostaglandin Metabolism. *American Thoracic Society* 125, abstract.

MONJUKOWA, N. K.; FRADKIN, M. J. (1935). New Experimental Observations on the Pathogenesis of Cataracts. *Archiven der Ophthalmologie* 133:328-338.

MORISHIGE, F.; MURATA, A. (1978). Vitamin C for Prophylaxis of Viral Hepatitis B in Transfused Patients. *Journal of the International Academy of Preventive Medicine* 5:54-58.

MORISHIGE, F.; MURATA, A. (1978). Prolongation of Survival Times in Terminal Human Cancer by Administration of Supplemental Ascorbate. *Journal of the International Academy of Preventive Medicine* 5:47-52.

MUKHERJEE, D.; SOM, S.; CHATTERJEE, I. B. (1982). Ascorbic Acid Metabolism in Trauma. *Indian Journal of Medical Research* 75:748-751.

MURAD, S.; GROVE, D.; LINDBERG, K. A.; REYNOLDS, G.; SIVARAJAH, A.; PINNELL, S. R. (1981). Regulation of Collagen Synthesis by Ascorbic Acid. *Proceedings of the National Academy of Sciences USA* 78:2879-2882.

MURAD, S.; SIVARAJAH, A.; PINNELL, S. R. (1981). Regulation of Prolyl and Lysyl Hydroxylase Activities in Cultured Human Skin Fibroblasts by Ascorbic Acid. *Biochemical and Biophysical Research Communications* 101:868-875.

MURAD, S.; TAJIMA, S.; JOHNSON, G. R.; SIVARAJAH, A.; PINNELL, S. R. (1983). Collagen Synthesis in Cultured Human Skin Fibroblasts: Effect of Vitamin C and Its Analogs. *Journal of Investigative Dermatology* 81:158-612.

MURATA, A. (1975). Virucidal Activity of Vitamin C: Vitamin C for Prevention and Treatment of Viral Diseases. *Proceedings of the First Intersectional Congress of Microbiological Societies.* Science Council of Japan 3:432-442.

MURATA, A.; KITAGAWA, K. (1973). Mechanism of Inactivation of Bacteriophage J1 by Ascorbic Acid. *Agricultural and Biological Chemistry* 35:1145-1151.

MURATA, A.; KITAGAWA, K.; SARUNO, R. (1971). Inactivation of Bacteriophages by Ascorbic Acid. *Agricultural and Biological Chemistry* 35:294-296.

MYASNIKOVA, I. A (1947). Effect of Ascorbic Acid, Nicotinic Acid, and Thiamine on Cholesterolemia. *Voenno-Morskoi Med. Akad. Leningrad* 8:140 (in Russian).

MYLLYLÄ, R.; MAJAMAA, K.; GUNZLER, V.; HANUSKA-ABEL, H. M.; KIVIRIKKO, K. I. (1984). Ascorbate Is Consumed Stoichiometrically in the Uncoupled Reactions Catalyzed by Prolyl-4-Hydroxylase and Lysyl Hydroxylase. *Journal of Biological Chemistry* 259:5403-5405.

NANDI, B. K.; SUBRAMANIAN, N.; MAJUMDER, A. K.; CHATTERJEE, I. B. (1976). Effect of Ascorbic Acid on Detoxification of Histamine under Stress Conditions. *Biochemical Pharmacology* 23: 643-647.

*New York Times* (1985). Aspirin: Firms Agree to Use Warnings. January 12.

NEWMARK, H. L.; SCHEINER, J.; MARCUS, M.; PRABHUDESAI, M. (1976). Stability of Vitamin $B_{12}$ in the Presence of Ascorbic Acid. *The American Journal of Clinical Nutrition* 29:645-649.

NICOLÉ, C.; LEBAILLY, C. (1918). Quelque notions expérmentales sur le virus de la grippe. *Comptes rendus Acad Sci.* (Paris) 167:607-610.

OCHSNER, A. (1964). Thromboembolism. *The New England Journal of Medicine* 271:211.

OCHSNER, A.; DEBAKEY, M. E.; DECAMP, P. T. (1950). Venous Thrombosis. *Journal of the American Medical Association* 144:831-834.

OGILVY, C. S.; DOUGLAS, J. S.; TABATABAI, M.; DU BOIS, A. B. (1978). Ascorbic Acid Reverses Bronchoconstriction Caused by Methacholine Aerosol in Man; Idomethacin Prevents This Reversal. *The Physiologist* 21:86.

OGILVY, C. S.; DU BOIS, A. B.; DOUGLAS, J. S. (1981). Effects of Ascorbic Acid and Indomethacin on the Airways of Healthy Male Subjects with and without Induced Bronchoconstriction. *Journal of Allergy and Clinical Immunology* 67: 363-369.

OMURA, H.; FUKUMOTO, Y.; TOMITA, Y.; SHINOHARA, K. (1975). Action of 5-Methyl-3,4-Dihydroxytetrone on Deoxyribonucleic Acid. *Journal of the Faculty of Agriculture, Kyushu University* 19:139-148.

OMURA, H.; TOMITA, Y.; NAKAMURA, Y.; MIRAKAMI, H. (1974). Antitumoric Potentiality of Some Ascorbate Derivatives. *Journal of the Faculty of Agriculture, Kyushu University* 18:181-189.

OSMOND, H.; HOFFER, A. (1962). Massive Niacin Treatment in Schizophrenia: Review of a Nine-Year Study. *The Lancet* 1:316-322.

PAESCHKE, K. D.; VASTERLING, H. W. (1968). Photometrischer Ascorbinsäure-Test zur Bestimmung der Ovulation, verglichen mit anderen Methoden der Ovulationstermin-bestimmung. *Zentralblatt für Gynakologie* 90:817-820.

PANUSH, R. S.; DELAFUENTE, J. C.; KATZ, P.; JOHNSON, J. (1982). Modulation of Certain Immunologic Responses by Vitamin C. III. Potentiation of In Vitro and In Vivo Lymphocyte Responses, in *Vitamin C: New Clinical Applications in Immunology, Lipid Metabolism, and Cancer,* ed. A. Hanck, Hans Huber, Bern, pp. 35-47.

PAPPENHEIMER, A. M. (1948). *On Certain Aspects of Vitamin C Deficiency.* Charles C. Thomas, Springfield, Ill.

PASSMORE, R. (1971). That Man . . . Pauling! *Nutrition Today,* January-February, pp. 17-18.

PASSWATER, R. A. (1975). *Supernutrition.* The Dial Press, New York.

PASSWATER, R. A. (1977). *Supernutrition for Healthy Hearts.* The Dial Press, New York.

PATRONE, F.; DALLEGRI, F. (1979). Vitamin C and the Phagocytic System. *Acta Vitaminologica et Enzymologica* 1:5-10.

PAUL, J. H.; FREESE., H. L. (1933). An Epidemiological and Bacteriological Study of the "Common Cold" in an Isolated Arctic Community (Spitsbergen). *American Journal of Hygiene* 17:517-535.

PAULING, L. (1953). Protein Interactions: Aggregation of Globular Proteins. *Faraday Society Discussion,* pp. 170-176.

PAULING, L. (1958). The Relation between Longevity and Obesity in Human Beings. *Proceedings of the National Academy of Sciences USA* 44:619-622.

PAULING, L. (1960). Observations on Aging and Death. *Engineering and Science Magazine,* California Institute of Technology, Pasadena, Cal., May issue.

PAULING, L. (1961). A Molecular Theory of General Anesthesia. *Science* 134:15-21.

PAULING, L. (1968a). Orthomolecular Psychiatry. *Science* 160:265-271.

PAULING, L. (1968b). Orthomolecular Somatic and Psychiatric Medicine. *Journal of Vital Substances and Diseases of Civilization* 14:1-3.

PAULING, L. (1970a). *Vitamin C and the Common Cold.* W. H. Freeman, San Francisco.

PAULING, L. (1970b). Evolution and the Need for Ascorbic Acid. *Proceedings of the National Academy of Sciences USA* 67:1643-1648.

PAULING, L. (1971a). *Vitamin C and the Common Cold,* revised edition. Bantam Books, New York.

PAULING, L. (1971b). That Man . . . Pauling! *Nutrition Today.* March-April, pp. 21-24.

PAULING, L. (1971c). Vitamin C and the Common Cold. *Journal of the American Medical Association* 216:332.

PAULNG, L. (1971d). Vitamin C and Colds. *New York Times,* January 17.

PAULING, L. (1972). Preventive Nutrition. *Medicine on the Midway* 27:15-17.

PAULING, L.; ET AL. (1973a). Results of a Loading Test of Ascorbic Acid, Niacinamide, and Pyridoxine in Schizophrenic Subjects and Controls, in *Orthomolecular Psychiatry: Treatment of Schizophrenia,* eds. D. Hawkins and L. Pauling. W. H. Freeman, San Francisco.

PAULING, L. (1973b). *Vitamin C and the Common Cold,* abridged edition. Bantam Books, New York.

PAULING, L. (1974a). Early Evidence About Vitamin C and the Common Cold. *Journal of Orthomolecular Psychiatry* 3:139-151.

PAULING, L. (1974b). On the Orthomolecular Environment of the Mind: Orthomolecular Theory. *American Journal of Psychiatry* 131:1251-1257.

PAULING, L. (1974c). Are Recommended Daily Allowances for Vitamin C Adequate? *Proceedings of the National Academy of Sciences USA* 71:4442-4446.

PAULING, L. (1976a). On Fighting Swine Flu. *New York Times,* June 5.

PAULING, L. (1976b). Ascorbic Acid and the Common Cold: Evaluation of Its Efficacy and Toxicity. *Medical Tribune,* March 24.

PAULING, L. (1976c). The Case for Vitamin C in Maintaining Health and Preventing Disease. *Modern Medicine.* July, pp. 68-72.

PAULING, L. (1976d). *Vitamin C, the Common Cold, and the Flu.* W. H. Freeman, San Francisco.

PAULING, L. (1978). Robert Fulton Cathcart III, M.D., an Orthomolecular Physician. *Newsletter* 1: no. 4, fall issue. The Linus Pauling Institute of Science and Medicine, Palo Alto, Cal.

PAULING, L. (1984). Sensory Neuropathy from Pyridoxine Abuse. *The New England Journal of Medicine* 180:197.

PAULING, L.; WILLOUGHBY, R.; REYNOLDS, R.; BLAISDELL, B. E.; LAWSON, S. (1982). Incidence of Squamous Cell Carcinoma in Hairless Mice Irradiated with Ultraviolet Light in Relation to Intake of Ascorbic Acid (Vitamin C) and of D, L-$\alpha$-Tocopheryl Acetate (Vitamin E), in *Vitamin C: New Clinical Applications in Immunology, Lipid Metabolism, and Cancer,* ed. A. Hanck. Hans Huber, Bern, pp. 53-82.

PAULING, L.; NIXON, J. C.; STITT, F.; MARCUSON, R.; DUNHAM, W .B.; BARTH. R.; BENSCH, K.; HERMAN, Z. S.; BLAISDELL, E.; TSAO, C.; PRENDER, M.; ANDREWS, V.; WILLOUGHBY, R.; ZUCKERKANDL, E. (1985). Effect of Ascorbic Acid on the Incidence of Spontaneous Mammary Tumors in RIII Mice. *Proceedings of the National Academy of Sciences USA* 82:5185-5189.

PEAR, R. (1985). Lower Nutrient Levels Proposed in Draft Report on American Diet. *New York Times.* 23 September: 1, 17.

PEARSON, D.; SHAW, S. (1982). *Life Extension: A Practical Scientific Approach.* Warner Books, New York.

PELLETIER, O. (1977). Vitamin C and Tobacco, in *Re-evaluation of Vitamin C,* ed. A. Hanck. Hans Huber, Bern, pp. 139-148.

PETROUTSOS, G.; POULIQUEU, Y. (1984). Effect of Ascorbic Acid on Ulceration in Alkali-Burned Corneas. *Ophthalmic Research* 16:185-189.

PFEIFFER, C. C. (1975). *Mental and Elemental Nutrients: A Physician's Guide to Nutrition and Health Care.* Keats Publishing, New Canaan, Conn.

PFISTER, R. R.; KOSKI, J. (1982). Alkali Burns of the Eye: Pathophysiology and Treatment. *Southern Medical Journal* 75:417-422.

PHILLIPSON, B. E.; ROTHROCK, D. W.; CONNOR, W. E.; HARRIS, W. S.; ILLINGWORTH, D. R. (1985). Reduction of Plasma Lipids, Lipoproteins, and Apoproteins by Dietary Fish Oils in Patients with Hypertriglyceridemia. *The New England Journal of Medicine* 312:1210-1216.

PHILPOTT, W. H. (1974). Maladaptive Reactions to Frequently Used Foods and Commonly Met Chemicals as Precipitating Factors in Many Chronic Physical and Chronic Emotional Illnesses, in *New Dynamics of Preventive Medicine,* ed. L. R. Pomeroy. Intercontinental Medical Book Corp, New York, pp. 171-198.

PINNELL, S. R. (1982). Regulation of Collagen Synthesis. *Journal of Investigative Dermatology* 79:73s-76s.

PITT, H. A.; COSTRINI, A. M. (1979). Vitamin C Prophylaxis in Marine Recruits. *Journal of the American Medical Association* 241:908-911.

POHL, F.; KORNBLUTH, C. M. (1953). *The Space Merchants.* Ballantine Books, New York.

PORTMAN, O. W.; ALEXANDER, M.; MARUFFO, C. A. (1967). Nutritional Control of Arterial Lipid Composition in Squirrel Monkeys. *Journal of Nutrition* 91:35-44.

PORTNOY, B.; WILKINSON, J. F. (1938). Vitamin C Deficiency in Peptic Ulceration and Haematemesis. *British Medical Journal* 1:554-560.

PRIESTMAN, T. J. (1977). *Cancer Chemotherapy—An Introduction.* Montedison Pharmaceuticals Ltd., Barnet, England.

PRINZ, W.; BORTZ, R.; BRAGIN, B.; HERSCH, M. (1977). The Effect of Ascorbic Acid Supplementation on Some Parameters of the Human Immunological Defence System. *International Journal of Vitamin and Nutrition Research* 47:248-256.

PRINZ, W.; BLOCH, J.; GILICH, G.; MITCHELL, G. (1980). A systematic study of the effect of vitamin C supplementation on the humoral immune response in ascorbate-dependent mammals. I. The antibody response to sheep red blood cells (a T-dependent antigen) in guinea pigs. *Int J Vitam Nutr Res.* 50(3):294-300.

PRITIKIN, N. (1983). *The Pritikin Promise: 28 Days to a Longer, Healthier Life.* Simon and Schuster, New York.

PUGH, D. M.; SHARMA, S. C.; WILSON, C. W. M. (1975). Inhibitory Effect of Ascorbic Acid on the Yield of Prostaglandin F from the Guinea-Pig Uterine Homogenates. *British Journal of Pharmacology* 53:469P.

RABACH, J. M. (1972). *Vitamin C for a Cold.* Dell Publishing, New York.

RAFFEL, S.; MADISON, R. R. (1938). The Influence of Ascorbic Acid on Anaphylaxis in Guinea Pigs. *Journal of Infectious Diseases* 63:71-76.

RAMACHANDRAN, G. N.; REDDI, A. H. (1976). *Biochemistry of Collagen.* Plenum Press, New York.

RAPAPORT, S. A. (1978). *Strike Back at Cancer: What To Do and Where To Go for the Best Medical Care.* Prentice-Hall, Englewood Cliffs, N.J.

RAUSCH, P. G.; PRYZWANSKY, K. B.; SPITZNAGEL, J. K. (1978). Immunocytochemical Identification of Azurophilic and Specific Granule Markers in the Giant Granules of Chediak-Higashi Neutrophiles. *The New England Journal of Medicine* 298:693-698.

*Reader's Digest Family Health Guide and Medical Encyclopedia* (1976). The Reader's Digest Association, Pleasantville, N.Y.

RÉGNIER, E. (1968). The Administration of Large Doses of Ascorbic Acid in the Prevention and Treatment of the Common Cold. Parts I and 11. *Review of Allergy* 22:835-846, 948-956.

RHOADS, G. C.; GULBRANDSEN, C. L.; KAGAN, A. (1976). Serum Lipoproteins and Coronary Heart Disease in a Population Study of Hawaiian Japanese Men. *The New England Journal of Medicine* 294:297.

RICH, A.; CRICK, F. H. C. (1961). The Molecular Structure of Collagen. *Journal of Molecular Biology* 3:483-506.

RIMLAND, B. (1973). High-Dosage Levels of Certain Vitamins in the Treatment of Children with Severe Mental Disorders, in *Orthomolecular Psychiatry: Treatment of Schizophrenia,* eds. D. Hawkins and L. Pauling, W. H. Freeman, San Francisco, pp. 513-539.

RIMLAND, B. (1979). Nutritional Medicine vs. Toxic Medicine. *Let's Live,* March, 127-128.

RIMLAND, B.; CALLAWAY, E.; DREYFUS, P. (1977). The Effect of High Doses of Vitamin $B_6$ on Autistic Children—A Double Blind Crossover Study, in *Diet Related to Killer Diseases. V. Nutrition and Mental Health.* Hearing before the Select Committee on Nutrition and Human Needs of the United States Senate. Government Printing Office. Washington, D.C., pp. 276-279.

RINEHART, J. F.; GREENBERG, L. D. (1956). Vitamin $B_6$ Deficiency in the Rhesus Monkey with Particular Reference to the Occurrence of Atherosclerosis, Dental Caries, and Hepatic Cirrhosis. *American Journal of Clinical Nutrition* 4:318-327.

RINGSDORF, W. M., JR.; CHERASKIN, E. (1982). Vitamin C and Human Wound Healing. *Oral Surgery* 53:231-236.

RITZEL, G. (1961). *Kritische Beurteilung des Vitamins C als Prophylacticum und Therapeuticum der Erkältungskrankheiten. Helvetica Medica Acta* 28:63-68.

RITZEL, G.; BRUPPACHER, R. (1977). Vitamin C and Tobacco, in *Re-evaluation of Vitamin C,* ed. A. Hanck. Hans Huber, Bern, pp. 171-184.

ROBIN, E. D. (1984). *Matters of Life and Death: Risks vs. Benefits of Medical Care.* W. H. Freeman, New York.

ROSS, W. S. (1971). Vitamin C: Does It Really Help? *Reader's Digest* 98:129-132.

RUSKIN, S. L. (1938). Calcium Cevitamate (Calcium Ascorbate) in the Treatment of Acute Rhinitis. *Annals of Otology, Rhinology, and Laryngology* 47:502-511.

SABISTON, B. H.; RADOMSKI, N. W. (1974). Health Problems and Vitamin C in Canadian Northern Military Operations. *Defence and Civil Institute of Environmental Medicine Report No. 74-R-1012.*

SALOMON, L. L.; STUBBS, S. W. (1961). Some Aspects of the Metabolism of Ascorbic Acid in Rats. *Annals of the New York Academy of Sciences* 92:128-140.

SAMBORSKAYA, E. P.; FERDMAN, T. D. (1966). The Problem of the Mechanism of Artificial Abortion by Use of Ascorbic Acid. *Bjulleten Eksperimentalnoi Biologii i Meditsinii* 62:96-98.

SAYED, S. M.; ROY, P. B.; ACHARYA, P. T. (1975). Leukocyte Ascorbic Acid and Wound Infection. *Journal of the Indian Medical Association* 64:120-123.

SCHAUMBERG, H.; CAPLAN, J.; WINDEBANK, A. (1983). Sensory Neuropathy from Pyridoxine Use: A New Megavitamin Syndrome. *The New England Journal of Medicine* 309:445-448.

SCHEUNERT, A. (1949). Der Tagesbedarf des Erwachsenen an Vitamin C. *Internationale Zeitschrift für Vitaminforschung* 20:371-386.

SCHLEGEL, J. U. (1975). Proposed Uses of Ascorbic Acid in Prevention of Bladder Carcinoma. *Annals of the New York Academy of Sciences* 258:432-438.

SCHLEGEL, J. U.; PIPKIN, G. E.; BANOWSKY, L. (1967). Urine Composition in the Etiology of Bladder Tumor Formation. *Journal of Urology* 97:479-481.

SCHLEGEL, J. U.; PIPKIN, G. E.; NISHIMURA, R.; DUKE, G. A. (1969). Studies in the Etiology and Prevention of Bladder Carcinoma. *Journal of Urology:* 101:317-324.

SCHLEGEL, J. U.; PIPKIN, G. E.; NISHIMURA, R.; SCHULTZ, G. N. (1970). The Role of Ascorbic Acid in the Prevention of Bladder Tumor Formation. *Journal of Urology* 103:155-159.

SCHMECK, H. M., JR. (1973). Research Funds and Disease Effects Held Out of Step. *New York Times.* February 10.

SCHORAH, C. J. (1981). Vitamin C Status in Population Groups, in *Vitamin C (Ascorbic Acid),* eds. J. N. Counsell and D. H. Hornig. Applied Science Publishers, London.

SCHRAUZER, G. N.; RHEAD, W. J. (1973). Ascorbic Acid Abuse: Effects of Long Term Ingestion of Excessive Amounts on Blood Levels and Urinary Excretion. *International Journal of Vitamin and Nutrition Research* 43:201-211.

SCHWARTZ, P. L. (1970). Ascorbic Acid in Wound Healing—A Review. *Journal of the American Dietetic Association* 56:497-503.

SCHWARZ, R. I.; MANDELL, R. B.; BISSELL, M. J. (1981). Ascorbate Induction of Collagen Synthesis as a Means for Elucidating a Mechanism for Quantitative Control of Tissue-Specific Function. *Molecular and Cellular Biology* 1:843-853.

SCHWERDT, P. R.; SCHWERDT, C. E. (1975). Effect of Ascorbic Acid on Rhinovirus Replication in WI-38 Cells. *Proceedings of the Society for Experimental Biology and Medicine* 148:1237-1243.

SELTER, M. (1918). Zur Aetiologie der Influenza. *Deutsche medizinische Wochenschrift* 44:932-933.

SHARMA, S. C. (1982). Interactions of Ascorbic Acid with Prostaglandin, in *Vitamin C: New Clinical Application in Immunology, Lipid Metobolism, and Cancer,* ed. A. Hanck. Hans Huber, Bern, pp. 239-256.

SHUTE, E. V. (1969). *The Heart and Vitamin E.* The Shute Foundation for Medical Research, London, Canada.

SHUTE, W. E.; TAUB, H. J. (1969). *Vitamin E for Ailing and Healthy Hearts.* Pyramid House, New York.

SHUTE, W. E. (1978). *Vitamin E Book.* Keats Publishing, New Canaan, Conn.

SIEVERS, M. L.; HERRIER, R. N. (1984). Sensory Neuropathy from Pyridoxine Abuse. *The New England Journal of Medicine* 310:198.

SMITH, W.; ANDREWES, C. H.; LAIDLAW, P. (1933). A Virus Obtained from Influenza Patients. *The Lancet* 225:66-68.

SMITHELLS, R. W.; SHEPPARD, S.; SCHORAH, C. J. (1976). Vitamin Deficiencies and Neural Tube Defects. *Archives of Disease in Childhood* 51:944-950.

SOKOLOFF, B.; HORI, M.; SAELHOF, C. C.; WRZOLEK, T.; IMAI, T. (1966). Aging, Atherosclerosis, and Ascorbic Acid Metabolism. *Journal of the American Geriatric Society* 14:1239-1260.

SPERO, L. M.; ANDERSON, T. W. (1973). Ascorbic Acid and Common Colds. *British Medical Journal* 4:354-359.

SPITTLE, C. R. (1971). Atherosclerosis and Vitamin C. *The Lancet* 2:1280-1281

SPRINCE, H.; PARKER, C. M.; SMITH, G. G. (1977). L-Ascorbic Acid in Alcoholism and Smoking Protection against Acetaldehyde Toxicity as an Experimental Model, in *Re-evaluation of Vitamin C,* ed. A. Hanck. Hans Huber, Bern, pp. 185-218.

STARE, F. J. (1969). *Eating for Good Health.* Cornerstone Library, New York.

STEFANSSON, V. (1918). Observations on Three Cases of Scurvy. *Journal of the American Medical Association* 71:1715-1718.

STEFANSSON, V. (1964). *Discovery.* McGraw-Hill, New York.

STELLAMOR-PESKIR, H. (1961). On the Therapy of Alkali Burns of the Eye. *Klinische und Mikrobiologische Augenheilkunde* 139:838-841.

STONE, I. (1965). Studies of a Mammalian Enzyme System for Producing Evolutionary Evidence on Man. *American Journal of Physical Anthropology* 23:83-86.

STONE, I. (1967). The Genetic Disease Hypoascorbemia. *Acta Geneticae Medicae et Gemellologiae* 16:52-60.

STONE, I. (1972). *The Healing Factor: Vitamin C against Disease.* Grosset and Dunlap, New York.

STRAUSS, L. H.; SCHEER, P. (1939). Über die Einwirkungen des Nikotins auf den Vitamin C-Haushalt. *Zeitschrift für Vitaminforschung* 9:39-48.

SUBRAMANIAN, N. (1978). Histamine Degradative Potential of Ascorbic Acid: Considerations and Evaluations. *Agents and Actions* 8:484-487.

SYDENSTRICKER, V. P.; CLECKLEY, H. M. (1941). The Effect of Nicotinic Acid in Stupor, Lethargy, and Various Other Psychiatric Disorders. *American Journal of Psychiatry* 98:83-92.

SZENT-GYÖRGYI, A. (1937). *Studies on Biological Oxidation and Some of Its Catalysts.* Szeged, Hungary.

TAJIMA, S.; PINNELL, S. R. (1982). Regulation of Collagen Synthesis by Ascorbic Acid: Ascorbic Acid Increases Type I Procollagen mRNA. *Biochemical and Biophysical Research Communications* 106:632-637.

TAYLOR, T. V.; RIMMER, S.; DAY, B.; BUTCHER, J.; DYMOCK, I. W. (1974). Ascorbic Acid Supplementation in the Treatment of Pressure-Sores. *The Lancet,* September 7, pp. 544-546.

TORREY, J. C.; MONTU, E. (1931). The Influence of an Exclusive Meat Diet on the Flora of the Human Colon. *Journal of Infectious Diseases* 49:141-176.

TSAO, C. S. (1984a). Equilibrium Constant for Calcium Ion and Ascorbate Ion. *Experimentia* 40:168-170.

TSAO, C. S. (1984b). Ascorbic Acid Administration and Urinary Oxalate. *Annals of Internal Medicine* 101:405.

TSAO, C. S.; MIYASHITA, K. (1984). Effects of High Intake of Ascorbic Acid on Plasma Levels of Amino Acids. *IRCS Medical Science* 12:1052-1053.

TSAO, C. S.; SALIMI, S. L. (1984a). Effect of Large Intake of Ascorbic Acid on Urinary and Plasma Oxalic Acid Levels. *International Journal of Nutrition and Vitamin Research* 54:245-249.

TSAO, C. S.; SALIMI, S. L. (1984b). Evidence of Rebound Effect with Ascorbic Acid. *Medical Hypotheses* 13:303-310.

TSAO, C. S.; SALIMI, S. L; PAULING. L. (1982). Lack of Effect of Ascorbic Acid on Calcium Excretion. *IRCS Medical Science* 10:738.

TUKE, J. B. (1881). Insanity. *The Encyclopedia Britannica.* 9th ed., vol XIII. 95-113. Charles Scribner's Sons, New York.

TURKEL, H. (1972). *New Hope for the Mentally Retarded—Stymied by the FDA.* Vantage Press, New York.

TURKEL, H. (1977). Medical Amelioration of Down's Syndrome Incorporating the Orthomolecular Approach, in *Diet Related to Killer Diseases* V. *Nutrition and Mental Health.* Hearing before the Select Committee on Nutrition and Human Needs of the United States Senate. U.S. Government Printing Office, Washington, D.C, pp. 291-304.

TURLEY, S. D.; WEST, C. E.; HORTON, B. J. (1976). The Role of Ascorbic Acid in the Regulation of Cholesterol Metabolism and in the Pathogenesis of Atherosclerosis. *Atherosclerosis* 24:1-18.

TYRRELL, D. A. J.; CRAIG, J. W.; MEADE, T. W.; WHITE, T. (1977). A Trial of Ascorbic Acid in the Treatment of the Common Cold. *British Journal of Preventive and Social Medicine* 31:189-191.

VALIC, F.; ZUSKIN, E. (1973). Pharmacological Prevention of Acute Ventilatory Capacity Reduction in Flax Dust Exposure. *British Journal of Industrial Medicine* 30:381-384.

VALLANCE, S. (1977). Relationships between Ascorbic Acid and Serum Proteins of the Immune System. *British Medical Journal* 2:437-438.

VANDERKAMP, H. (1966). A biochemical abnormality in schizophrenia involving ascorbic acid. *Int J Neuropsychiatry.* Jun;2(3):204-6.

VANE, J. R. (1971). Inhibition of Prostaglandin Synthesis as a Mechanism of Action for Aspirin-like Drugs. *Nature (New Biol.)* 231:232-235.

VARMA, S. D.; KUMAR, S.; RICHARDS, R. D. (1979). Light-Induced Damage to Ocular Lens Cation Pump: Prevention by Vitamin C. *Proceedings of the National Academy of Sciences USA* 76:3504-3506.

VARMA, S. D.; CHAND, D.; SHARMA, Y. R.; KUCK, J. F., JR.; RICHARDS, R. D. (1984). Oxidative Stress on Lens and Cataract Formation. *Current Eye Research* 3:35-57.

VARMA, S. D.; SRIVASTAVA, V. K.; RICHARDS, R. D. (1982). Photoperoxidation in Lens and Cataract Formation: Prevention Role of Superoxide Dismutase, Catalase, and Vitamin C. *Ophthalmological Research* 14:167-175.

VIRNO, M.; BUCCI, M. O.; PECORI-GIRALDI, J.; MISSIROLI, A. (1967). Oral Treatment of Glaucoma with Vitamin C. *The Eye, Ear, Nose, and Throat Monthly* 46:1502-1508.

VOGELSANG, A. (1948a). Effect of Alpha Tocopherol in Diabetes Mellitus. *Journal of Clinical Endocrinology* 8:883-884.

VOGELSANG, A. (1948b). Cumulative Effect of Alpha Tocopherol on the Insulin Requirements in Diabetes Mellitus. *Medical Record* 161:363-365.

VOGELSANG, A.; SHUTE, E. V. (1946). Vitamin E and Coronary Heart Disease. *Nature* 157:772-773.

WALKER, H. M. (1980). *Chelation Therapy: How to Prevent or Reverse Hardening of the Arteries.* M. Evans, New York.

WATNE, A. L.; LAI, H.-Y.; CARRIER, J.; COPPULA, W. (1977). The Diagnosis and Surgical Treatment of Patients with Gardner's Syndrome. *Surgery* 82:327-333.

WAUGH, W. A.; KING, C. G. (1932). Isolation and Identification of Vitamin C. *Journal of Biological Chemistry* 97:325-331.

WEINHOUSE, S. (1977). Problems in the Assessment of Human Risk of Carcinogenesis from Chemicals, in *Origins of Human Cancer: Book C, Human Risk Assessment,* eds. H. H. Hiatt, J. D. Watson, and J. A. Winsten. Cold Spring Harbor Laboratory, Cold Spring, N.Y.

WHELAN, E.; STARE, F. J. (1975). *Panic in the Pantry.* Atheneum, New York.

WHITE, P. L. (1975). Editorial: Megavitamin This and Megavitamin That. *Journal of the American Medical Association* 233:538-539.

WILLIAMS, R. J. (1951). *Nutrition and Alcoholism.* University of Oklahoma Press, Norman, Okla.

WILLIAMS, R. J. (1956). *Biochemical Individuality, the Basis for the Genetotrophic Concept.* University of Texas Press, Austin, Tex.

WILLIAMS, R. J. (1959). *Alcoholism, the Nutritional Approach.* University of Texas Press, Austin, Tex.

WILLIAMS, R. J. (1967). *You Are Extraordinary.* Random House, New York.

WILLIAMS, R. J. (1971). *Nutrition against Disease.* Pitman, New York.

WILLIAMS, R. J. (1973). *Biochemical Individuality.* University of Texas Press, Austin, Tex.

WILLIAMS, R. J. (1975). *Physician's Handbook of Nutritional Science.* Charles C. Thomas, Springfield, Ill.

WILLIAMS, R. J.; DEASON, G. (1967). Individuality in Vitamin C Needs. *Proceedings of the National Academy of Sciences USA* 57:1638-1641.

WILLIAMS, R. J;. KALITA, D. K., EDS. (1977). *A Physician's Handbook on Orthomolecular Medicine.* Pergamon Press, New York.

WILLIS, G. C.; FISHMAN, S. (1955). Ascorbic Acid Content of Human Arterial Tissue. *Canadian Medical Association Journal* 72:500-503.

WILLIS, R. A. (1973). *The Spread of Tumours in the Human Body,* 3d ed. Butterworth, London.

WILSON, C. W.; LOH, H. S. (1973). Vitamin C and Colds. *The Lancet* 1:1058-1059.

WILSON, C. W.; LOH, H. S.; FOSTER, F. G. (1976). Common Cold Symptomatology and Vitamin C. *European Journal of Clinical Pharmacology* 6:196-202.

WINITZ, M.; GRAFF, J.; SEEDMAN, D. A. (1964). Effect of Dietary Carbohydrate on Serum Cholesterol Levels. *Archives of Biochemistry and Biophysics* 108:576-579.

WINITZ, M.; SEEDMAN, D. A.; GRAFF, J. (1970). Studies in Metabolic Nutrition Employing Chemically Defined Diets. I. Extended Feeding of Normal Human Adult Males. *American Journal of Clinical Nutrition* 23:525-545.

WINITZ, M.; ADAMS, R. F.; SEEDMAN, D. A.; DAVIS, P. N.; JAYKO, L. G.; HAMILTON, J. A. (1970). Studies in Metabolic Nutrition Employing Chemically Defined Diets. II. Effects on Gut Microflora Populations. *American Journal of Clinical Nutrition* 23:546-559.

WITTES, R. E. (1985). Vitamin C and Cancer. *The New England Journal of Medicine* 312:178-179.

WOLFER, J. A.; FARMER, C. J.; CARROL, W. W.; MANSHARDT, D. O. (1947). An Experimental Study in Wound Healing in Vitamin-C-Depleted Human Subjects. *Surgery, Gynecology, and Obstetrics* 84:1-10.

WOOLLEY, D. W. (1962). *The Biochemical Bases of Psychoses.* Wiley, New York.

WYNDER, E. L. (ED.) (1981). *The Book of Health.* Franklin Watts, New York.

YANDELL, H. R. (1951). The Treatment of Extensive Burns. *American Surgeon* 17:351-360.

YEW, M. S. (1973). "Recommended Daily Allowances" for Vitamin C. *Proceedings of the National Academy of Sciences USA* 70:969-972.

YONEMOTO, R. H.; CHRETIEN, P. B.; FEHNIGER, T. F. (1976). Enhanced Lymphocyte Blastogenesis by Oral Ascorbic Acid. *Proceedings of the American Association for Cancer Research* 17:288.

YONEMOTO, R. H. (1979). Vitamin C and the Immunological Response in Normal Controls and in Cancer Patients (in Portuguese). *Medico Dialogo* 5:23-30.

YUDKIN, J. (1972). *Sweet and Dangerous.* Peter H. Wyden, New York.

YUDKIN, J.; EDELMAN, I.; HOUGH, L. (EDS.) (1971). *Sugar: Chemical, Biological, and Nutritional Aspects of Sucrose.* Daniel Davey, Hartford, Conn.

ZAMENHOF, S.; EICHHORN, H. H. (1967). Study of Microbial Evolution Through Loss of Biosynthetic Functions: Establishment of "Defective" Mutants. *Nature* 216:456-458.

ZUCKERKANDL, E.; PAULING, L. (1962). Molecular Disease, Evolution, and Genic Heterogeneity, in *Horizons in Biochemistry,* eds. M. Kasha and B. Pullman. Academic Press, New York, pp. 189-225.

ZUSKIN, E.; LEWIS, A. J.; BOUHUYS, A. (1973). Inhibition of Histamine-Produced Airway Constriction by Ascorbic Acid. *Journal of Allergy and Clinical Immunology* 51:218-223.

ZUSKIN, E.; VALIC, F.; BOUHUYS, A. (1976). Byssinosis and Airway Responses Due to Exposure to Textile Dust. *Lung* 154:17-21.

# Afterword

The Linus Pauling Institute of Science and Medicine was founded by Pauling and located in California from 1973 to 1996. At that time, the institute, now known simply as the Linus Pauling Institute, moved to Oregon State University. The institute's mission is to determine the function and role of micronutrients and phytochemicals (plant chemicals that may affect health) in promoting optimum health and preventing and treating disease and to determine the role of oxidative and nitrative stress and antioxidants in human health and disease. This work is designed to help people achieve a healthy and productive life, full of vitality, with minimal suffering, and free of cancer and other debilitating diseases.

Linus Pauling wanted to update *How to Live Longer and Feel Better*, but his illness in the early 1990s intervened. He recognized that much research had been published since the first edition of his book in 1986 on substances that had begun to attract a lot of attention, such as coenzyme Q10, carotenoids, and carnitine, and that this information should be part of a new edition. Of course, the scientific and medical literature on vitamins, especially vitamins C and E, also continued to expand rapidly. After Pauling's death, the Linus Pauling Institute tried unsuccessfully to arrange for a revision of *How to Live Longer and Feel Better*, carefully aligned with his expressed wishes. We finally concluded that a resource LPI established in 2000, the Linus Pauling Institute Micronutrient Information Center (MIC), has become, in effect, an update of *How to Live Longer and Feel Better*. The MIC serves as a continually updated on-line resource of accurate information on micronutrients, including vitamins and nutritionally relevant minerals; phytochemicals like carotenoids and flavonoids; and constituents of the diet, such as nuts, tea, cruciferous vegetables, alcohol, garlic, coffee, alpha-lipoic acid, L-carnitine, coenzyme Q10, and omega-3 fatty acids. Every article in the MIC is peer-reviewed and represents the latest status of the scientific and medical knowledge of particular micronutrients and other dietary substances and how they affect health and disease. The MIC can be accessed on the Internet at http://lpi.oregonstate.edu/mic. In 2003, *An Evidence-based Approach to Vitamins and Minerals: Health Benefits and Intake Recommendations* by Jane Higdon collected the on-line sections on vitamins and minerals into a book available from Thieme Medical Publishers. A second volume, *An Evidence-based Approach to Dietary Phytochemicals*, will be published in 2007 and features chapters on foods rich in phytochemicals, such as fruits and vegetables, legumes, nuts, coffee, and tea; and sections on glycemic index, essential fatty acids, and specific phytochemicals, such as carotenoids, chlorophyll, fiber, flavonoids, soy isoflavones, and indole-3-carbinol. Both books feature appendices with drug-nutrient and nutrient-nutrient interactions, a glossary, and a comprehensive index.

Additionally, the semi-annual Linus Pauling Institute Research Newsletter, available on-line at http://lpi.oregonstate.edu/research-newsletter, offers detailed information on research in this field. The Research Newsletter features original articles on discoveries made by LPI faculty that influence the direction of research in orthomolecular medicine, especially in aging, heart disease, cancer, and neurological diseases. The National Library of Medicine, through Medline, also provides an excellent on-line, searchable resource for retrieving abstracts of the vast biomedical literature (http://www.ncbi.nlm.nih.gov/pubmed), consisting of thousands of journals and millions of entries over the last five decades. Using "vitamin C" in its most permissive configuration as the search term, about 31,500 papers dating to 1949 are retrieved, although abstracts are not available for most of the older entries. About 16,000 of these were published since the first edition of *How to Live Longer and Feel Better* in February 1986, illustrating that intense research on vitamin C continues.

A short biography of Linus Pauling is posted on the LPI Web site (http://pauling.library.oregonstate.edu), and more information on his scientific work and life is available from the Ava Helen and Linus Pauling Papers, a special collection at Oregon State University that archives over 500,000 items, including research notebooks, manuscripts, medals and awards, and correspondence with many of the 20th century's leading cultural, political, and scientific figures (http://scarc.library.oregonstate.edu/coll/pauling).

•  •  •

*How to Live Longer and Feel Better* remains an outstanding classic that presents with utter clarity the basis of orthomolecular medicine. We decided that the book stands tall as a historical document that covers the older clinical literature often neglected today and should be republished with as few changes as possible. We have annotated some statements that may be modified in light of scientific and medical evidence accumulated since the 1980s (see the following pages), but Linus Pauling's main thesis—varying the concentration of molecules normally present in the body to attain optimum health and to prevent and treat disease—survives powerfully intact. The Linus Pauling Institute continues today as a working tribute to a great American hero, who was, as Linus Pauling's grandson, Alexander Kamb, once said, "a force of nature."

*Stephen Lawson*
Linus Pauling Institute

Page 8: No serious toxicity has been reported for vitamin C. In 2000, the Food and Nutrition Board set the tolerable upper intake level (UL) for adults at 2,000 mg/day based solely on the possible laxative effect or gastrointestinal disturbances in some people at higher intakes.

Page 8: In 2000, the Food and Nutrition Board set the tolerable upper intake level of vitamin E for adults at 1,500 IU/day of *d*-alpha-tocopherol based on a possible risk of hemorrhage at higher intakes.

Page 8: In 2001, the Food and Nutrition Board set the tolerable upper intake level of preformed vitamin A for adults at 10,000 IU/day based on the possible risk of hypervitaminosis A at higher intakes, leading to mild symptoms in most people but also to liver damage or hemorrhage in others.

Page 10: The RDAs given in the table are different from current RDAs.

Page 11: The current RDAs are different from the ones given in the chart.

Page 12: When revising the Dietary Reference Intakes for antioxidants in 2000, the Food and Nutrition Board considered the available evidence in the scientific and medical literature. The Board found that the evidence for systemic conditioning, or the rebound effect, was inconsistent.

Page 13: In the case of vitamin E, the natural form, *d*-alpha-tocopherol or *RRR*-alpha-tocopherol, is twice as effective as the synthetic form, *dl*-alpha-tocopherol or *all rac*-alpha-tocopherol. A vitamin E transfer protein (characterized in 1991) made in the liver preferentially recognizes *d*-alpha-tocopherol for transport to tissues.

Page 61: Most fish also do not synthesize acsorbic acid and require it as a vitamin.

Page 79: The Food and Nutrition Board set the RDA of vitamin C in 2000 at 15 mg for children 1-3 years old, 25 mg for children 4-8 years old, 45 mg for children 9-13 years old, 65 mg for girls 14-18 years old, 75 mg for boys 14-18 years old, 75 mg for adult women, 90 mg for adult men, and somewhat higher for smokers and pregnant or breastfeeding women.

Page 89: Recent pharmacokinetic studies at the National Institutes of Health indicate that circulating cells in blood become saturated with vitamin C at a dose of about 400 mg/day. The NIH studies involved only healthy young men and women, and the situation may be different in older or ill people. A model proposed in 2004 by the NIH group suggests that maximal, consistent concentrations of vitamin C in the blood may be attained with repeated oral doses (e.g., 2.5 g four times daily).

Page 101: Up-to-date information on the roles of vitamins and other constituents of the diet in preventing and treating disease is available from the Linus Pauling Institute Micronutrient Information Center (http://lpi.oregonstate.edu/mic) and the LPI Research Newsletter (http://lpi.oregonstate.edu/research-newsletter).

Page 148: Infection with the bacterium *Helicobacter pylori* is now believed to be responsible for most peptic ulcers.

Page 158: It has been found that the type of fat that one consumes is important in determining the risk of heart disease. A high intake of saturated fat or *trans* fat (partially hydrogenated vegetable oil) has been found to adversely affect blood lipid profiles and to increase the risk of heart disease. *Trans* fat, in particular, lowers levels of the good HDL cholesterol and raises the bad LDL cholesterol. Its effect on heart disease risk is greater than that of saturated fat. Monounsaturated and polyunsaturated fats, including omega-3 fatty acids, provide some protection against heart disease.

Page 165: See annotation for page 13.

Page 167: In 2000, the Food and Nutrition Board set the tolerable upper intake level for adults at 1,500 IU/day of *d*-alpha-tocopherol based on the possible risk of hemorrhage at higher intakes. Results from recent studies on vitamin E and heart disease treatment have been inconsistent, possibly due to the form of vitamin E ingested, how it was taken (with or without fatty food for absorption), dose, duration, and the "polypharmacy" (multiple drugs) of patients in the studies. Vitamin E may affect the metabolism of drugs taken by heart disease patients, such as cholesterol-lowering statins and blood pressure-lowering drugs.

Page 173: EDTA chelation therapy for atherosclerosis remains controversial and unproven. A clinical trial is currently (2006) being conducted by the National Center for Complementary and Alternative Medicine under the auspices of the National Institutes of Health.

Page 176:  Dr. Ewan Cameron died in 1991.

Page 176: An updated and expanded edition of *Cancer and Vitamin C* was published in 1993, featuring a new preface by Linus Pauling and new appendices discussing epidemiological studies and the anticancer micronutrient regimen developed by Dr. Abram Hoffer. Dr. Hoffer's observations are thoroughly discussed in the book, *Vitamin C & Cancer*, which he co-wrote with Linus Pauling.

Page 185: Work done by researchers at the Linus Pauling Institute of Science and Medicine, the National Institutes of Health, and by others has demonstrated that vitamin C is selectively toxic to cancer cells *in vitro*, probably by generating hydrogen peroxide. Structural characteristics of the vitamin C molecule and derivative substances may also play a role in cancer cell toxicity.

Page 189: Another critical difference between Cameron's work and the two Mayo Clinic studies concerns the mode of administration of vitamin C. Cameron typically gave 10 grams/day of vitamin C by intravenous infusion for about 10 days to his cancer patients, followed by equivalent oral dosage continued indefinitely. The Mayo Clinic researchers gave vitamin C only by mouth and for a limited time. Recent pharmacokinetic studies have found that the peak blood concentration of vitamin C after intravenous infusion is about 70 times greater than that achieved by oral administration (220 μmol/L [oral] vs. 14,000 μmol/L[IV]). The high concentrations attained by intravenous infusion are similar to those found in cell culture studies to selectively kill cancer cells.

Page 199: The current RDA of vitamin $B_3$ (niacin) is 16 mg for adult men and 14 mg for adult women.

Page 206: Dr. Henry Turkel died in 1992.

Page 207: The Institute for Child Behavior Research has been known as the Autism Research Institute since 1990.

Page 213: The name of the *Journal of Orthomolecular Psychiatry* was changed in 1986 to the *Journal of Orthomolecular Medicine.*

Page 223: The current RDA of vitamin $B_6$ is 1.3 mg for most adults. The tolerable upper intake level for adults is 100 mg/day based on possible sensory neuropathy at larger doses (generally over 1,000 mg/day).

Page 224: Dr. Karl Folkers died in 1997.

Page 225: Norman Cousins died in 1990.

Page 257: See annotation for page 189.

Page 277: In 1997, the Food and Nutrition Board eliminated the RDA of vitamin D and replaced it with the Adequate Intake (AI). The AI of vitamin D is 200 IU/day for adults 19-50 years old, 400 IU/day for adults 51-70 years old, and 600 IU/day for adults over 70.

Page 278: The current RDA of vitamin A is 3,000 IU for adult men and 2,333 IU for adult women. The tolerable upper intake level for adults is 10,000 IU/day.

Page 278: The current RDA of vitamin $B_1$ (thiamin) is 1.2 mg for adult men and 1.1 mg for adult women.

Page 278: The current RDA of vitamin $B_2$ (riboflavin) is 1.3 mg for adult men and 1.1 mg for adult women.

Page 279: The current RDA of vitamin $B_3$ (niacin) is 16 mg for adult men and 14 mg for adult women.

Page 279: The current RDA of vitamin $B_6$ is 1.3 mg for adult men and women 19-50 years old, 1.7 mg for men 51 and older, and 1.5 mg for women 51 and older.

Page 280: The current RDA of folic acid is 400 micrograms (mcg) for adult men and women. For vitamin $B_{12}$ the current RDA is 2.4 mcg for adult men and women. Adequate Intakes (AI) have replaced RDAs of pantothenic acid (5 mg/day for adult men and women) and biotin (30 mcg/day for adult men and women).

Page 281: There are eight stereoisomers of vitamin E. Synthetic vitamin E is *all racemic* (*all rac*)-alpha-tocopherol, also called *dl*-alpha tocopherol. Natural vitamin E is *RRR*-alpha-tocopherol, also called *d*-alpha tocopherol.

Page 282: The current RDA of vitamin E is 22.5 IU of *d*-alpha-tocopherol (*RRR*-alpha-tocopherol) for adult men and women.

Page 287: Of three large-scale, long-term epidemiological studies (1996, 1999, 2004), only one found a slightly increased risk of kidney stones in men who consumed at least 1,000 mg of vitamin C per day. High-dose intravenous vitamin C may cause kidney stones in susceptible patients with renal problems of undergoing dialysis.

Page 292: See annotation for page 12.

# Name Index

## Subject Index

References to figures and tables
are set in italic.